THE MAUDSLEY
Maudsley Monographs

MAUDSLEY MONOGRAPHS

HENRY MAUDSLEY, from whom the series of monographs takes its name, was the founder of The Maudsley Hospital and the most prominent English psychiatrist of his generation. The Maudsley Hospital was united with the Bethlem Royal Hospital in 1948 and its medical school, renamed the Institute of Psychiatry at the same time, became a constituent part of the British Postgraduate Medical Federation. It is now a school of King's College, London, and entrusted with the duty of advancing psychiatry by teaching and research. The South London & Maudsley NHS Trust, together with the Institute of Psychiatry, are jointly known as The Maudsley.

The monograph series reports high quality empirical work on a single topic of relevance to mental health, carried out at the Maudsley. This can be by single or multiple authors. Some of the monographs are directly concerned with clinical problems; others are in scientific fields of direct or indirect relevance to mental health and are cultivated for the furtherance of psychiatry.

Maudsley Monographs number forty-eight

Mad Tales from Bollywood
Portrayal of Mental Illness in Conventional Hindi Cinema

Dinesh Bhugra

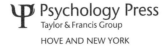

Psychology Press
Taylor & Francis Group
HOVE AND NEW YORK

First published 2006
by Psychology Press
27 Church Road, Hove, East Sussex BN3 2FA

Simultaneously published in the USA and Canada
by Psychology Press
711 Third Avenue, New York, NY 10017

First issued in paperback 2015

*Psychology Press is an imprint of the Taylor & Francis Group,
an informa business*

Typeset in Times by Garfield Morgan, Mumbles, Swansea
Cover design by Lisa Dynan

British Library Cataloguing-in-Publication Data
A catalogue record for this book is available from the British Library

Library of Congress Cataloging in Publication Data
Bhugra, Dinesh.
  Mad tales from Bollywood : portrayal of mental illness in
conventional Hindi cinema / Dinesh Bhugra.
      p. ; cm. – (Maudsley monographs ; no. 48)
  Includes bibliographical references and index.
  ISBN 1-84169-646-3 (hbk)
1. Mental illness in motion pictures. 2. Motion pictures–India.
  [DNLM: 1. Mental Disorders–India. 2. Attitude to Health–India.
3. Hinduism–India. 4. Motion Pictures–India. WM 140 B575m
2006] I. Title. II. Series.
  PN1995.9.M463B48 2006
  791.43'6561–dc22

                                                    2006003490

ISBN13: 978-1-138-88151-8 (pbk)
ISBN13: 978-1-84169-646-1 (hbk)

ISSN: 0076-5465

The Narangs—Chander, Shashi, Rajiv, & Sanjiv

Contents

List of figures and tables

FIGURES

TABLE

Preface

Hindi cinema has been the staple source of entertainment for millions of people over the past century and more. While, both technically and performance-wise, Hindi cinema has come a long way, its portrayal of mental illness has remained remarkably poor.

As a practising psychiatrist, I have always been intrigued by the way characters with mental illness are brought into focus and abandoned in Hindi films. Notions of "the other" in the Indian psyche are well ingrained, be they based on gender, caste, age, or even other characteristics. "The other" plays a key role in releasing the venom, adding the spice of humour, or providing a counterpoint mostly to the main protagonist and the way he or she functions.

This book starts by focusing on some basic aspects of cinema, including how to view a film, how Indian cinema developed, the interaction between culture, mental illness, and cinema, and then covers films according to chronology.

My hypothesis is that the portrayal of mental illness in Hindi films has been influenced by social, political, and economic factors over the past 50 years or so. Independence was followed by the idealism of the 1950s and 1960s, when the portrayal of mentally ill people was gentle, as in films such as *Funtoosh, Karorpati, Pagla Kahin Ka, Khamoshi,* and *Raat aur Din.* In the 1970s, people with mental illness started being shown as rough and violent, as in *Sholay.* This tinge of psychopathy became a full-blown personality disorder in later films, including *Khalnayak, Baazigar, Anjaam, Darr, Dastak,* and *Daraar*. During the 1990s, women joined in psychopathic activities in films such as *Kaun* and *Gupt*. The role of the family in managing mental illness and electroconvulsive therapy (ECT) in curing the illness has been quite useful and films have reflected this: sometimes successfully, but mostly as stereotypes.

Many sources of film reviews were used and these are indicated in the Appendix. The Selected Filmography is confined to Hindi films and is selective, focusing only on films with significant mental illness. For ease of understanding chronological changes, these are presented in the order in which they were released. The diagnostic categories used should be seen as directive and portrayal by various actors does not reflect on their personal lives.

I have deliberately stayed away from the issues of alcohol and substance misuse, and bereavement and the resulting trauma. When I embarked upon this study, I knew of very few Hindi films that dealt with mental illness. As I went along, I discovered many more. My selection of films for this book is a matter of personal choice and focuses on psychoses. There are more films out there and, one day, I hope to get back to them. Personally, I don't like using the words "Bollywood" and "mad", but these are well recognized and understood and there is a journalistic licence in their use. This book is the culmination of a number of strategies and strands; not all may have been successful and I acknowledge that.

Dinesh Bhugra
September 2005

Acknowledgements

I am grateful to many colleagues and friends who took time off for discussion and offered names of films for review. Satyendra and Mridula Tyagi, Monisha Wadhwa, Reenu Mehra, Raj Brahmbhatt, Vihang Vahia, Rajesh Mishra, Cleo van Velsen, Peter Byrne, Rachel Dwyer, Geetha Oommen, Govind and Swati Jog, Professor N. N. Wig, and Mohan Agashe were among those who gave me their time freely. I thank you all.

My discussions with Richard Dyer, Rachel Dwyer, and Simon Cohn were extremely helpful in guiding me in the right directions. A course organized by Harvinder Nath and Pushpinder Chowdhury whose *Tongues on Fire* gave me an opportunity to link up with Girish Karnad, Nasreen Kabir, and others. My thanks. Rohan Sippy pointed me in the right direction, thanks. Martin Guha, Clare Martin, and Sarah Bentley at the Institute of Psychiatry library were unstintingly and unfailingly helpful. I really appreciate your help.

I am grateful to the Wellcome Trust for funding my sabbatical to allow me to research the subject. I acknowledge the valuable assistance and advice received from the Wellcome Institute of History of Medicine, especially from the late Roy Porter, Chris Lawrence, Michael Naeve, Trevor Turner, and Sally Bragg.

The staff of National Films Archives of India in Pune went beyond the call of duty in their help. The director, Mr Sashidharan, and his staff, in particular Mrs Aarti Karkhanis, Mrs Lakshmi Aiyar and Mrs Urmila

Joshi, were superb and ungrudging in their help: I am grateful. Thanks also to Tony David and Joanne Forshaw for their patience and support.

Rebecca Schilling, Sarah Sheppard-Wright and Andrea Livingstone gave the book shape—I am grateful.

Rahul Bhintade worked as an unpaid research assistant, travelling, chasing and finding reviews, references, and stills. I am thankful.

Mike as ever put up with it all: books, DVDs and papers on the dining table, sitting room, and everywhere else. How can mere thanks convey it all?

CHAPTER ONE

Cinema's culture

Cinema as an art form not only reflects the society it is set in, but also acts as a reflector to that society. Some films leave their mark on society; and society, in turn, reacts to these films in a variety of ways. The key question, which is somewhat difficult to answer at times, is whether films influence society more than the other way round. The way certain characters are portrayed in films, and perhaps the consistency of this portrayal, may bring about changes in society's perceptions over a period of time.

WHY STUDY CINEMA?

Cinema has been the most powerful medium since the early twentieth century. The images projected in cinema allow individuals to look into the workings of another family through a storyline that lets them forget their own worries for a while. Films encourage people to look at events in a fresh manner, suggest possible solutions to their own problems, and confirm their views and, perhaps, prejudices.

Going to the cinema may reflect a desire to pry into other people's lives and get the vicarious pleasure of gossiping without really losing anything of one's own. It is less dangerous than theatre because one can look in, but cannot be looked at. It is always fun to watch or gossip about someone who is different, and to feel smug about oneself. Also, film provides a sense of fun and entertainment; especially in the case of Hindi films, the viewer knows that by and large everything will turn out to be all right in the end.

Viewers also feel that their problems are not as bad as those of the people on the screen. The yearnings that these films give rise to among the audience reflect a psychological existence which is on the margins of the two utopias. As Nandy (1998, p. 5) notes, one of these utopias harks back to the rural idyll of the past, which would make the viewer yearn for the political and cultural self-expression of the relatively less well-off. The other utopia refers to the future, the fantasy being that of materialistic gain such as riches and success. Hence, in order to be successful, popular films should ideally have everything: from the classical to the folk in terms of music and story, from the sublime to the ridiculous in terms of execution, from the terribly modern to the incorrigibly traditional, from clearly written plots to those that never get resolved, and from cameo roles to the stereotypical characters which never get developed (p. 7).

Murthy (1980) proposes that, if we accept cinema as an art form, we have to study it as we study any other art form, as well as its impact on society. He illustrates the influence of society on cinema, using the example of the appearance of gangster films in Hollywood in response to the Great Depression of 1929. In depicting human interaction, film can borrow from any element and medium, serving as a sociocultural mirror. Murthy goes on to observe that filmmakers who become too esoteric in their outlook fail to communicate with their audiences. Thus, the team behind the director plays an important role in formulating the look and shape of the film, attempting to ensure that the producer/director ends up with a film that pleases the crowd. At the same time, cinema also holds up a mirror to society by indicating what is going on. There remains a gulf between those who look upon cinema merely as a medium of entertainment and those who would like to see it as a medium for communicating cultural and social values, and thus as a tool for bringing about a better social order (Murthy, 1980). The latter goal, however, may be better achieved through documentaries rather than mainstream commercial cinema.

Film is a unique medium in that it can use subjective and objective viewpoints alternatively. It is likely that the direct and indirect suggestions made in films will have both an overt and covert impact on the viewer. Furthermore, film has a captive audience that is compelled to see what has been edited into it: It shows only what the director chooses us to see. Even though a film is the product of many contributors and is shot according to a specific screenplay, the editor and director can still change its shape and message. As the camera is mobile, the viewpoint keeps shifting, leaving scope for emphasis, counteremphasis, reinforced statements, and so on. The final soundtrack, together with the original sound and the background music, gives its own tinge to the visual experience. The process of editing the exposed film results in a further manipulation of the image, introducing a meaning not originally captured by the camera.

The degree of accessibility provided by film, a largely visual medium, is unmatched by other media. The close-up can exaggerate the physical dimension, breaking down the barrier between the actor (as "the other") and the viewer. The capacity of the medium to animate images imparts a kinetic force to the film, making it possible to communicate at a level usually not possible through the media of books and paintings. Because there is a collaborative effort involved, the influence of social, political, and cultural factors is far more implicit than would be in the case of a one-person effort.

Film relies on the mental state of the viewers, who are "trapped" in a dark hall, waiting to be excited, frightened, cheered up, entertained; to get their money's worth. The employment of images, words, and music together create an atmosphere that the audience absorbs. Each viewer may take home the same or different message after watching the film once or several times. In addition, the viewer can look in and gasp at the culture, customs, mores, dialogue, and marvels of modern technology portrayed in the film, and yet empathize at several levels with what is happening on the screen.

Shifting focus from the content of the film, Mitra (1999) studies the structures that hold the film together; that is, the properties that sustain the narrative. By studying the film narrative, we can examine the logic of the story, look at the stereotypes portrayed, and delve into the several layers of meanings and interpretations. The text itself can be read at various levels of complexity. According to Mitra (p. 49), two primary semantic units can be used in the categorization of films: the place and the character. When we study the portrayal of madness in films, therefore, we have to do so both in the context of the place as well as the character. The meanings the author, the director, or the actor attribute to madness may not be the structures that an audience views in the same manner.

Mayer (1972), in his landmark publication on the sociology of the film, uses the term "participation mystique" to understand the psychological mechanism of the film or television experience. Following on from the theory of Lévy-Bruhl, who suggested that human beings were prelogical (this being more visible in primitive societies), Mayer proposes that participation mystique, or "mythical participation" as he calls it, is a useful term because it allows adults to see the theatrical or cinematic performance as "play". Thus, prelogical societies (traditional or kinship-based societies such as India) can and do have this mythical participation in the cinema. Such a participation therefore allows the Indian viewer to see cinema at multiple levels: that of simple entertainment, occasionally educational, confirming prejudices, and feeling detached or involved. This participation relies on a number of factors such as age, gender, and education. Folk theatre in India, as typified by the staging of *Ramayana* and other street theatre such as puppet shows, allows the individual to observe and be involved; this interplay is also seen in the cinema, but the degree of involvement differs. There are differences between staged dramas and films, although historically films were often literal filmings of stage plays.

Monaco (2000, p. 48) suggests that the most salient difference between staged drama and film drama lies in the fact that in the latter we see what the filmmaker wants us to see. Films have, no doubt, been influenced by theatre and the unit of construction in both is the basic scene. Hindi cinema has been influenced by Parsi theatre, which is what makes it loud and slapstick, particularly in its early days. Unlike theatre, the viewers of a film cannot "enter" the milieu; they are merely surrounded by it, and yet can lose themselves in it. Music plays a key role in this process: Tunes, songs, and background music can all raise expectations as to what is about to happen, what is on its way (the music of the film *Jaws* is an excellent example), and what has already occurred (repeating tunes that have already been played).

Films convey meaning both through denotative and connotative means. A film can convey a more realistic or closer approximation to reality, and can communicate precise knowledge; written or spoken language can seldom do this. Language systems are often abstract, whereas films can be seen in a concrete way. Further, cinema can use other art forms to create various effects, as well as record them. As a film is the product of the culture it is set in, the diagesis (the sum of its denotations) expresses something beyond the film. The way in which the scenes are constructed, the characters defined and delineated, and the manner in which the story moves forward with the help of music and symbols, lends the film a certain cultural edge.

The Hollywood formula was said to be based on certain elements recognizable to a public that had to know, in general terms, what to expect at the cinema every week. The primary ingredient of the formula was the star, an ideal for the audience to identify with, who was embodied in a constant personality from film to film (Roffman & Purdy, 1981, p. 3). The star's presence gave the public a clear idea of what type of film they were about to see. The genre film also had its own conventions.

The dramatic conflict hovered around the polarization of good and evil, with a clearly defined hero and villain. Unlike heroes in Hindi films, Hollywood heroes had some moral traits that were slightly tainted. An essential area of wish fulfilment was romance and true love. Womanhood was represented by two extremes—the virgin heroine and the sexual vamp. The resolution of the film was positive, that is, it had a happy ending. Conventionally, the emphasis was placed on the individual and the underlying assumption was that anyone could aspire to success (Roffman & Purdy, 1981, p. 6). Hindi films have followed the same formula, and in some cases copied Hollywood films scene by scene. The star cast in the 1950s and 1960s clearly identified the roles the heroes and heroines would play, and the cinema-going public would reject the film if its expectations were not fulfilled. In both America and India, the audience ranged from the rich to the poor living largely in the cities. In India, however, a proportion of the audience is poorly educated, often having migrated from poor rural areas to slums in the cities.

A key factor in cinema's contribution to society is the immense possibilities it holds for disseminating good or ill, given its widespread influence on the juvenile as well as the adult mind. Added to the films themselves are the various sources of information appended to them such as fanzines, other periodicals, and media coverage, including film reviews, and interviews with directors, actors, and other professionals linked with pro-duction. Shah (1950/1980, p. 4) asserts that the social power of the film lies in the subtlety of its propaganda rather than in any particular theme or story. Shah states that one of the most significant effects of cinema is that it makes for a similarity of outlook among people of different occupations, incomes, or classes and, to a lesser degree, among nations; it produces an increased awareness of various themes and issues among the audience. In this context, it becomes crucial to examine the way people portray mental illness and how it is seen by the reviewer.

Roffman and Purdy (1981) have identified in the Hollywood of the 1930s the gangster cycle, and also the woman's cycle and the prison cycle, which presented the individual as a victim. This was followed by a period in which the individual was redeemed. Next came the influence of fascism, followed by the optimism of the postwar Hollywood film, and then films showing violence with sci-fi thrown in. These trends bring out the cyclical nature of films. In Hindi films, too, the cycle has gone through mythological, social, crime, and romantic films. The social films of the 1960s were seen again in the 1990s under a slightly different modified and perhaps more modern and retrotraditional guise.

Roffman and Purdy (1981, p. 257) point out that, until the mid-1940s, alcoholism was rarely dealt with in a serious fashion by Hollywood; pro-hibition as a cause of crime was the context in several films. Since this volume does not aim to tackle alcoholism and its portrayal in Hindi films, the subject will not be discussed here.

Hollywood also shied away from mental illness for a long time and it was only in the 1940s, with the acknowledgement of the emergence of psychoanalysis, that psychology and psychotherapy made their appearance in various films. However, mental illness was seen and projected as being similar to physical illness. It was curable, like physical illness, provided you had a good white-coated psychoanalyst who would fix the broken pieces of the mind. The first serious exposition of mental illness in Hollywood came in 1948 with *The Snake Pit* (Roffman & Purdy, 1981, p. 260). Messages were often conveyed about the treatment of, and physical space afforded to, mental patients, as well as about staffing problems and shortages. The genre of films depicting social problems did hold up a mirror to society: These films suggested that the ugly truth is not really so ugly, and that individuals can rise above the problems facing them and their families if they deal with them with professional help. Although several directors in Hindi cinema, such as V. Shantaram and Guru Dutt, looked at social problems, more often than not their films won critical acclaim but had little success at the box office.

Rodowick (1991) urges that the most productive way to use Freud in film theory is to derive a theory of signification from the Freudian theory of fantasy. Looking at both male and female bodies thus becomes second nature to the viewer. The association of heroes or heroines with certain specific genres allows the spectator to indulge in fantasy without any guilt. It is interesting to note that it is the image that transcends and illuminates the fantasy. The language used to describe "identity" as a different form, conforming to an image of gender, class, or race, is intrinsically tied to the mechanics of power. Such power is multilayered and multifaceted. The producer, the director, and the distributor all dictate to the actors what is expected; the spectators also have power as in their sexual gaze see the image as sexual.

Carroll (1980) observes that the latent content of the dream is of great interest to the psychoanalyst and this inference (which derives from the psychoanalytic theory) abstracts the analysis from the subjective experience. The study of phenomenology qua theory, according to Carroll, notes that viewers know that they are not witnessing reality perceptually, but the coding of the images becomes important. Lebeau (1995) refers to the point in Freud's account of the favourable circumstances in which a female patient was able to "capture" an unconscious fantasy in the process of making its way to the conscious fantasy life or daydream.

The psychological determinant in films is therefore introspective. The relationship between the world and the work (the film) reflects the connections between the work and the artist which, in turn, affects what the work communicates to the observer. Monaco (2000, p. 32) suggests that psychological analysis of the film centres around the connection between the artist and his work, which varies with his psychological states. Interestingly, as films are both capital-intensive and labour-intensive, they also have to be seen as economic products. Monaco (p. 68) points out that once the work of art has been completed, it has a life of its own and is an economic product waiting for exportation and exploitation. The end product is political, and it is up to the viewer how to interpret the political component. Both the political and social conditions that are prevalent may determine the context of "art". The utility of art (in this case, films) lies in the fact that it is useful and enjoyable: Its usefulness is governed by the political doctrine, and its enjoyability by psychological factors.

The portrayal of mental illness, mental distress or disability, and physical disability in Hindi films has broadly paralleled the cycles seen in Hollywood films. Occasionally, Hindi films on mental illness showing its cure and its impact on both the sufferer and others around that individual, have been inspired by Hollywood and have reflected social, political, and economic factors prevalent at that time.

Films may be limited in their appeal because of the time constraint involved, as well as the limits to the geographical access and emotional access they have. The information contained in novels is controlled by authors and we see/hear/read what they want us to, though we may read *into* the characters, situations, and actions according to our own knowledge, experience, and attitudes. On the other hand, even though the auteur of the film is controlling what we see, the scenes are far richer on the screen than in the novel. The driving tension of the film is between the materials of the story and the objective nature of the image, and the viewer can participate in the experience much more actively.

DEFINITIONS

Film draws on other arts for its connotative power: Films use neologisms. Wollen (1969/1972) suggested that cinematic signs are of three orders:

(1) *The Icon*: A sign in which the signifier represents the signified mainly by simulation of it, i.e., its likeness.
(2) *The Index*: This measures a quality, not because it is identical but because it has an inherent relationship with it.
(3) *The Symbol*: An arbitrary sign in which the signifier has neither a direct nor an indexical relationship with the signified.

A scene may have a paradigmatic connotation, i.e., if a person is shot from above, his/her stature will seem to be lower than if he/she is photographed from below. Further, the connotation may be syntagmatic, i.e., the meaning of the shot adheres to it because it is comparable with other shots that we see. After the filmmaker has decided to shoot a scene, the next decisions are how to shoot it (paradigmatic) and how to present it (syntagmatic). To understand the cinematic signs, it is essential that we understand what phenomena are, how they exist, and how they are defined and understood in psychiatry and psychology.

SIGNS, SYMBOLS, OR PHENOMENA

Persson (2003) suggests that in the world of phenomena (this is relevant to understanding the mental phenomena in psychiatry and psychology, too), we perceive and categorize entities, called objects, that have certain properties such as colour, weight, and position. In the phenomenal world, things not only exist but also happen. In addition, there are clear distinctions made between living and nonliving matter. Events and social situations are seen as coherent routines and habitual activities, which proceed in a temporal chain. It is when these activities lose their normality and are replaced or overwhelmed by unreal events, that thoughts and experiences are changed by phenomena, causing the individual to develop mental distress or illness. It is essential to highlight that cultural, religious, and personal rituals play an important role in the phenomenal world, giving meaning to the world. These rituals also provide a channel for formalized interactions, which is what is expected of the individual in terms of behaviour. The creation of narratives and fictional worlds, whether in literature or cinema, involves some degree of fantasy (which could be called unreality), and this influences the way the participants or observers respond and behave.

It is through our emotions that we relate to and make sense of the world by which we are surrounded. Our emotions, and other people's reactions to our emotions, are experiences that regulate and synchronize our behaviour with others. Under the circumstances, we enter the world of the phenomena portrayed on the screen, however temporarily. Interestingly, and not surprisingly, our entry into the disjointed and unreal world of an individual who is mad is chaotic, frightening, and perhaps too close to the bone, more so if no previous exposure exists. The portrayal of madness in films is generally unsympathetic; madness is either shown as frightening, in a psychotically violent way, or it provides comic relief to give the audience a break and sense of relief. Thus, an individual watching another's madness, even if it is somewhat distant, gets drawn into feelings of bewilderment, to which he or she responds with fear or a sense of comic relief.

The world of phenomena is part of one's consciousness and philosophy. Another approach to the phenomena is through culture. The components of culture, such as its artefacts, tools, technology, rituals, images, and language are the key mechanisms by which we experience the world of phenomena (Cole, 1996). It is through interaction with these artefacts that the members of a culture develop practices, conventions, norms, and codes (Persson, 2003). Thus, there is little doubt that the introduction of new technologies alters the individual's view of the world of phenomena. The use of e-mails, the internet, and SMS texts has already redefined the way messages are communicated to friends and has changed the nature of the friendships. Shared phenomenal worlds make personal and mass communication possible. Thus, watching a film at home on television, DVD, or video is a remarkably different experience compared with watching it in the cinema hall with an audience. A film or genre of films is likely to be influenced by new technologies (e.g., use of digital technology in cartoon films). It may also introduce new ways or conventions in the daily lives of its audience. Another point worth emphasizing is that such changes can occur not only through the film itself, but also through its trailers, the broadcast of its songs on television, its publicity, and discussions of it in the print media. Changes in the sociocultural environment affect the phenomenal world more quickly than do changes in the physical-perceptual environment (Persson, 2003). The phenomena can be understood at different levels through various approaches, as indicated above. To understand this, it is helpful to understand visual perception.

There is little doubt that culture influences visual perception of individuals. Segall, Campbell, and Herskovits (1966) observe that experimental psychologists in general have been extremely reluctant to concede that groups of individuals perceive things differently. An analysis of the stimulus dimensions of a typical photograph helps explain how it might be perceived by one not familiar with it. Segall et al. point out that, when looking at a photograph, its strongest contours are its rectangular edges, which constitute its boundaries as a solid thing. Within these boundaries the most striking thing is the white border around the edge. But nearly 40 years after this observation photographs have changed because of the advent of colour and the virtual abolition of white borders with the development of digital photography. In digital photography the whole shape and viewing of the photograph has altered dramatically. When looking at a photograph it is clear that something large is being represented as quite small. Films similarly portray a three-dimensional world in two dimensions, which are being viewed as such but are being interpreted as three-dimensional. These conventions are invariably ethnocentric, which is why some films do well in some cultures and not in others. Combined with the visual perception is the auditory one. In any language sounds are organized into sets of phonemes, used for distinguishing meaningful vocal symbols. In addition to phonemes, each language contains many irrelevant, meaningless sound variations. These also rely on acquired distinctions of cues. Language also influences cognitive behaviour and vice versa. The role of cognitions across cultures has not been developed as much as one would have expected. Thus, a combination of visual perception, language differences, and cognitions would indicate the way in which a culture communicates and will be heavily influenced by that particular culture. For example, French cinema has its own style and the viewer knows what to expect. Similarly, Hindi musical films have a certain language style, both in spoken and visual manner, and the success of these films will depend upon how the audience interprets these.

Segall et al. (1966) also illustrate the cultural difference in colour perception and its colour vocabulary. They cite research which indicates that classicists had noted the lack of explanation of various colours in different languages, thereby indicating that most non-Europeans lacked a colour vocabulary due to an (inherent) defective colour recognition. There was a belief that human colour sense had evolved only relatively recently, i.e., within the last 3000 or so years. However, there may be an underlying suspicion that the colonized were inferior because they lacked a sense of colour, thereby explaining the innate superiority of the imperialist power. Subsequent studies disposed of such a hypothesis to a large degree. The point here is that although some languages may lack a vocabulary to describe various colours it is unusual to find that any culture lacks terms for major or primary colours.

Perceptual capacity has also shown itself to be differing across cultures. Thoulees (1933) noted that oriental artists produce strikingly flat, perspective-free drawings because "they see objects in a manner much further from perspective than do the majority of Europeans—they tend not to see shadows" (p. 330). Segall et al. (1966) emphasize that this is not the case. However, once again this illustrates that colour, composition of the picture, and perceived depth may be influenced by cultural differences. In addition to these cultural differences, personal differences are also likely to play a role. Following a study across different cultures, Segall et al. demonstrated that cross-cultural differences are not the same for all illusions. They conclude (p. 213) that:

> Perception is an aspect of human behaviour and, as such, it is subject to many of the same influences that shape other aspect of behaviour. In particular, each individual's experiences combine to determine his [sic] reaction to a given stimulus situation. To the extent that certain classes of experience are more likely to occur in some cultures, including differences in perceptual tendencies, great enough to even surpass the ever-present individual differences within cultural groupings.

These findings indicate in the viewer's mind the perception of various pictures from the same cultural background and the conversion of three-dimensional settings into two-dimensional images, and the interpretation of these in to three dimensions, thereby making it likely that interpretation is culturally influenced. Viewers look for the symbols they recognize, identify with, and can take away with them in their mind. These symbols will include archetypes that are culturally influenced and predominantly wrapped up in that culture. In addition, communication styles and the use of songs and situations will be determined by the culture. The archetype of the good, long-suffering mother, devoted sister, errant daughter-in-law, and wayward younger son have been exploited time and again by Hindi filmmakers. When these archetypes changed, largely in response to the changing political social and economic climates, it was inevitable that the reflection of these archetypes would be dictated by the society at large. Filmmakers will often state that they are simply reflecting the state of society.

Compared with psychology or psychiatry, the field of cinema is limited. Branches of psychology and psychiatry, using social, cultural, and cognitive concepts, attempt to understand individuals and their responses both in the context of individual cognitive schemata as well as social and cultural phenomena. Psychoanalytical studies of cinema focus on numerous factors. It is by understanding the behaviour of an individual and the processes taking place within them that the clinician can make sense of the individual's responses. Therefore, it becomes important to understand the phenomenal world too. It would be an understatement to say that the phenomenal world is complex; It is multilayered and multifaceted. To understand what the individual is going through, one must understand the interaction between the organism and the environment. This relationship is the basis of survival and understanding of the process of survival.

Understanding is the process by which we come to "have a world", and this forms the basis of our physical, cultural, social, and ethical behaviour in the world (Persson, 2003). Thus understanding may be seen as a "clinical" process involving perception and cognition, but it also involves complex emotions and feelings. Persson emphasizes that understanding does not operate in a void and has to be seen along with mental structures.

Mental structures that have "models" (e.g., cognitive schema and image schema) are thought structures influenced by culture and other related factors, such as education and social class. Within these mental "models" we have hypotheses, commonsense knowledge, the background knowledge of the individual, and the context. This conglomerate of beliefs is culturally obtained and culturally processed. Thus, the viewing of cinema and the understanding of its processes cannot be seen in a vacuum. These complex mental models form the basis for everyday reasoning. They may be influenced by previous experiences and culturally specific and culturally modified knowledge, which are generated from different domains. Human beings behave in certain ways due to intentions, emotions, sensations, perceptions, and beliefs. How these mental states are given causal status and how people reason around these depend upon the complex and culturally specific models of folk psychology (Dennett, 1981; Persson, 2003; van den Broek, Bauer, & Bourg, 1997). This makes the understanding of the portrayal of mental illness in cinema all the more interesting. It is then that it starts to make sense why some films depict the use of folk healers in their treatment and management of the mentally ill. Mental structures also encompass abstract phenomena, such as the people's image of politics, morals, righteousness, individual freedom, responsibility of the state, modernity (which is influenced by industrialization and urbanization), and religious thoughts (incorporating the concepts of fate, death, old age, life, etc.). The role of cognitive schema cannot be underestimated. Cultures dictate the individual's image perceptions.

Persson (2003) proposes that the parameters of an individual's disposition are important because they guide the encoding of information, bringing coherence to incoming stimuli and structure to their experiences. When individuals sit in front of the television or cinema screen, these parameters come into play. An individual's disposition includes certain assumptions that they place within the context of what is being shown and what is being understood. Obviously, if individual dispositions are shared, less information is required to be communicated explicitly. In addition, shared assumptions are oral, written, or image-based, making communication more effective, more efficient, and less ambiguous, but perhaps also more stereotypical.

When reading a book or viewing a film, a person treats the book or film as an object. A film acquires meaning only through its interaction with the spectator's knowledge of the world, morals, and dispositions that are being played on the screen.

Understanding of cinema discourse, according to Persson (2003), can work at many levels. In trying to understand how the audience views cinema, it is helpful to look at Persson's levels. These levels are also similar to the way mental illness is seen.

- Level 0 is the most basic level, at which all types of cinematic discourse are taken as formal patterns, independent of the content or the representational nature. Here the cinematic meanings are equivalent to the verbatim form and level of natural language. At this level, the viewer can identify patterns, movements, and various sounds, but these do not represent anything in his or her mind. In the context of mental illness, this level illustrates the basic problems of communication.
- At level 1, the viewer is able to see things in three dimensions, even though they are being portrayed in two dimensions. Here, the viewer enters the domain of representation or *mimesis*. The viewer sees mental illness as representative of something else.
- At level 2, perceptual meaning becomes more sophisticated and abstract; the viewer can recognize and identify a character across its various appearances. At this level, meaningless observations are given recognition and even the meanings attached to them by the viewer start to become more complex. The auditory and visual stimuli tend to come together in the viewer's mental structure. When applied to seeing mental illness on the screen, the experience becomes more personal for the viewer.
- Level 3 is marked by the introduction of situational or inferential meaning. The viewer can now understand the behaviour being

portrayed in terms of character psychology. Causal relationships can be understood and moral judgements made. It is at levels 2 and 3 that comprehension or narrative interpretation come in and possible explanations for mental illness can be made and understood by the viewer.

- Level 4 is one of more abstract meanings. The viewer's understanding of the temporal, causal, and spatial relations between different situations starts to become clearer. The viewer can make thematic inferences and explicit meanings, and use these to make sense of the moral of the story. These meanings can then establish symbolic relationships within the diagesis of the narrative. The behaviour of a mentally ill individual is understood in the narrative context, but at the next level sheer horror of the experience is interpreted. Understanding at each level depends upon the sophistication and the interest of the viewer. For mental illness this level can be understood in the context of what mental illness does to individuals and those around them.
- Level 5 includes the meanings understood at level 4, but the viewer's comprehension and interpretations include emotional reactions and attitudes towards the film. At this level the reactions of others to mental illness can be studied.

Persson (2003) suggests that levels 1 and 2 may be of interest to those concerned with special effects; levels 3 and 4 to scriptwriters; level 4 to reviewers; and level 5 to students of history.

A parallel set of factors that influence the viewer's understanding of a film are the assumptions they have formed about it. If the viewer assumes that the theme of the story is "X", for example, it will affect their perception and comprehension. The viewer may have formulated such high-level hypotheses at the beginning of the film or through the contextual sources (i.e., by reading the story in a film magazine, the book on which the film is based or reviews, by talking to others who have already seen the film, or by knowing who the stars and directors are and what genre of films they make).

Thus, according to Persson's (2003) description of levels, in trying to understand the portrayal of mental illness, the viewer has to go beyond the visual or auditory image. This is where the problem begins, because the mental image of the viewer is quite different from that of the characters. The reviewer's observations may be of little or no consequence in a country where the rates of literacy are low and few would read the reviews. However, an interesting new development in India is the proliferation of television channels, most of which telecast several programmes a day showing songs and/or trailers of forthcoming films. These mental representations may shift the viewer's perceptions and expectations from level 0 to 1 or even 2 or higher. If a trailer focuses on the violent consequences of mental illness, then viewers are likely to go to the cinema hall expecting precisely that. In the 1950s and 1960s, this was certainly not an issue, but over the past decade or so, it has become a major development. Recent releases, such as *Kyunki*, *Tere Naam* and *Aetbaar*, highlight the role of the (psychotic) hero, thereby priming the audience to expect certain kinds and levels of behaviour. It would be extremely interesting to explore the impact of film trailers on the viewer's attitudes, not only towards the film, but also towards specific psychiatric conditions.

There is no doubt that the discourse of cinema is influenced heavily by the media, fiction, narratives, legends, and folk tales. Such a discourse influences the audience in how they view a film and how they interpret it. These discourses are of two types: constructivist (building meaning) and detectivist (finding meaning), both of which will be influenced by the viewer's expectations, dispositions, cognitive and visual schema, cultural models, and clues from the images and representations of images, as well as by other stimuli such as songs. The viewer may be seeing what the director is showing, but, in addition, he or she interprets the background of such behaviours and internally translates the perception of the behaviours into mental images. The viewer also watches the characters interacting with each other and interprets their actions in a way that makes sense. Mental health professionals, too, can see only what is being shown while viewing the character (the patient), but they have to look beyond the character's behaviour to interpret and make sense of the mental image being projected. In a clinical setting, the mental health professional tries to understand the patient's distress on a one-to-one basis, and the clinical interaction allows both parties to determine and consolidate shared knowledge; in cinema, the viewer's gaze follows the film character's gaze onto the mentally ill person. The viewer's gaze may thus shift from one character to another, and this is where the deception comes in. In cinema, an individual's action or behaviour may simply be used to deceive the viewer, including the mental health professional.

As noted earlier, cultures determine how the viewer looks at something and how he or she interpret the film's gaze at the mentally ill and the mental images used to portray mental distress. In this context, it can be argued that psychiatry may look at the patient in a manner not too dissimilar from the way the general viewer does. The viewer's gaze at the mentally ill individual gets even more intriguing at another perhaps higher level. The actor is "playing" the role of the mentally ill individual according to his or her individual experiences and behaviours. This means that, to make sense of the portrayal, the viewer has to understand the circumstances (however dramatic they may be) and personality traits of the actor playing the mentally ill individual. Similarly, the viewer's gaze will also interpret the gaze of the other characters on the said mentally ill individual. The other characters' reactions and the messages contained in their gaze are bound to influence the viewer's gaze. The portrayal of the extent of stigmatization of the mentally ill individual depends on the way the writer perceives such a condition (i.e., where his or her knowledge comes from), how the director has developed such a character, and how the actor has interpreted the mental condition and the character. Although it may be crucial that the viewer should know about the stigma attached to mental illness, its portrayal in the film is not necessarily meant for education. It is more likely meant to provide entertainment, thereby making the character less believable.

Somaaya (2004) cites the case of *Hum Kisise Kam Nahin*, directed by David Dhawan. The hero, Sanjay Dutt, is a patient suffering from paranoia. The actor Amitabh Bachchan was originally due to play a psychiatrist, but was told by the filmmakers that as the audience would not be able to identify with the complexity of such a character, it would be safer for him simply to don a white coat and use a stethoscope. In this film, Somaaya compares the diagnosis of anxiety by simply checking the pulse using a stethoscope with the perception that all mental illnesses are alike and patients with different illnesses behave in the same way. She also gives the example of *Rakhwala*, in which Shabana Azmi plays the role of a mentally retarded woman. When the actress was asked what disorder she was supposed to be portraying, her response was unsatisfactory: She said that she had played the role as it would be perceived by the audience of commercial cinema (i.e., as the viewer may not be able to differentiate between different mental illnesses, a stereotype of mentally ill can be used as a shortcut).

The interpretation of the emotions of the characters through the director's eyes and the cameraman's lens and viewer's gaze is an interplay of many factors. Cultural factors determine which emotional expressions are to be highlighted and which suppressed. Yet viewers can understand some universal emotions and behavioural responses, which may influence their own responses, views, and attitude, and confirm their prejudices. To understand the mental state of film characters, the viewer has to assume that the characters themselves possess an ability to attribute these experiences to mental phenomena (Persson, 2003). What happens in the mental landscape of a given character is often related to the mental landscape of other characters, and the viewer has to be able to interpret this. As seen above, scriptwriters, actors, and directors may be reluctant to portray complex mental illness in case they do not make the grade in the eyes of viewers. The role of the viewer thus becomes frightening, even though the film is aimed at the viewer. Writers and directors focus on entertaining rather than educating by keeping the portrayal of mental illness at a very simple level. The causality of narrative is a psychological causality. Such causality, often attributed to "logic", distinguishes a list of events from narratives. For the narrative to succeed, the viewer has to be able to make sense of it, and, therefore, popular perceptions of madness have to fit in quite neatly into the narrative. Mental attribution and cognition thus acquire a very significant role.

To help the viewer make sense of the discourse on mental illness, the writer and director not only simplify what is going on, but also focus on less common or esoteric conditions, such as trance, possession states, "split personality", or multiple personality. Some of these conditions are culture-specific; others are not.

The state of society and its reflection of political and economic factors determine the way mental illness is used in the narrative. Quite often, mental illness is brought into the narrative either as a peg for hanging the story or to provide comic relief. The latter gives the audience the freedom to laugh at the mentally ill and feel relieved that this is not happening to them. Viewers have often rejected films that depict severe mental illness. For example, *Raat aur Din* did not succeed commercially, even though it was the last film of the noted actress Nargis and won several awards. *Funtoosh*, too, was unsuccessful in commercial terms, in spite of the fact that it starred the very popular Dev Anand. However, *Khilona* did succeed: Perhaps the songs and some light entertainment helped (see Chapter 14).

VIEWING THE FILM

Monaco (2000) offers some definitions of the icon, the index, and the symbol as denotative. However, these categories are not mutually exclusive. The link between denotation and connotation appears in a continuum; much of the connotative power of the film depends upon devices that are indexical. Metonymy is a figure of speech in which the associated detail or notion is used to convey an idea or represent an object. The synecdoche is a figure of speech in which the part stands for the whole or the whole stands for the part, e.g., an automobile can be referred to as a motor or a set of wheels. Both these concepts can be used as cinematic shorthand and are seen in old Hindi films. For example, blasts and mountains falling represent a burden on the individual, "the sky falling in". The pages of calendars falling or flipping into the wind are used to denote the passage of time.

Monaco (2000) asserts that the film has no grammar, but this does not mean that there are no rules. Although they may be vaguely defined, rules are present and systematic arrangements lead to the development of the syntax. Unlike written and spoken language systems where syntax deals with the linear aspect of construction, cinema includes spatial composition as well. The film syntax develops both in time and space (Monaco, 2000, p. 172). Roberts and Wallis (2002, p. 3) argue that, at a basic level, the study of a film has four points of focus: the text; the makers; the institutions; and the social, political, and historical context of the text. The narrative can be linear or episodic, and cause and effect may link events. The narrative structure in Hindi cinema includes emotional scenes, comedy subplot, and song and dance sequences held together by a thin thread of main storyline (Kasbekar, 1999). A popular Hindi film is thus radically different in narrative form and content from the Hollywood model of entertainment. Film syntax includes both development in time and development in space: The modification of the scene is called *mise-en-scène*, "putting in the scene", and the modification of the time is called montage, i.e., the signifier is more optical, whereas the signified is more mental.

Mishra (2002, p. 16) notes that in an India in which modernity is no longer something that "belongs" to a specific group and the "condition" of the state, "an etiquette of modernity from the point of view of eternal India", is most clearly found in the trans-India and universalistic agenda of Hindi commercial cinema. However, this critique is often subdued and subtle (as subtle as can be in Hindi cinema), but the criticism is also couched in family values and gender roles, rather than purely in religion. The role of melodrama indicates that renunciation and the mother contribute to the melodrama in the way that society allows them to. If we take Mishra's theory one step further, especially in the context of madness, the voluntary renunciation of reality indicates that, when combined with melodrama, the portrayal has to be over the top. The use of melodrama leads straight to bereavement, not necessarily as tragedy, but as a sentimentalized act. This allows the viewer and the performer to be involved, but at the same time gives them permission to detach themselves. The melodrama in two Hindu epics, the *Mahabharata* and the *Ramayana*, is discussed elsewhere in this volume. It can also be argued that melodrama allows the hero/heroine to reach a level of functioning where he or she can define his or her self and place this social self in the context of family and kinship. If the psychosis splits this self, it would mean that the social self is more vulnerable, especially because of the stresses of love and loss. The two points of view—that of the spectator and that of the director—allow spectators to modify their own view of the self and their identity. Thus, "the other" seen on the screen may become "the other" in their psyche, thereby making it impossible for them to accept the psychotic individual because that would reflect a fear of losing control. Metz (1982) sees the viewer as the voyeur, and viewing the madness may also provide a sense of relief: "Thank goodness it is not me." The moral of such stories then becomes amply clear, especially where a character says to another, "don't be mad", "you are crazy", "you are insane", and so on.

According to Mishra (2002), Metz (1985) identifies the specularity (in the audience's mind) with the Lacanian stage in which a child reads his or her own image as one another's image, but internalizes it as an "I". Mishra (p. 93) argues that the economy of the mirror image is incomplete in the specularity of cinema: One's own image does not appear, as the screen is not an image, and he asserts that there is no complete voyeurism either. There are two problems: First, the whole purpose of watching a Hindi film is to be entertained (and not necessarily to be educated), and to obtain a view of rich houses, luxurious lifestyles, and foreign locales of which the individual may only dream. Second, the voyeur is looking for personal titillation, whether it is sexual or materialistic. The voyeur's gaze focuses on what is personally relevant. This reflects one's own identity and notion of the self. The bad, represented by "the other", is not dissimilar to the mad. But whereas the former, the bad, gets resolved following appropriate punishment, the latter, the mad, remains more ambiguous. The concept of the mad may get confused with the sad, because both may be seen to be suffering, not always because of their own doing, but owing to an external set of circumstances.

READING THE IMAGE

Reading an image in the manner depicted in Figure 1.1 is similar to the interaction between patient and therapist, where the expression of mental disorder is being understood by the therapist.

The image of the film is experienced as both an optical and a mental phenomenon. The optical pattern is used saccadically, while the mental experience is the result of the sum of cultural determinants and is formed by them. The signifier is more optical than mental, and the signified more mental than optical. All three levels of reading—saccadic, semiotic, and cultural—then combine with each other in various ways to reduce the meaning either to essentially denotative or essentially connotative (Monaco, 2000). The image has to be studied and understood in a context, be it social, cultural, or political. The individual viewer, therefore, does so in different permutations and combinations.

In recent times, an increased attention by anthropologists to varied forms of visual culture, i.e., visual anthropology (films, video and television, and popular image production), allows us to understand visual expressions that form strands in larger cultural systems, which MacDougall (1998) calls "braids". In turn, visual media also becomes a means of exploring social phenomena and expressing anthropological knowledge. Films can be seen as ethnographic accounts of certain subcultures and cultural groupings. Although these film theories are developed in the west, it is useful to have a brief look at these because of their implications for Hindi cinema.

Gopalakrishnan (1995) acknowledges that Hollywood remains a big influence in world cinema today and, in America, it represents *the*

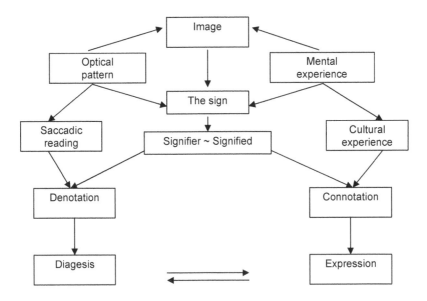

Figure 1.1 Reading an image

entertainment industry. He suggests that the difference between Hollywood and Indian cinema is related to the fact that the western mind likes to have things clear and compartmentalized. He objects to the dubbing of American films in Indian languages because of the mismatch of the two languages.

Chakravartee (1995) points out that cinema has enabled culture to be transmitted through a mechanical medium, which projects a totality of effect. The medium of films is a very sophisticated one when it comes to influencing cultural constructs. It is the breakdown of rural culture, and the acculturation resulting from industrialization and urbanization, that makes cultural transformation achievable. As assimilation proceeds simultaneously with adaptation, films have become the most expedient means for the export and import of culture. The influence of films on people belonging to the age group of 18–25 years is greater than on any other age group. For a film to have any bearing on culture, it is imperative that the psychology of identification should be operative, if such a process of identification begins to bring the distant closer and also creates and reinforces stereotypes. The portrayal of mental illness relies on this identification, which may be frightening to the viewer. In addition, stereotypes confirm this fear and colour the viewer's vision of mental illness in many ways.

The visual element acquired greater power in modern civilization with the visual arts, but became entrenched with the introduction of cinema.

This was the case for nearly a century before television (and now the internet) took over and added further elements to the visual understanding of culture. Gusdorf (1953) argues that whereas primitive man found equilibrium at the level of myth, modern man finds himself alienated from the myth as well as from the intellect: a double infidelity to the human condition. He suggests that such alienation is related to the demythization of our existence: a process that only accelerates with advances in technology. The alienation from the intellect contributes to anaesthetizing our fundamental values. The interaction between cinema and culture therefore has to be seen as bidirectional: cinema affecting culture and in turn culture affecting cinema.

Mayer (1972) posits that the media represents information and instruction, and not only reflects the trends prevalent in society but also goes on to influence cultural attitudes and beliefs. A good example of culture influencing cinema is the recent reworking of *Romeo + Juliet* by Baz Luhrmann. The setting has been moved to Venice Beach in the USA, with the Capulets and Montagues representing two competing business interests. The star-crossed lovers are placed in an extremely violent society, with startling images of guns and revolvers, police helicopters buzzing overhead, and a television newscaster providing a commentary, all of which reflect the social milieu of the late twentieth century. The fact that the film was such a huge hit in the USA and the UK in spite of its Shakespearean genesis suggests that it conveys some clear universal and visual values in consonance with the existing social mores.

On the basis of his study of the British audience and its views on cinema, Mayer (1972) suggests that the nature of the influence of cinema on its audience is also a moral one. He argues that such an effect, although exerted on all classes of British society, varies differently across class. Given the easy access to cinema (and now television and the internet), together with the uprooting of the traditional structures of life, the nuclear cinemagoer seeks a "participation mystique" in the story and the events unfolding on the screen, according to Mayer. The mystique of the myth among the Indian audience is discussed later in this book (see Chapter 5).

As noted above, the distinction between folk theatre and professional cinema is an interesting one. In India, folk theatre was largely subsidized and supported by sponsors. These were either the maharajas, nawabs, or rajas (the rulers), or the feudal landlords. Audiences could watch the plays or musical performances for free. The performances sometimes continued for days and contained an important element of improvization. After the British colonized India, a different pattern emerged and audiences had to start paying money to attend the theatre. Performances became more focused and one or two shows would be staged in a day, against the earlier practice of performances going on for days. Later, with the development of cinema halls, sections of the audience demanded greater comfort and privacy, which resulted in differential rates for entry. The financial aspects of going to the cinema, theatre, or internet café are minor inconveniences compared with the visual joy or observation that works as an eye into someone's life. The difference between theatre and cinema also allows the viewer to see things in three dimensions or two dimensions respectively, but the interpretation related to cognitive schema remains three-dimensional whether visual stimulation is bidimensional or tridimensional.

Living in this era of visualization leads to a consequence of the modern, rationalized structures of our lives. The key questions here are: Where does such a rationalization originate from, and why does it influence us so? It can be argued that, as a society becomes modern and rational, it still has an inherent need to escape into myths or folklore, which can change one's world-view. Although the rationalization is arguably scientific, irrational views of science and the impact of this nonetheless influence it. There is some truth in Simmel's (1908) observation that, compared with small towns, large cities are more visual than auditory. He suggests that modern communications, with their ever-increasing tendency towards pure visual-mindedness, produce something that concerns by far the greater proportion of the finer relationships between man and man. Mayer (1972) states that the impact of modern cinema on contemporary life is confirmation of Simmel's observations. This distinction also makes an interesting point about differences between the rural and urban audience and their expectations. Thus there are numerous differences in the way films are viewed.

Unlike the daydreamer walking through the streets, the viewer may impose an unconscious fantasy life on the screen, imagining what his or her life could be and also wishing for things to change. Lebeau (1995) argues that a fantasy made public through a dramatic spectacle, according to Freud's view, is reliant upon the writer's personal daydreams. The fantasy thus becomes embedded in a reality that is not necessarily that of the spectator. These daydreams can be benevolent (also communal and dramatic) through the creative gifts of the writer and a more silent, less speakable participation in the fantasy structure.

Kakar (1983) points out that popular Hindi films should be seen as a collective fantasy containing unconscious material and the hidden wishes of a vast number of people, as well as of the creators; though motivated by the goal of making money, through their marketing and product placement the creators of film also increase the needs and desires of the viewers. The films, therefore, have to be singular enough to fascinate and excite but general enough to excite many. Kakar's view is that Hindi films emphasize the central features of fantasy—the wish fulfilment and humbling of enemies and competitors. The underlying message, of course, is that the struggle in life is inevitable but, if one faces life's hardships and its many often unjust impositions with courage and steadfastness, eventually one will emerge victorious. Kakar points out that, in the end, both in fairy tales and films, parents are happy and proud, the princess' hand won, and villains are either ruefully contrite or dead. Evil too may be in temporary ascendance but its failure and defeat in the long run are inevitable. Evil in Hindi films is related to narcissism and the attractions of licentiousness in sex and alcohol. Another point, according to Kakar, is the oversimplification of situations, and the elimination of detail as in fairy tales. The characters are always stereotypical without any unnerving complexity of real people. Kakar criticizes the rationalist critics of Hindi films who dismiss these films as being unrealistic and unbelievable by pointing out that their condescending judgement is usually based on a very restricted version of reality. Their description of the external world may be seen as flawed, but their grasp of the topography of desire is sure-footed and confident.

The origins of fantasy may be a result of unavoidable conflict between many of our desires related to environment and environment's inability to fulfil these, but the power of fantasy comes to fruition by extending or withdrawing the desire beyond what is possible or even reasonable. Nandy (1981) confirms that the Bombay film is a spectacle, not an artistic endeavour. In a spectacle black is black and white is white—all shades of grey must be scrupulously avoided. Any change in the story has to be dramatic. Nandy notes that spectacle has to be an overstatement with predictable climax, with its storyline being synchronic and ahistorical. Thus typecasting, where certain characters are played by well-known actors who will rarely change the type they play, makes sense. This is linked with the fantasy of the viewers; if viewers go to see a Bruce Willis film, they have certain expectations, e.g., they would wish to see action and not comedy, although some actors manage to straddle more than one genre.

Theatre reflects the prevailing social and political climates more spontaneously and has a sense of immediacy, something that cinema can only sometimes provide. The satirization of political leaders and political philosophies is again more pertinent and immediate in theatre than in cinema. This may be related to the fact that the development of a cinematic project is more complicated and cumbersome; getting the story and script right is likely to take longer, and identifying the director and other personnel is a time-consuming task. On the other hand, a play is initially a one-person job and, even though putting it together on stage may take some time, once it has been handed over to the impresario it is more immediate in terms of improvization of recent happenings.

The growth of cinema can also be linked with the development of capitalism in American society. This relationship is important, but its impact on the audience that "purchases" the product is beyond the scope of this study. However, the growth of capitalist society allows a specific directional development of cinema. As India has opened its doors to globalization, not only has the number of films increased, but the technical quality has also improved.

CONCLUSIONS

In summary, we can say that cinema has caught the imagination of people all around the world, in spite of their different cultural traditions. Various cultures influence the storytelling and the visual understanding of the story differently. The ways we look at a story, interpret the visual coda, and note the signifier and signified are determined by a number of factors, such as education, social status, and past historical knowledge. This mode of looking at cinema is parallel to the mode by which clinicians see mental illness. The optical and mental aspects of any visual stimulation determine what is seen in the story. The iconic representation within the film and the iconic status of the film stars influence the message that each viewer derives from the story, and this message is different for different people.

CHAPTER TWO

Culture and mental illness

The World Health Organization (WHO) defines health as well-being and not merely as an absence of illness. Mental health and mental illness are often seen as exclusive to each other, and the criteria for health include medical, personal and social factors.

Mental illness, on the other hand, is seen as a condition with certain positive features. It is a term derived from the medical model of mental disorder, and is used to describe a number of behavioural patterns that disrupt the smooth and orderly conduct of life. The term is often used as a catch-all to include many psychiatric conditions, varying from anxiety, depression, and phobias (also known as common mental disorders) to psychoses such as mania, schizophrenia, and depressive psychoses. The use of a definition to medicalize problems arising from social maladjustment, and personal, emotional, and motivational problems, makes the conditions seem broad, generalized, and too nonspecific. The label of mental illness can be extremely stigmatizing and frightening, not only for the sufferer, but for the carers as well.

The study of mental disorders (psychopathology) entails knowledge of certain statistical, physiological, psychoanalytical, behavioural, and humanistic norms. Any deviation from these norms (which may well be defined by the society, family, or specific individuals, for example community or religious leaders) can help in the recognition of abnormality, but not necessarily in a diagnosis of mental illness.

There are, of course, problems with such statistical approaches in defining abnormality and the interested reader is directed to other works including that of Davis and Bhugra (2004) and Sims (1999). According to the statistical norm, it is assumed that people who diverge from the majority are abnormal. The physiological paradigm assumes the existence of an underlying physiological or organic defect. Thus, psychopathological states can be likened to medical diseases and, like diseases, they manifest themselves as a set of symptoms. A diagnosis is made on the basis of this group of signs and appropriate interventions may be put into place.

This approach has contributed to important advances, such as the discovery that general paresis of the insane is caused by uncontrolled syphilitic infection and that there may well be a genetic predisposition to schizophrenia. Therefore, the therapies associated with this paradigm often include biological interventions to address the presumed physical or biological disorder. Mental illness is also defined in cultural and social norms.

The psychoanalytical paradigm for mental illnesses relies largely on the theories of Sigmund Freud, who proposed that mental disorders arise from repressed and unresolved conflicts in childhood, and from the relationships the patient had as a child with parents and others. Central to Freud's theories is the idea that individuals undergo four phases of development of psychosexual urges: oral, anal, phallic, and genital. Each highlights a specific part of the body that is presumed to be more sensitive to erotic gratification than the other parts. A satisfactory resolution of each stage helps the individual cope successfully with stress and demands later on in life. On the other hand, when these underlying conflicts remain unresolved and misunderstood, psychiatric problems may well emerge during adulthood.

According to the behavioural paradigm of the development of human beings, an individual is more likely to repeat actions that are rewarded than those that are not. Society determines which of these actions are "normal" and which are "deviant". Principles from classical conditioning, operant conditioning, and cognitive psychology are used to explain how the individual develops, learns, and deals with subsequent pressures and stresses.

The humanistic paradigm relies on an innate drive for fulfilment and growth. According to this, man's basic nature is good and, when this is denied, human beings develop psychological distress.

Each of these paradigms has something to contribute to the understanding of human distress and psychiatric illness, and none by itself can adequately explain the origins of distress. Thus, in understanding and managing psychiatric distress we need to take more than just one model into account. Depending on the model being used, society will still define, to a large extent, what is normal and what is not.

One of the prominent antipsychiatrists, Thomas Szasz (1962, 1981), has argued extensively against the concept of mental illness on the basis that, as the mind does not exist, neither does mental illness. His rather simplistic view is that psychiatrists cannot demonstrate mental illness simply because they are not able to define it. He argues that mental illness exists only in the eyes of those who believe in imaginary illnesses or causes, and that even though mental illnesses are related to the brain and not to the mind, there is no clear biological evidence to demonstrate them. Superficially, this view is extremely attractive, but one of its major problems is the denial of the distress that patients and their carers suffer, irrespective of the causation of this distress and the various factors that contribute to it.

Although developed for local use, the Diagnostic and Statistical Manual Test–Revised (DSM-IV-TR; American Psychiatric Association, APA, 2000) has been used around the world and defines mental disorder in many ways (either as distress, dysfunction, dyscontrol, disadvantage, disability, inflexibility, irrationality, syndromal pattern, aetiology, or statistical deviations). Mental disorder is a combination of one or more of the above. It is conceptualized as a clinically significant behavioural or psychological syndrome or pattern that occurs in an individual. It is associated with present distress (e.g., a painful symptom), disability (impairment in one or more important areas of functioning), a significantly increased risk of suffering death, pain, or disability, or with an important loss of freedom. Thus, a manifestation of a behavioural, psychological, or biological dysfunction can be construed as mental distress. According to this approach, neither deviant behaviour (for example, political, religious, or sexual) nor conflicts that are primarily between the individual and society can be called mental disorders, unless the deviance or conflict is a symptom of a dysfunction in the individual.

It is inevitable that the classification of symptoms into disorders can lead to a classification of individuals rather than of conditions. Making a diagnosis and using a more categorical approach is problematic, especially across cultures. No category can be bound by absolute boundaries, although in the two major classification manuals, the International Classification of Diseases–Version 10 (ICD-10; WHO, 1992) and DSM-IV-TR (APA, 2000), there are sincere attempts to reach diagnoses that are bound by operational criteria. Thus, it is important that all individuals who suffer from the same condition should not be seen as being alike in every way. The use of cultural, ethical, and clinical judgements is essential for the development and employment of any diagnostic criteria.

Eisenberg (1977) suggests that even the models adopted by psychiatric clinicians for diagnosing and managing disorders are often pluralistic. Helman (2000) lists the possible factors affecting the standardization of psychiatric diagnostic aspects across cultures. These include a lack of hard physiological data, the vagueness of diagnostic categories, the range of explanatory models available and used by the clinician and the patient alike, the subjective aspect of diagnosis, and the influence of social, cultural, and political forces on the process of diagnosis. Such factors create a situation in which the clinician and society can interchangeably dub the diagnosis as mad or bad and vice versa, depending upon the context.

The perceptions of a person's social behaviour may depend on how controlled or uncontrolled it is, and how far it conforms to or deviates from the norm. Helman (2000) postulates that a particular society's perceptions of social behaviours and the fluid nature of such an acceptance allows individuals to develop these behaviours in view of their personality, motivation, experience, emotional state, or physiology. The normality, like the social definition of sickness, depends upon a range of factors such as age, gender, occupation, social rank, and social distance. Anthropologists have defined the rules (where rigid codes of moral behaviours are deliberately flouted or inverted) as sites of several and symbolic inversions (Babcock, 1978). These acts of explosive behaviour invert, contradict, abrogate, or, in some fashion, present an alternative to the commonly held cultural codes, values, and norms, be they linguistic, literary or artistic, religious, social, or political. In this way, illness can be inverted into a form of fun. Thus, visual or written portrayal can be taken to a logical extreme without social sanction. As for spirit possession and trance states, they can be seen as reversals and regressions into childhood behaviours. However, they still fall within certain taboos, social, political and economic contexts, and implicit cultural norms. In normative terms, they are still identified as odd or abnormal, and help is sought. This allows the individual not only to become "the other", but also to deal with the "dangerous" other in a socially acceptable way.

The development of a disease pattern depends on several factors. The first step has to be recognition of the symptoms by the sufferer and his or her carers, in that they have to recognize as abnormal either the phenomena being experienced by the sufferer or the resulting behaviour. The recognition of these behaviours or experiences as abnormal may be confined to that particular society, although sometimes experiences across cultures and societies may well contribute to the definition of abnormality. For example, when Malaysia was under the British rule, "amok" was identified as a culture-bound syndrome and, ever since, the term has been used to identify a mentally ill individual. Prior to colonial times, the state of being amok was seen as an acceptable form of the expression of distress. It is only when the British changed the law to identify amok behaviour as criminal that the condition was not only medicalized and pathologized, but also criminalized. On the other hand, when individuals in the USA suddenly start shooting at random and without provocation, they are treated differently and are not said to be running amok, even though the two phenomena are the same. More abnormal physical investigations underlying the clinical condition have been reported (for further discussion see Bhugra & Jacob, 1997; Levine & Gaw, 1995).

According to Wig (1994), there are often wide divergences between what is described under European and North American classifications (probably because these systems of classification have emerged from these countries and were based on original observations on these populations), and other countries and cultures. For example, a far greater number of cases of acute psychosis are reported from India than are cases of schizophrenia along with ill-defined somatic complaints, which do not fit into organic pathology, but are without doubt a significant cause of distress. Therefore, the role of culture in the development of psychopathology and help-seeking cannot be underestimated. These models are worth noting as they are portrayed in films in culturally specific ways.

The key questions that need to be linked with the aetiological models of mental illness are whether these models themselves are influenced by culture and cultural expectations, and the way the individuals themselves influence the models. Wig (1994) raises the possibility that the essential core of psychiatric illness differs across cultures and that sociocultural factors act as modifying factors, influencing the presence of symptoms.

However, a new movement within psychiatry called New Cross-Cultural Psychiatry led by, among others, Kleinman (1977) and Littlewood (1990), denies the universality of psychiatric symptoms. Littlewood argues, "Psychiatry at present lacks any rigorous theory for dealing with the dialectical interplay of biology and human society or for examining the relationship between psychopathologies and its own procedures of research and practice."

Wig (1994) suggests that this view indirectly casts a doubt on the whole approach of structured interviews and defined operational criteria on the grounds that the methods are as biased as the phenomena they are supposed to study. The uniqueness of each culture and society may be subsumed under the similar threads running across different cultures, especially as a result of globalization through the media, i.e., the easy access to films, television, the written media, and now the internet. The frustration experienced by clinicians who try to fit square pegs into round holes may be due to their failure to understand the impact of acculturation and the media. The portrayals can never be straightforward and changes in such portrayals are commonplace.

Wig (1994) posits that drastic positions on the uniqueness of each culture and subculture might do more harm than good, in that they obscure similarities across cultures and mental illnesses. He points out that,

Although the scientific method may be universal, the topics chosen for scientific study and the particular instrumentation are determined by scientists, who are themselves prone to personal and cultural bias like any other group of human beings. Yet without some degree of generalization and categorization, it is very difficult to proceed in modern science.

Such a paradox means that not only professionals are caught between generalization and categorization, but also lay people will find it confusing.

Definitions and perceptions of mental illness have a bearing on the effectiveness of the practitioners of psychiatry, who try to help those seeking help from them. If individuals see mental illness as a physical condition, they will seek help from physicians. On the other hand, if they see it as a spiritual trance or possession state, the chances are that they will first approach religious or faith healers, especially if these are close by. Often, however, the reality is that individuals use pluralistic models of explanation and help-seeking. Wig (1994) suggests on the basis of his own clinical experience that people know for which conditions modern treatment is effective and for which it is not. For example, people in rural societies of India turn to modern (western/allopathic) services for the treatment of epilepsy, psychosis, severe depression, and acute anxiety. However, people often seek traditional healers for dissociative or somatoform disorders. Another factor influencing the perception of mental illness and, consequently, the success of the practitioner, is the way the subject is portrayed in the media. On the whole, the kind of help provided by the practitioner, as well as its success, depends on what is required and accepted by the people.

The cultural dimension of psychiatric classification acquires maximum importance in the case of low-income countries, where the role of metaphysical, spiritual, and philosophical factors in the treatment and management of psychiatric disorders must be taken into account. Therefore, the definition of mental illness and mental distress depends very heavily on the norms, be they statistical, biological, psychological, or social. Of these, the social norms may be more abstract and more difficult to define and test, whereas the biological and psychological ones are easier to define, test, and treat. What is intriguing is that individuals suffer from disease, but it is illness which affects others around them, and it is the illness which is often portrayed in the cinema.

Eisenberg (1977) draws the distinction between disease and illness. It is important to bear this distinction in mind because it is the illness that needs to be studied and often portrayed, while the disease is what the clinician tends to focus on. The clinician's perception, labelling, interpretation, and treatment of a condition focus on a specific pathology. For example, in the case of a patient complaining of excessive thirst, polyuria, and weight loss, the physician will look for evidence to determine whether the patient is suffering from diabetes mellitus. Through physical examination and investigations, the clinician can show the illness process to be a disease. The clinician thus constructs a new social reality: The interpretation of the disease and the patient's understanding of it will undoubtedly influence the way the members of the society think of and handle their illnesses. From the biomedical viewpoint, a disease is an abnormality in a biological structure or function that generates the symptoms of illness (Kleinman, 1986).

Kleinman (1986) suggests that illness has several meanings: overt, covert, subtle, cultural, and subjective. Individuals, their families, and society understand these meanings. The cultural meanings of illness are quite significant, in that they partly define and influence perceptions and the monitoring of bodily processes, as well as the very behaviours that constitute illness as a life experience. Culturally marked disorders can be said to "bring" these meanings to patients and their social networks.

The illness, suggests Kleinman (1986), also takes on peculiar meanings which differentiate our personal lives and interpersonal situations from each other. Bodily processes are mediated by our understanding of them as meaningful events and their relations in our lives. He goes on to argue that a person simultaneously has a sick body (which separates the individual from the real individual), and is the sick body (the sickness is the individual). Illness meanings so viewed are physiological as well as social, indicating that illness is also viewed in different ways.

The sick person is seen as different beings with different meanings by those who surround him or her. For example, the sick person's spouse may see the sick person as being a bad parent; the sick person's parents may see the sick person as not being a good child; the physician may make an assessment in terms of pathology, and so on. Thus, the illness process itself may lead to differential identification of the patient's distress. The process also "empowers" the sick individual to take a break from routine tasks. At the same time, when an individual's functioning is affected by illness, it may well erode his or her power as an individual.

The arts, which include cinema, represent sickness and sick or ill individuals in different ways, which are in turn influenced by stages of the culture. The role of the sick individual in providing for the family in spite of the illness, the role of continuing to hold that particular job, the stresses leading to or a consequence of the illness can all be seen as and reflected as narrative points in the film. Pinney (2001) uses the term "cultural agency" to indicate a whole domain of potential interventions in the world through cultural practices, representational declarations, or cosmological hypotheses. Cultural agency is seen as indicating the political consequences of films (e.g., if the film depicts decay of the state it influences the voting patterns) and becomes a way of conceptualizing diverse domains that share the common positioning of the individual and collective.

In order to make the discourse on mental illness within the context of the film easier (more understandable), the author and the producer/director simplify the concepts of mental illness, often confusing symptoms and lumping various psychiatric conditions together (Bhugra, 2005). The psychiatric conditions portrayed in films are therefore exotic and esoteric.

The relationship between the healer, doctor, or shaman and the patient is of crucial importance in understanding how a particular culture deals with the ill individual, as well as the condition. Moreover, there is no doubt that clinicians and patients often share the language of illness and its meaning, but the interpretation of the language is different in the minds of the two individuals. The interplay between the clinician and the patient, like the interplay between disease and illness, is a complex one.

PSYCHOSES AND THE WESTERN PERSPECTIVE

As psychosis, as a clinical condition, is often misunderstood, feared and made dramatic by the lay person, it offers an attractive option for the authors and directors of the films to utilize to make dramatic points. Therefore, it is important for the reader to know a bit more about the condition.

Psychosis is not a heterogeneous entity but can be broadly defined as a mental illness in which the individual loses touch with reality, and his or her mood may be elevated, depressed, or blunted. The patients may suspect that people are against them or are plotting to harm them. They may feel that forces or powers external to them are interfering with their thoughts and bodies. The person may hear voices, see things, or smell odd smells without any source to explain these experiences.

There are different kinds of psychoses, including mania, depressive psychosis, schizophrenia, and schizoaffective psychosis. The recent revision of the DSM-IV-TR defines schizophrenia as being characterized by delusions, hallucinations, disorganized speech, grossly disorganized or catatonic behaviour, or negative symptoms, i.e., affective flattening, alogia (difficulty in speech) or avolition (lack of volition) for less than 1 month (APA, 2000, p. 298). The other dysfunctions include social/occupational dysfunctions. There are various subtypes of schizophrenia. In mania, the patient is elated, expansive, or irritable for at least 1 week, with one or more additional symptoms, such as grandiosity, decreased need for sleep, excessive talking, flight of ideas, distractibility, and excessive involvement in pleasurable activities. The mood disturbances are sufficiently severe to cause marked impairment in occupational functioning (p. 362). It is sometimes difficult to make a diagnosis and the clinician may have to rely on third-party information, investigations, and observations.

Cultural factors have an extremely important influence on the development of symptoms and the outcome, and are essential for studying help-seeking. The attitude of the carers reflects on how they identify pathways for the care of a mentally ill individual. In this context, how the symptoms are perceived, i.e., whether they are seen as abnormal, threatening or non-threatening, and the stigma attached to the patient's condition by the larger community, become significant factors. Of course, the role played by the carer is also determined by the interventions available locally.

The overall western view of psychoses needs to be understood, largely because it is those ideas which are carried into India (and consequently into Indian cinema).

Several major international multicentre studies have looked at the rates of schizophrenia and the possible socioeconomic factors involved. The International Pilot Study of Schizophrenia (IPSS), conducted by WHO in 1974, studied cases of schizophrenia at 11 sites across nine countries; three sites were in developing countries. This was followed by a WHO-sponsored study titled Determinant of Outcome of Severe Mental Disorder (DOSMED; Jablensky et al., 1992). These studies found that the rates of schizophrenia were broadly similar across the developing and developed countries, but cultural differences were ignored in the interpretation of the data. In the IPSS studies, nine centres were involved to ascertain whether the main study (DOSMED) was possible. Using standardized inclusion criteria and assessments (covering a 1-year follow up), the DOSMED study identified some factors that could influence the formation of attitudes in rural Chandigarh. For example, a joint family or extended family was the norm and 50% of the sample was uneducated. (A joint family has been described by Karve, 1953, as "a group of people who generally live under one roof, to eat food cooked at one hearth, who hold property in common and participate in common family worship and are related to each other as kindred".) However, as the studies recruited patients from healthcare centres, which rely on personal/social, professional and kinship views, the individual differences in the findings were ignored. Cohen (1992) argued that although data were collected on the structural elements of the culture and the distinct treatment modalities, they were not correlated with other findings. He also pointed out that the vast majority of cases were recognized only in the settings of western-type psychiatric facilities. In developing countries, the proportion of cases involving acute onset was twice as high as that in developed countries. This may indicate significant differences in the cultural manifestations of schizophrenia. Further, Karno and Jenkins (1993) observed that the better prognosis in developing countries might well be related to family networks, which would make the family an ideal unit for research. We can also say that the importance of the family unit in these countries and the resultant differences in mental illness (especially schizophrenia) leads to different pathways to care as well as differences in the outcome.

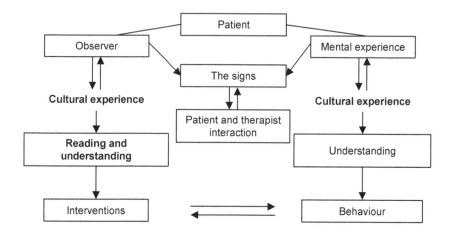

Figure 2.1 The relationship between culture and symptoms

The forms an experience takes in different social systems need to be translated into a universal language if there is to be a cross-culturally valid science of human behaviour and clinical work (Kleinman, 1977). A society's attitudes to illness of any kind are embedded in its local context and the prevalent hierarchy of the individual, family, kinship, and society at large. The local cultural system systematically relates the person (agency) to the social structure, bridging physiological processes and social relations (Kleinman, 1977). The interaction between the therapist and the patient illustrates the relationship between culture and symptoms (Figure 2.1).

It is clear that culture can influence the development and treatment of mental illness by defining what is normal or deviant, how the treatment is sought, and the sources used for treatment. Cultural mechanisms can be beneficial in creating preventive strategies. Culture allows individuals to use various cathartic emotional strategies, which may well be culture-specific. In addition, cultural factors influence mental health by providing mechanisms that reduce the impact of stressors by social adaptation and by creating social roles. Cultures can create and sustain gratifying environments through the use of socioeconomic organization, political control, and leadership. Culture influences child-rearing patterns, which in turn may determine personality traits, especially if genetic factors are involved in the aetiology of personality disorders. By fostering unhealthy practices, such as mating within the ingroup, cultures have a bearing on what the individual becomes vulnerable to. Cultures also influence how an individual "sees" certain things. It may be added that these perceptions affect how the arts and cinema deal with culture-specific norms. Culture has an effect on nonverbal communication as well, and constitutes the medium for the transmission of certain patterns. Considering all of the above, any portrayal of mental illness is bound to be affected by various cultural and subcultural patterns.

CONCLUSIONS

There is little doubt that cultures influence mental illness in a number of ways. Cultures provide idioms of distress to allow the individual to express underlying emotions in a culturally appropriate way. Cultures can produce psychopathology, can cover up psychopathology, and can facilitate the development and perpetuations of psychopathology, as well as providing means by which any therapeutic intervention is sought and delivered. Thus, it would appear that although schizophrenia as an illness may exist in different cultures, the symptoms that form this illness and the possible aetiological factors may well vary. The portrayal of mental illness, the pathway into care, and the outcome are likely to differ across cultures.

CHAPTER THREE

Cinema, emotions, and psychiatry in India

The Hindu personality and its basic nature, in terms of narcissism, confusion, and paradoxical compartmentalizations, have been discussed by many at length (Lynch, 1990; Spratt, 1966). Here, the focus is on specific emotions and how they fit into or portray the psyche of the Hindu individual. As most of the data looks at Hindu individuals, although occasionally the term Indian is used, the psyche described is Hindu.

Lynch (1990) suggests that emotion means different things in India than in its western counterparts. He argues that the social construction of emotion in India differs from the physicalist theory based on the writings of Descartes. According to Descartes, emotions are the registering in the soul of particular feelings caused by primary sensations associated with some ideas or perceptions. Similarly, William James suggested that bodily changes directly follow the perception of an exciting fact and "our feeling of the same changes as they occur is the emotion" (1890/1902, p. 261). Behaviourism, psychoanalysis, and cognitive approaches further expanded these theories. The cognitive approach dates back to *Aristotle's Rhetoric* (Lynch, 1990).

When we talk of social construction of emotions, we mean that emotions are appraisals and judgements of situations made on the basis of cultural beliefs and values. Lynch (1990) suggests that emotional appraisals are constitutive for the individual and deeply involve or even move the self in its relationships to social "others", things, and events. As cultural appraisals, emotions are learned or acquired through society, and do not arise naturally. They are, therefore, culturally relative. They are identified by the intention of the object. However, the viewer may misunderstand the emotions and the cultural influences on these.

Bedford (1986) defines emotion similarly, suggesting that emotions presuppose concepts of social relationships and institutions, and concepts belonging to the prevalent systems of judgement: moral, aesthetic, and legal. It is through emotions that behaviours can be understood and fitted into the complex background, making human actions intelligible.

In India, the "rasa" theory of emotion developed from a poetic, dramatic, and aesthetic tradition laid out in the Treatise on Dramaturgy (called *Natyasastra*) and is seen as cathartic. It lists eight primary emotions that are inherent in all human beings: love, humour, courage, disgust, anger, astonishment, terror, and pity. In addition, there are 33 transitory emotions, which include envy, jealousy, despair, and anxiety.

The rasa theory draws upon elements in the Ayurvedic texts. The physical or gross body ("sthula sarira") and the inner subtle body ("linga sarira") are the physiological and psychological predicates, respectively. The Ayurvedic texts do not posit any dichotomy between the mind and the body. Residing in the linga sarira is the "manas" (mind or heart; the mind is said to be situated in the heart), which is the centre for reason and judgement as well as emotion.

The rasa theory was reinterpreted by the Vaishnavites, the exponents of the medieval devotional (*bhakti*) movement, according to which the aesthetic experience becomes the vehicle of religious experience itself (Wulff, 1985). *Bhakti* was conceived of and was meant to be experienced as an emotion through which the individual attains a state of bliss. The Vaishnavites reduced the eight primary emotions to the following five:

- *Santa bhava*: repose, calm, grace.
- *Dasya bhava*: the humility and obedience of a servant towards the master.
- *Sakhya bhava*: the friendship between friends.
- *Vatsalya bhava*: the love of a mother for her child.
- *Madhurya or sringara bhava*: the erotic love of lovers.

A knowledge of the emotions in literature and poetry is helpful to understand how these are portrayed in cinema.

Lynch (1990) emphasizes that the emotions outlined by the Vaishnavite sects are based on real human relationships. It is interesting to note that in most Hindi films the underlying predominant theme involves one or more of these emotions. The religious emotions are part of everyday life in India, largely because religion and spirituality are an integral part of the Indian way of life. Emotions also have a very strong and clear moral influence on how everyday actions and life are conceived and evaluated.

On the basis of his supposition that the personality traits of the adults reflect on the way their children are brought up, Boss (1969, p. 67) argues that the development of aggressive traits in children in India is curtailed by the way infants are pampered by the many women belonging to the clan group. The link of this observation with emotions is discussed further in the following chapters, when we start to look at the portrayal of mental illness in Indian cinema. The ways emotions are felt, expressed, and understood are influenced by culture.

The interactions within different systems generate both pathological and modifying processes, and protective and preventive processes. The risk for illness, its onset, and psychological distress are, to a great extent, the result of factors present in the place one lives in and particularly one's relationships, i.e., the local cultural macro- and microsystems.

Spratt (1966) discusses literary descriptions of the behaviour of individuals suffering from material and maternal deprivation. Such a loss may be linked with a sign of guilt but, in the emotional sense, descriptions of grief are drawn from observations of the typical reactions of the less cultivated type of narcissist. Spratt observes that nearly all the heroes and heroines in different myths pine away and grow pale, not due to unrequited love, but due to the pain caused by separation. They lie on their beds, are afflicted by fever, and sandal paste and fanning increase their heat rather than cooling them. The convention in these stories is that it is the intensity of emotions that kills the protagonists, and not that they actually commit suicide. The heroes and heroines in these stories are emotional individuals and stories are portrayed with emotions that are understood in specific cultural formats by the listeners and viewers. The personality of the Hindu is seen as being ascetic and leading on to deprivation of material belongings.

Restraining one's emotions resembles restraining the public expression of one's emotions, especially in response to spouses. Once the dam bursts, it becomes extremely difficult to control one's emotions. Related to deprivation is the concept of tapasya, which may include inflicting pain and deprivation on oneself in order to obtain a boon from a god. Anger is often used for rebelling against the father, and the son's self-castration or self-abnegation allows him to obtain his father's blessings. There are countless examples of this in Hindu mythology and the association between power and chastity occurs commonly. Pain and material deprivation may divert the libido inward, towards the ego, and may accentuate narcissistic trends in individuals.

According to the narcissistic principle, when the struggle for supremacy is between a son and his father, the son may succeed; when it is between father and daughter, the father must succeed. The youngest son too has a special place in such psychology because he is treated more indulgently and his conflicts with his parents may be more muted.

In Hindi cinema, the mother often plays a key role in the life of the hero. Marriage and motherhood are shown as the pinnacle of desire for even the most educated and modern woman. The roles allocated to women within marriage and family are clearly demarcated. Vasudev (1988) remarks that one of the paradoxes of Hindi films is that the woman, on the one hand, is victimized as a wife and, on the other, venerated as a mother. This mother figure occupies a prominent place in the cast of characters of most films. The mother–daughter relationship is handled by few Hindi films and is treated as less significant than the mother–son relationship. The strong tie between the mother and son can lead to maltreatment of the daughter-in-law. For the young daughter-in-law, salvation lies in producing a child, preferably a male heir. The relationship between sons and overinvolved mothers in Hindi films reflects the Indian psyche's desire to be helpless and be looked after. More often than not, male characters tend to manipulate this maternal affection and responsibility.

Hindu society reflects the Hindu personality. For example, the people are passive in their relationship with leaders. The case is similar in relationships with members of other minority groups and religions.

A note of caution is necessary in understanding the influence of Hindu psyche on the Hindi cinema. Das Gupta (1995, p. 242) bemoans that the higher class, more intelligent audience stopped patronizing films, leaving behind the lower class audience. In order to cater to the latter, filmmakers take their films to an even lower level, thus reinforcing the trend. They fail to take into account that understanding of film does not necessarily mean involvement. Just because a viewer understands the film, it does not follow that he or she would become involved in its proceedings or vice versa. In their attempt to make the film understandable at the lowest common denominator, filmmakers may well exclude a large section of the audience. Currently, Hindi cinema is in the process of being pulled down to its lowest possible level of understanding, though there have been similar episodes in the past.

In contrast to the Hindu or Indian expression of emotions, European values have been quite different, for instance in identifying abnormal emotions.

The impact of Hindi cinema and its popularity has taken many of its stars to the Rajya Sabha, "the upper house", as nominated members. Many, including Amitabh Bachchan, Rajesh Khanna, Vinod Khanna, Sunil Dutt, Raj Babbar, Shatrughan Sinha, Jayaprada, and Dharmendra have stood in elections for the Lok Sabha, "the lower house", and often have won and then even gone on to become ministers. The reasons for their success are many and beyond the scope of this study.

In Europe, with his *The Birth of the Clinic*, Foucault (1973a) dared to look with a critical eye at medicine and its consequences, such as the establishment of hospitals, teaching hospitals, and other medical institutions. The fantasy or the imagination of the doctor, the advances in scientific tests and investigations, and the patients and their carers influence a number of interactions. These interactions are related to the situation and attitudes towards the illness. The gaze of the viewer, as perceived by Foucault, is the key signifier; for Descartes (who spoke of the mind–body dichotomy, thereby placing mental illness at a different level), to see was to perceive. The individual became an object, with its own particular qualities and its impalpable colour, and its unique transitory form acquired weight and solidity. It is this formal reorganization in depth that makes the clinical experience possible for the patient. The doctor–patient relationship and the resulting therapeutic encounter, therefore, has to be seen in this particular context. Seeing such an encounter on the screen allows the viewer to be an observer, without actual participation or modifying any part of it. Yet, he may be influenced by it in a way that might be quite unpredictable. His type of observation is more like that of a peeping tom than that of a scientific or detached observer. The outsider in this encounter, therefore, is not only the character who is seeing the doctor or the psychiatrist, but also the viewer.

As mentioned in the first chapter, the signifier and signified are autonomous, and their importance lies both in their individual characteristics as well as their joint interaction. When we talk about the thoughts of others, we analyse the signified, whereas analysis of the commentary itself may prove to be more appropriate and helpful. Foucault (1985) goes on to propose that the history of ideas was initially linked with the aesthetic method, involving analogy (and charted in time or in historical space), and the denial of contents, from which emerges psychoanalysis. Any configuration of disease and the localization of illness are therefore linked with a fundamental system of relations between the patient and the therapist.

The doctor, for example, gazes at the patient, but not at the concrete body (that viable whole). The doctor gazes at the intervals in nature, lacunae, and distances: the signs that differentiate one disease from another. Similarly, the viewer sees the screen in terms of components. The difference may be that, whereas doctors and patients maximize their differences, as do the viewer and the auteur, the latter dyad is at a physical distance, which may provide an element of "protection".

The analogy between the clinic and the cinema can be extended further, as both represent something to the dyads. However, the space provided for the interaction between the participants may be more objective in the cinema and more subjective in the clinic. Yet, the observer status of the viewer (participant) may cause within them a sense of knowledge of alienation, depending upon the type of cinema. Another similarity is that the system of classifying diseases may not be universally applicable (as discussed in the previous chapter), as is the case with cinema, which also is culturally influenced. Thus, even if a Hindi film is a direct copy of a Hollywood film, it is heavily Indianized as, for example, *Chori Chori* (Raj Kapoor–Nargis), which was modelled on *It Happened One Night*.

Foucault (1985) argues that like civilization the hospital is an artificial locus, in which the transplanted disease runs the risk of losing its essential identity. The disease has the same natural locus, the family, as the natural locus of life. In India, where the family has always been a key component of society, placing the individual self in a particular context, the portrayal of family life in Hindi cinema becomes an even more potent factor. The expression of love, spontaneous care and a common desire for cure assists nature in its struggle against illness. In the Hindi films discussed later, the family plays a very significant role, and has a strong presence in managing patients, as well as their attitudes to what has been termed as *baawrapan*, *paagalpan*, *zunoon*, and *divanapan* (also called *deewangi*), all synonyms for madness.

The hospital doctor sees only distorted, altered diseases and a whole range of extreme pathology, whereas the family doctor and the family are at the forefront while dealing with the disease before any complications arise, and in supporting and helping them understand problems and solutions. Unlike in Europe, and contrary to Foucault's assertions, the health-care system in India is needs-based and pluralistic. Patients and their families think nothing of seeking help from an astrologer, vaid, temple priest, shaman, or homoeopath at the same time as seeking help from a western physician or healthcare worker.

Using France as an example, Foucault (1973a) proposes that lunatic asylums were developed because of the sense of power and control that one set of individuals wanted to impose on another. He argues that confinement, initially used as a tool by the police, began being used as a means of preventing mendicancy and idleness as a source of all [mental] disorders. In western Europe, at least, confinement was used as a way of dealing with the economic crisis afflicting the western world at the time: It was a question of not only confining those out of work, but also of giving work to those who had been confined, thus making them contribute to the prosperity of all.

The development of the asylum is based on the eighteenth-century economic analysis. As private nursing homes in India are often more accessible, more expensive, and possibly less threatening, the split between the patient and the carers, and between them and the doctors may be less intimidating. Foucault (1985) argues that though diseases vary from one period to another and from one place to another, they are related to the overall poverty of a nation, but only in economic terms. Given the wars and famines characterizing the Middle Ages, the sick were prone to suffer from fear and exhaustion (apoplexy fever). This gave way to a period of relaxation in the sixteenth and seventeenth centuries. The consequence was greater lust and gluttony, and the spread of venereal diseases. When the eighteenth century dawned, the search for pleasure was carried over into the imagination and, consequently, theatre and literature flourished. This, according to Foucault, meant that one stayed up at night and slept during the day, leading to the emergence of hysteria, hypochondriasis, and so on.

As Foucault (1985) noted, not only the prevalence of different illnesses changed over the decades; the medical conditions that emerged and are presented in cinema and literature also changed according to social, political and economic climates. Also, the symptoms with which patients go to the clinic are equally influenced by cultural norms.

The first task of the doctor, according to Foucault (1985), is political: The struggle against disease must begin with a war against bad governance. Man will be totally and definitely cured only if he is first liberated. In this polemic, Foucault is right in linking poverty and riches with different types of illnesses, but his argument that liberty will somehow cure all diseases does not hold water. Liberty, whether of society or of the individual, places a different set of responsibilities and stresses on the individual. Foucault's notion that if inequalities were reduced and concord reigned, the doctor would have no more than a temporary role to play is nothing but a utopia. Medicine would then embrace a knowledge of healthy man, that is, the study of nonsick man, and a definition of a model man. So under this vision of Foucault's, how can the doctor's role be temporary?

The cultural differences between India and Europe are many, not only in terms of importance of emotions and how these are expressed, but also how emotional distress is identified by lay and professional people alike. How the society creates the sickness and places where sickness is treated, and how these clinics are created, is essential in understanding the role sickness plays in that society and culture.

The prevailing notions of health and normality are important in our understanding of the portrayal of any illness, but perhaps more so in case of mental illness, as are definitions of normality and deviance. In modern medicine, pathology and normality are often polarized, and this emphasis on diagnosis determines what the doctors do.

Foucault (1985) further argues that social and pathological spaces should be understood together if medicine is to make any sense. The convergence between medical technology and political ideology is an important factor in making sense of the individual's experiences. Hospitals were developed to look after sick people who had no family, or those who were very poor. Foucault (1973b) suggests that as the family was bound to the state by the notion of collective social duty, it was the state's responsibility to provide assistance. Thus, it is important to make sense of the family's as well as the nation's gaze on the illness.

The principles advocated by Foucault (1985) cannot be blindly applied to other cultures and societies, especially India, where the concept of "the other" is quite different. His argument that asylums were religious domains without religion, but domains of pure morality and ethical uniformity, ignores nondenominational institutions. It is worth highlighting some of his ideas on asylums simply to emphasize the differences between Europe and India. Foucault (1973a) holds that, in asylums, all signs of the individual's old life (outside the asylum) are obliterated. The asylum represents the great continuity of social morality and the values of family and work reign there. These came to the fore in two ways: First, these values are at the heart of madness, lying beneath the violence and disorder that characterize insanity. Second, the asylum reduces differences between individuals, represses vices, eliminates irregularities, and denounces everything that opposes the essential virtues of society. This needs to be remembered when we talk of films where asylums are being shown.

Foucault (1973a) argues that the asylum generates an indifference (among those outside it) if the law does not reign universally because there are men who do not recognize a class of society that lives in disorder, negligence, and almost illegality.

In French asylums, Pinel organized the life of the inmates so as to allow moral syntheses to function. Of these, silence, the absence of language, was a fundamental structure of asylum life. The second was fostering recognition of oneself through the mirror: The inmates were made to observe themselves. The third was perpetual judgement, which Foucault (1973a) links with the law and the legal system. Medical help was the fourth factor guiding the running and development of asylums; the physician played an important role in the "diagnosis" of mental disease.

The medical factor gave rise to the possibility of the development of a new relationship between doctor and patient, and also between insanity and medical thought. This is what ultimately came to guide the modern ideas regarding madness; the asylum has been converted into a medical space. Further, the doctor–patient dyad has become a madness–disorder (or should it be order–disorder?) dyad. The branch of medicine dealing with the mind has assumed almost complete autonomy. There is now an eagerness to discover the origin of madness, whether in organic factors or hereditary dispositions.

In Europe, the positivism imbibing the study of medicine and psychiatry gave the psychiatrist more and more power, verging on the miraculous. The doctor became powerful because the authority he borrowed from order and morality became his. His seemingly magical potential reached an even greater height with the development of psychoanalysis in the nineteenth century.

For a variety of reasons we need to create "the other", an individual who stands for something quite opposite of what we stand for. How "this other" and "the other" get defined, identified, vilified, criticized, made fun of, or rejected outright, is crucial in understanding of our functioning in relation to the individual.

"THE OTHER" IN THE INDIAN CONTEXT

The process of describing "the other" in the Indian context is a complex one. Traditionally, in a sociocentric society, "the other" is not one individual against one individual, but perhaps against the entire kin group. The way "the other" is viewed fulfils the need for demonization, especially if "the other" is more threatening to the individual's kinship and family than to the individual. The derogation of "the other", who is sociocentric, is by emphasizing the failure of "the other's" family and kinship. "The other" is essential because such a concept performs several functions. Being an outsider, she or he can be heaped with blame for doing wrong. She or he is easy to target and easy to hate, so such ill feelings become acceptable, especially from a distance.

It would appear that if the said "other" does see mental illness as a visitation, it mitigates his or her responsibility and it becomes easier for others to accept the mental illness. It was under the British rule that asylums developed in India in the eighteenth and nineteenth century. Foucault's hypothesis does not seem to be entirely applicable to conditions in India. First, in India, "the other" and the disorder in society were related to a very strongly hierarchical class- and caste-based society, which gave rise to the possibility that individuals who were outsiders were rejected more readily. Language and exposure through confession were key elements in Europe, but such factors (especially confession) did not exist in the Indian tradition. The same logic thus cannot be applied in the Indian context. Furthermore, the creation of space for the mentally ill was unnecessary in India because the individual may have found it in a more spiritual and religious context, rather than in a medical one. Medical personage, in the traditional psychiatric sense, remains a relatively modern development. For a considerable period, the British did not allow the natives to become doctors (Bhugra, 1999). As Ernst (1988) avers, the Raj looked after its own mentally ill individuals; when its own employees and the white soldiers became mentally ill, they were sent back to the UK.

Two aspects of the development and role of the asylum are worth examining. One is the institutionalization of mental illness, i.e., its being taken out of the family, kinship, and local folk systems. The other is how it promoted professionalization. Both are necessary for understanding the portrayal of mental illness in Hindi cinema.

The British developed lunatic asylums in India following exactly the same models as in Britain, importing the architects and architecture intact, without taking local needs or climate into account. Victorian buildings were

constructed as almost exact replicas. The development of professionalization of alienists led to the development of a new discipline. Both these
approaches meant that the traditional models of looking at emotions and
mental illness were seen and identified as backward. Thus, the portrayal
of mental illness had to be professional and urban.

The Ayurvedic system of medicine, which has its roots in ancient India,
is one of the three great non-western traditions of medicine. By including a
theory of the self and of social behaviour, the system not only complements
the previously existing theories of philosophy and metaphysics but also
those of health and illness. The kind of understanding that the ancient texts
display of madness/insanity and the sympathetic attitude of the healers
indicates a degree of acceptance of the mentally ill not evident elsewhere in
the world. Haldipur (1984) dwells on some such issues. Like other authors,
he notes that there is no mention of special mental hospitals or asylums in
the ancient traditional medical texts. Fabrega (1991) assumes that the
family and community provided for the immediate and long-term care for
the psychiatrically ill. He also assumes the existence of areas of confinement
in the concerned homes and the clinical facilities of practitioners (although
this has not been discussed in any text).

The emergence of asylums meant not only ignoring, but also positively
denigrating the traditional Indian systems of medicine. The British set up
the East India Company on 31 December 1600 and, incidentally, it was a
doctor who managed to get the company its first trading rights. The influence of the British on the development of psychiatry in India can be considered under three points: the establishment of the Indian Medical Service,
the development of asylums, and the influence of the Royal Medico-
Psychological Association.

It is said that the last known asylum in India before the British came was
in existence in Madras in the ninth century (Somasundaram, 1987). The
early establishment by the British of mental hospitals in India reflected the
needs and demands of European patients in the country (Sharma & Varma,
1984). The growth of asylums runs parallel with the turmoil that accompanied the decline of the Mughal empire in India, the resurgence of the
nationalist Sikh and Maratha movements, and the fight for supremacy
between the British and French in south India. It is significant that the first
asylums were established in the three major cities that the British helped
develop: Calcutta, Bombay, and Madras. Bombay had an asylum in 1745,
Calcutta in 1787, and Madras in 1794, with subsequent expansions in 1799
and 1807.

The first Lunacy Act, passed in 1858, set out the procedures for the
admission of mental patients, as well as guidelines for establishing mental
asylums. It also gave the police the power to round up all wandering
lunatics and all those noted to be dangerous. These people were presented

before a magistrate and, if they were certified insane by the civil surgeon, they would be ordered to be removed to an asylum. Alternatively, they could be discharged and entrusted to the care of their relatives.

In cases in which there was a doubt about the sanity of the patient, the magistrate could order detention for 10 days (extendable to 14 on medical certification) in an asylum. In Presidency towns, a relative of the patient could apply for detention, provided two physicians agreed (Ewens, 1908).

The asylums in India were built for the same reason as those in other countries. The idea was to protect the community, and segregating the patient was in answer to popular demand (Shaw, 1932). The structure and functioning of these asylums were clearly based on British concepts (Burdett, 1891). Early data suggest that the number of patients in Indian asylums was relatively lower than that in asylums in the UK in spite of a larger population. Ewens (1908) attributed this difference to the greater simplicity of life in India, the effect of the climate and tradition, and training rendered.

The construction of mental hospitals, in terms of their layout and architecture, was in the hands of Shaw, who, in 1932, suggested that a "pantlion" or "block" arrangement of buildings would be suitable. He held that Europeans and persons with European habits should not, as a rule, be treated in the same mental hospitals as Indians, not on grounds of sentiment, but because the accommodation and amenities necessary for the one were unsuited to the other.

Shaw blamed Gandhi and the Indian freedom movement for obstructing the progress of psychiatry. He felt the Ayurvedic and other indigenous systems of medicine were backward, compared with the system of medicine practised by Galen. It is important to understand the role of colonialism if we are to gain a complete understanding of the Indian psyche, as well as the social and cultural developments in the country. The task becomes more complicated still because of the high degree of heterogeneity and the variable impact of cultural factors in India.

Traditionally, the figure of the householder is an important one. Das (1999) points out that, while studying everyday life in India, we cannot place it solely within some universal notion of the family, but must also be aware of the particularity of Hindu civilization and tradition (Madan, 1987).

Urbanization, education, and social/cultural change in India have contributed to cultural adaptation. Cohn (2000) points out that few of the cultural and structural changes that have taken place, whatever their source, are not distinctively Indian. He mentions that in colonial times, as a response to colonization, some writers took on the mission of trying to purify Hindu thought and culture. They wanted to rediscover the country's past. These writers felt that, somewhere along the line, degradation had set in as a result of occupation, marring the rationality, monotheism, simple democracy, and sexual equality that reigned during the golden age. As the ideology of the western-influenced elite took hold, ambivalence towards, and then rejection of, the colonial masters grew.

Indian culture has seen many changes over the past 50 years. Cohn (2000, p. 112) suggests that to understand such a complex culture, one needs to penetrate the "bewildering proliferations of social forms and cultural expressions in India", which include a well-established hierarchical system. This hierarchy extends from the family to kinship and lineage. Even the greetings used symbolize the hierarchy central to the social structure. One's position in the social group too is symbolized at many levels. Any study of films or the visual media must take this hierarchical system into account.

Cinema is a medium reflecting cultural values. If one looks at the films of the 1930s to 1950s, they clearly reflect the prevalent mores and attitudes, although Murthy (1980) argues that they also reflect a fantasy which may bear no relationship to reality. However, the fantasy, too, is influenced by several factors such as folk tales, religiomagical preoccupations, and society's perceptions. Thus, the portrayal of madness is coloured by many factors, the predominant one of which may be the identification of "the other".

Desai (2004) observes that with the changes in the country's mood following Independence, the leading actors of post-Independence India, too, started to change. In the late 1980s and 1990s, caste and communal strife became more pronounced, which was reflected in the films of the time. We shall discuss later how the changes in the portrayal of characters in Hindi films corresponded with the changes that each decade brought. With the changes and fragmentation of society, the portrayal of madness changed accordingly, from gentle to extreme psychotic to psychopathic. The psychotic breakdown of society, leading to the fragmentation of the ego ideal, is well illustrated in many films in which men become increasingly and irrationally possessive about their women, and rationality goes out of the window. On the other hand, early heroes, played by Dilip Kumar, Dev Anand, and Raj Kapoor, are idealists, though as Desai points out, the portrayal of the characters differs according to the persona of the star and their place in the market.

Another important feature of Indian culture is the purity–pollution continuum, which is manifested in the hierarchy involved in the categories of food, and in the process of giving and receiving food. In this context, Cohn (2000) mentions five types of food: raw food (purest), food fried in oil, food boiled in water, food obtained from garbage, and, lastly, carrion. The purity of food varies, as does the degree of pollution. The purity–pollution concept also figures in the perception of madness. Coming in contact with "the other" (indicated by madness) is linked with a fear of pollution. Films deal with this in a paradoxical and ambivalent manner, with the family being split about the way the mentally ill individual should be dealt with. In this context, the film *Khilona* provides an interesting example (see later).

It is likely that, in Hindi films, madness is envisaged in a patchy way because the distinction between the good guy and the bad guy has always been black and white, with no room for grey areas apart from a few honourable exceptions. Because of this, the villain or the vamp becomes "the other" and no clear role is attributed to the mad people. There have been exceptions, of course, and over the past two decades or so the characters of the hero and the villain have started to merge.

As India remains a group-based society (although this is beginning to change as a result of urbanization), most of an individual's actions and behaviour are related to a sociocentric identity and concept of functioning. Cohn (2000) compares the concept of belonging to groups to the layers of an onion, reflecting the collectivist or kinship-based society.

The family to which the male belongs is related genealogically to other families, which live close by. Though relations between them may be hostile, the ties binding males to a lineage remain strong and colonization has not diluted these links. Getting an idea of these social ties, obligations, and rights, together with duties, is helpful in understanding the Indian psyche. It is also vital to make sense of the individual's links with the group and kinship. These ties are not equally or constantly operative; they are situational and contingent.

Caste is another essential aspect of the Hindu identity; certain occupations are bound up with certain castes. For example, for a considerable period of time, no Hindu woman (of any caste) played the role of the heroine in Hindi films. Instead, initially men dressed in female attire used to play the heroine in early films. Then Anglo-Indian women, followed by Muslim women (from the singing/dancing communities), started to do so. It is only in the past 50 years or so that Hindu women have emerged as heroines. Similarly, for a long time the occupation of nursing was considered suitable only for people of the lower castes and Anglo-Indian Christians.

The recent changes in the political system related to caste and kinship systems have had a strong influence in many spheres. Certainly, the portrayal of these systems in Hindi cinema also changed after Independence. In an increasing number of situations, one's caste has ceased to matter much. This is particularly true of the modern urban economy at least, in which roles now tend to be achieved rather than ascribed. It is still not unusual, however, for people to be put at a disadvantage due to discrimination and prejudice in certain areas, in rural as well as urban conurbations.

CONCLUSIONS

Personality is the sum total of what makes an individual behave and respond in a particular way. A person's behaviour and responses are likely to be influenced both by genetics (i.e., the accident of birth) and his or her upbringing (familial, social, and cultural environment). It is possible that different cultures ensure the development of culture-specific traits in the personality. When one talks of psychopathy or an antisocial personality, it is worth bearing in mind that some behaviours may well be more acceptable in certain cultures than in others. The role of culture-bound syndromes has already been alluded to. Although clinical research in this field is inadequate, anecdotal observations suggest that some types of clinical behaviours and personality traits are more common in some cultures than in others. It is also likely that bad behavioural actions are perceived differently.

CHAPTER FOUR

Attitudes towards mental illness

Attitudes to mental illness and mentally ill individuals are a result of multiple factors, both at the societal and personal levels. Interestingly, these attitudes do not always turn into behaviours. An "attitude" is defined as a tendency to react in a certain way towards specific events, people, ideas, or objects. An attitude has three components: thoughts or beliefs (cognitive), feelings (emotions), and behaviour. A knowledge of attitudes is not only germane to those concerned with the origins and maintenance of disturbed behaviour, but can also be used to develop means of primary prevention and early intervention, as well as community treatment of psychiatric patients (Bhugra, 1989; Rabkin, 1974).

Psychiatry and mental illness have had a bad press for a long time now. Mentally ill persons have often been misunderstood, as has the role of psychiatry. It was felt that psychiatry and psychiatrists promised to deliver much, but failed miserably in their attempt to deliver treatment or care. The tendency to confuse mental illness with religious possession, witchcraft, and sorcery, and to confuse psychiatric treatment modalities with mesmerism and hypnotism, signified the failure of modern science in the mind of the public. Furthermore, even now, when "modern" technologies such as brain scans are available and used extensively, the failure to determine precisely where the pathological lesions are makes it difficult for society at large to understand mental illness.

Throughout human history, mental illness and the treatment of mentally ill individuals have been emotive issues, and public attitudes have mirrored the prevailing social and cultural factors. For example, reactions to the taboo group or "the other" depend upon several factors. These include the frequency of the actual or anticipated behavioural events and, more importantly perhaps, the place that the said behaviour occupies in the hierarchy of taboos. Additional factors are the visibility of such behaviour, together with its intensity. The visibility of such behaviour in public places depends on the geographical location and the "abnormality" inherent in it, in addition to the actual drama and circumstances surrounding such behaviours (Fracchia et al., 1976).

At a personal level, attitudes towards mental illness and the mentally ill determine the source of help. At a community-based level, they determine the resources put into the delivery of mental health care, as well as the recruitment of staff for delivering those services. Mental illness is often still considered a product of the individual's lack of moral fibre or moral will. The existence of such attitudes means that more often help will be sought at nonmedical or religious places, where the stigma attached to the problem may be lower, especially in countries where psychiatric services are poor.

In a community survey of attitudes in India, Verghese and Beig (1974) found that nearly 10% of the 1887 subjects interviewed felt that witchcraft was the best treatment for mental illness. A majority would refuse a marital alliance with someone suffering from mental illness, yet 25% felt that marriage would improve the patient's mental state. However, social representations are considered as sets of concepts, statements, and explanations that are created and diffused within the society. Loaded with unspoken information, social representations inform us about individuals' theories regarding their shared experiences, which are strengthened and changed during the course of communication. Although these findings are over 30 years old, they are unlikely to have changed dramatically.

Encountered events as represented by insanity or madness are defined and categorized in terms of social functioning. The latter are prescriptive in nature, in that they impose themselves upon us with an irresistible force. Moscovici (1984) suggests that when social phenomena are investigated, we come across explanations at the level of the individual, such as attributions, dissonance and attitudes. Moscovici goes on to say that the function of social representations is to make the unfamiliar familiar.

Waxler (1974), dwelling on contemporary Sri Lanka, offers an overview of the prevalent attitudes towards mental illness. Although the attitudes and beliefs regarding mental illness cannot be said to exclusively reflect Ayurvedic theories and practice, and although help-seeking is pluralistic, the Ayurvedic system must have influenced, as well as reflected, lay or indigenous theories and practice. Her observations suggest that little, if any, psychiatric stigma exists in Sri Lanka. She attempts to explain this by using labelling theory of schizophrenia (which means that, once labelled, a patient with schizophrenia starts to behave like a schizophrenic) to explain the good outcome of this illness in Sri Lanka. She places the theory in the formulation that the identities of ill individuals are not changed and tarnished by the illness. Their families and kin continue to relate to them as before, accepting their identity and illness, and providing them with support and understanding. The idea that the illness undermines and/or alters the person's worth, capability, or capacity for continued productive involvement in social roles does not appear to hold currency. Waxler implies that the lack of stigma is an important factor in promoting improvement and making for a better prognosis. It is likely that similar views exist in India and influence attitudes.

If we aspire to modify people's attitudes towards mental illness, we must bear in mind that encountered objects and events are assigned meanings through comparisons with previous encounters. Thus, social representations that are in the realm of the familiar are used as a point of reference to decipher the unfamiliar. It is through a similar process that the observer tackles hypotheses as well. Eker and Öner (1999) argue that, during the process of converting the unfamiliar into familiar, social representations are created that serve to create and predict social reality in a continuous manner. Thus, longstanding new images of mental illness and the mentally ill individual will be required to produce any change in attitudes.

Social representations of mental illness in the cinema take on a completely different meaning for individuals. The author of the film is influenced by the concepts of mental illness already existing in society and also how these sets of explanations of mental illness influence these concepts, and then at an individual level how these social representations influence attitudes and attributions. The use of mental illness as a metaphor for the portrayal of "the other" in cinema takes on a negative meaning if the prevalent social attributions see mental illness as divisive. The use of mental illness as a counterpoint in the story allows the screen images of violence and bizarre, or even contradictory, behaviour to take precedence over the human being (who is suffering from the mental illness), and these further denigrate and marginalize the patient. The attitudes to psychosis and personality disorder are likely to be more negative.

It is worth emphasizing in some detail how personality disorders are diagnosed in different cultures. First, one must know how personality disorders are defined. A personality disorder is an enduring pattern of inner experience and behaviour that deviates markedly from the expectations of the individual's culture. The pattern is pervasive and inflexible. Its onset is in adolescence or early adulthood. It remains stable over time and causes distress or impairment.

Ten types of personality disorders are outlined in DSM-IV-TR (APA, 2000). Here, we need to focus on three: borderline, antisocial, and narcissistic.

Borderline personality disorder is a pattern of instability in interpersonal relationships, self-image, and affect, marked by impulsivity. A feeling of grandiosity, the need for admiration, and a lack of empathy characterize narcissistic personality disorder. A person with antisocial personality disorder has a disregard for others and violates the rights of others.

As described in DSM-IV-TR, the antisocial personality disorder is linked with disordered conduct, which is repetitive and persistent, and which violates the appropriate societal norms or rules, including the basic rights of others of age of majority. The specific characteristics of such behaviour include aggression towards people or animals, destruction of property, deceitfulness, theft, or the serious violation of rules. The pattern of behaviour is carried over into adulthood. The person may lie, cheat, use aliases, and disregard the wishes, rights, or feelings of others. He or she (more likely to be a he) will tend to be impulsive, failing to plan ahead. Being irritable and aggressive, the person may also get involved in physical fights, assaults, and so on. Such individuals will display a reckless disregard for the safety of others, will be similarly reckless about themselves, and are constantly and extremely irresponsible.

People with borderline personality disorder, other than what has already been described, make frantic efforts to avoid (real or imagined) abandonment. Their perception of impending separation or rejection, or fear of the loss of external structures, can lead to profound changes in self-image. Very sensitive to environmental stresses, such individuals experience intense fears of abandonment and inappropriate anger, even when faced with a realistically limited period of separation or unavoidable changes in plans.

Narcissistic personality disorder is characterized by a grandiose sense of self-importance, with a constant overestimation of ability and inflation of accomplishments. Such individuals often appear boastful and pretentious, and are often preoccupied with fantasies of unlimited success, wishing to mix with unique or special people only. They require excess admiration, expect recognition, and fish for compliments.

These personality disorders represent only a subgroup of the mentally ill, and such are the characters that are portrayed in films. These will be discussed further when we take up individual films.

CONCLUSIONS

Personal, social, and kinship factors explain the presence and perception of psychoses and personality disorders, especially psychopathic personality disorders. The attitudes towards mental illness and bizarre behaviours mean that resources will be allocated according to perceived or real stigma and a sense of curability. The role and description of "the other" and how it is used suggest that, across different cultural settings, attitudes and behaviour differ in a remarkable way. The role of family, carers, and the society at large reflects the way care is provided by the state for mentally ill individuals and also the manner in which help is sought. There is little doubt that the media influences public attitudes to mental illness.

CHAPTER FIVE

Socioeconomic factors and cinema in India

The choice of film and entertainment is influenced by social class in the context of cinema-going, especially in India. Cinema, as an imported art form in India, has been thoroughly indigenized according to the nationhood and identity of the people and their cinema-going habits. Thus, the stories and viewpoints of the characters in Hindi films have been modified according to sociopolitical factors in the country.

It is clear that the main target audience for films is the age group of 19–25 years. These young persons may have money and are also impressionable in terms of peer pressure and fashion. Patterns of cinema-going are influenced by several personal and external factors.

Shah (1950/1980, p. 1) observes that the little artificial world (created by cinema) of persons and personalities, facts and fantasies is a topic of conversation and a matter of journalistic discussion of which the public never tires. He argues that for good or for bad, cinema, by virtue of the subtlety of its nature, moulds the opinions of millions in the course of its apparently superficial business of merely providing entertainment. What was at one time the privilege of the few has now become the leisure/right of all. This growth in the entertainment industry (cinema, VCR, DVD, VCD, internet, and other media) is due to an increase in disposable income on the one hand, and easy availability of such products on the other. These trends may be linked to urbanization and industrialization. Shah (p. 2) raises the issue of how exactly cinema and other amusements have affected working-class life, and the gain or loss involved. The cinema has replaced the music hall in the west but, in cultures in which kinship and friendship are the mainstay, the exploitation of leisure for profit is to be expected. Leisure being unorganized, commercial concerns have standardized recreational activities for personal or corporate profit. In theory, entertainment may be the primary motive of the providers but, in reality, profit is the most significant motive. Cinema remains one of the cheapest and most easily accessible forms of entertainment.

Shah (1950/1980, p. 6) observes that ease of availability of entertainment does mean that the immense force of cinema, by the subtlety of its nature, moulds the opinion of millions in the course of its apparently superficial business of merely providing entertainment. The growth of leisure is due to economic and social changes brought about by industrialization, a reduction of working hours, an increased availability of gas and electricity, along with better wages, higher disposable income, and the development of faster communications. People go to the cinema because it is cheap entertainment, and motion pictures appeal to an individual's unconscious desires and means of self-identification and wish fulfilment. To many, films offer a release from the day's frustrations and compensate for the deficiencies of real life. In the course of watching a film, the spectator for a while not only loses his or her individual self-consciousness, but also identifies with a character—downtrodden or middle class—fantasy in the film.

Shah (1950/1980, pp. 116–118) classifies Indian films into the following categories:

(1) Love stories: the love element is predominant.
(2) Social: a social problem is explored and resolved.
(3) Mythological and folklore.
(4) Devotional and religious.
(5) Historical and biographical.
(6) Stunt and adventure.
(7) Crime.
(8) Melodrama.
(9) Comedy.
(10) War.
(11) Mystery and horror.
(12) Children's films.

Sometimes it is difficult to draw the boundaries between, for example, social and melodrama or love stories and social, but the predominance of one or the other will help identify the theme. Generally, films are built around the lives of young men and women, aimed at the age range of the audience who will have the same interests (see Valicha, 1988a).

Shah (1950/1980, p. 40) reported that in India the number of permanent cinema houses doubled from 121 in 1921 to 251 in 1927, and there was one cinema for 988,048 individuals compared with one for 5857 in the USA. Today, as in the past, the number of people attending a cinema is determined by such conditions as the locality in which the picture house is situated, the kind of picture showing, the weather conditions, etc.

Psychological effects of films include influencing fashion, dress, jewellery, hair styles, personal mannerisms, and speech, but the immediate response may include fear and jealousy as well as love and hero-worship of the film stars. Films no doubt also influence the conduct of individuals. The type of influence and the individual's response depend upon a number of factors, including social experiences and personal idiosyncrasies. Whether cinema affects delinquency and crimes, including antisocial behaviour, has not been resolved satisfactorily. As regards adolescents and young adults, all the evidence cited goes to show that motion pictures may affect their conception of life and courses of conduct, because the cinema presents an extensive range of experience, much of which is new and fascinating material to the average film-goer (Shah, 1950/1980).

National identity is to be seen at various interconnected levels: local, national, regional, and global (Dissanayake, 1994). The national identity of India is the basis of the diverse ethnic groups and the various religious affiliations coexisting within its geographical space. The multiple sedimentation of the country's history has also contributed to its identity. This identity is, therefore, complex and multifaceted and exists at many levels. Given this background, filmmakers consciously and unconsciously pick and choose the names of their characters (as indicative/nonindicative of the castes). Immediately after Independence, the actors as well as the characters they played were known by their first names only; surnames indicating the caste were hardly used. In the past 20 years or so, the characters as well as the actors have begun using their surnames. For example, Manoj Kumar never used his surname (Goswami), and the name of the hero in his later films was Bharat, whereas Manoj Bajpai uses his surname to emphasize his identity and caste. A similar observation has been made by Murthy (1980), who points out that, in the earlier days, the surnames of most heroes and heroines were not used in order to make them national characters. It is not clear whether he is referring to the characters played by the actors or the actors' real names; if he is referring to the former, that practice certainly has changed in that most films now have characters with surnames that clearly reflect their caste and culture. I believe this trend to be a result of the post-Mandal communal developments. People have since become very conscious about their roots and identity. Heroes in the 1950s and 1960s also used the same name, whichever character they played. For example, Guru Dutt played Vijay several times, as did Amitabh Bachchan subsequently. Salman Khan was called Prem and Shah Rukh Khan was Raj in several films.

The demands of a multilevel identity often conflict and compete with each other. Cinema is a powerful cultural institution, which reflects and intervenes in the identities of the people and the nation it represents.

CONCEPTS OF HINDU IDENTITY AND SELF

The Indian concept of working class as understood in the western demographic sense differs quite dramatically from its western counterpart. It contains two additional factors, caste and religion, apart from the usual economic factors. These play a major role in the attitudes of viewers and responses to commercial and parallel cinema.

Hinduism is extremely complex and encompasses almost every possible sort of religious belief and practice, from pagan superstition, to asceticism, to scholarly tradition (Gokulsingh & Dissanayake, 1998).

Hindus recognized two kinds of authoritative religious literature: *shruti*, "hearing", which is external and self-existent and divinely revealed; and *smriti*, "recollection" (also called memory), which is a product of human authorship and is thus at a lower level than *shruti*. The entire Vedic literature is said to be *shruti* (Singh, 1998). As the upbringing of Hindus is steeped in a plethora of religious, cultural, and spiritual rites, rituals, and ceremonies, these are central to the development of their personality. The Hindu personality and character traits are covered later in this book.

Although the tenets of Hinduism have changed over several millennia in various ways, the core spiritual values remain very significant to Hindus. The role of religion, spiritual values, and spirituality in the development of the individual's characterological traits is not entirely understood in this group. The Hindu pantheon starts with three Gods: Brahma, Vishnu, and Mahesh. Vishnu is the Supreme God, Brahma the God of Creation, and Mahesh (also known as Shiva) the God of Destruction.

Smart (1989) outlines seven dimensions of Hinduism (Table 5.1). The four thematic concepts that govern Hindu activity are: (1) *dharma* ("righteousness"), which is the basis of the universe and rules of social intercourse, and depends on status, inborn traits, and stages of life; (2) *arth* (economic/political goals), which is karma reflecting the grand design of life; (3) *kama* ("pleasure"); and (d) *moksha* (freedom from the cycle of birth, attained through knowledge and devotion).

Hindu philosophy is the subject of numerous texts, but its basic tenets are set forth in the *Vedas* and the *Upanishads*. The two major scriptures which have become an integral part of Indian folklore are the *Ramayana* and the *Mahabharata*. To fully understand the impact of the scriptures and

TABLE 5.1
Seven dimensions of Hinduism (after Smart, 1989)

Dimensions	Concepts
1. Ritual, practical	Yoga, worship, sacrifice, pilgrimage, austerity, bhakti, dhyana
2. Experiential, emotional	Bhakti, dhyana
3. Narrative, mythical	Gods
4. Doctrinal, philosophical	Rebirth, liberation
5. Ethical, legal	Reverence for animals, ethics of one's station
6. Social, institutional	Castes, varieties of sacred persons, family
7. Material, artistic	Holy places, temples

folklore on the individual's life and functioning, one has to have an understanding of how Indians see themselves.

Roland (1988) has categorized notions of the Indian self into four types: familial, individualized, spiritual, and expanding. The notion of the familial self encompasses symbiosis and reciprocity. Relationships are intensely emotional and intimate, and are characterized by interdependence. Such emotional connectedness produces a constant affective exchange through an outer ego which has permeable boundaries. These traits come strongly into play in different social contexts. Narcissistic configurations of we/self-regard (denoting self-esteem) are strongly identified with the reputation and honour of the family and others in the framework of hierarchical relationships, and they also figure in the relationships formed by the individual. The individualized self represents "I-ness". It has self-contained ego boundaries, and there is a sharp differentiation between the inner images of the self and of others (Roland, 1988). The inner spiritual reality characterizes the spiritual self. It is expressed through a complex structure of gods and goddesses, rites, rituals, taboos, and meditation. Roland emphasizes that in the traditional psychological make-up of an Indian, one can see varying degrees of integration of the familial self with the spiritual self, and very little of the more individualized self.

Another intriguing element involved in the understanding of the Indian psyche is the concept of time. Time has significant historical and mythological connotations, consisting of recurrent cycles that are represented by certain festivals and rituals. It is characterized by repetitive regeneration of and reintegration with the mythological and divine presence, and certain images and places are used to connect the earth with the divine.

Socially and emotionally, Hindus primarily can be seen to be enmeshed in the extended kinship group and, secondarily, in their community or caste. Their *gunas* ("qualities"), *shakti* ("power" or "energy"), *karmas* ("inclinations arising from past actions"), and *moha* ("attachments") influence their actions and interactions with others. Individuals are not equal to each other, but interact within a framework of hierarchical relationships through myriad transactions and exchanges of gross and subtle substances that transform effects on both the superior and the subordinate (Marriott, 1976).

Roland's (1988) caution that the Indian identity has to be understood in the context of British rule, which introduced new laws and a new economic, social, and educational infrastructure, is an important one. The British saw their institutions as inherently superior to anything that India had to offer. Their views of asylums in this context have already been discussed.

The Indian family remains an extended one in large parts of the country, especially in rural areas. The family gets together during festivals and rites of passage and mutual influential decisions may be taken on these occasions. The current literature and visual media, especially television, highlight some of these issues. In soap operas and serials, conflicts emerge within the joint family and often get resolved in religious contexts.

WORKING CLASS AND CINEMA IN INDIA

When films first arrived in India and were shown as a series of shorts—the very first screening was on 7 July 1896, only 7 months after the showing in Paris by the Lumière brothers—the cost of seeing a film was one rupee. However, within 3 weeks or so, two indigenous developments occurred: the introduction of differentially priced tickets; and reserved boxes for ladies, who followed the purdah system, and their families. The prices ranged from as low as four annas (a quarter of a rupee) to as high as two rupees. This wide range of prices, which has remained a permanent feature in India, has increased the range of appeal of cinema and also has contributed to its growth (Barnouw & Krishnaswamy, 1980; Fazalbhoy, 1939; Rangoonwalla, 1979). In the 1920s, the rates of tickets were divided into five grades rather than two, thereby making films more affordable for the working classes.

However, in spite of the introduction of low-priced tickets, members of the early audiences in Bombay consisted mainly of British residents and a few Indians of the upper and educated classes. Initially, films were shown in the Fort area of Bombay, where a large number of Europeans and rich Indians resided. Indians, especially Gujaratis and Maharashtrians, lived in what was called the native town and industrial areas, which gained access to cinema only later.

The middle classes in India have had a very ambivalent relationship with cinema. Several factors in the initial stages of the development of Indian cinema may have played a role.

TYPE OF FILM

The middle classes initially linked up with Indian cinema, which emerged in the beginning of the twentieth century, because it was a western invention and something that their colonial masters enjoyed. Subsequently, their attitude changed. It is important to bear in mind Mishra's (1985) assertion that any theoretical critique of Bombay cinema must begin with a systematic analysis of the grand Indian meta-text and founder of Indian discursivity, namely the *Mahabharata* and the *Ramayana*. As the earlier films were of the mythological variety, mainly centring around the tales from the *Mahabharata* and the *Ramayana* (or Tulsi Das' *Ramcharitmanas*), the audience could identify with them. The impact of these scriptures on Indian culture has been simply astounding. Folk theatre was strongly influenced by the *Ramayana* and reached a peak every year at the approach of the Dussehra festival (which marks the end of Lord Rama's war against and victory over the demon Ravana). This is still the case: Amateur actors enact Ram Leela (the story of Rama) and the entry is generally free even now. In the past, these activities were sponsored by the local landowners.

The *Mahabharata* revolves around the struggle between cousins who are fighting for the kingdom of Indraprastha. The Pandavas are five brothers who have Lord Krishna (a reincarnation of Vishnu) and dharma (the truth) on their side. They are married to the same woman, Draupadi. Their cousins, the Kauravas, win Draupadi in a gambling contest and subsequently war ensues. While facing his family on the battlefield, one of the Pandava brothers, Arjuna, starts to question the idea of fighting with and killing his family members. In response, Krishna, who is his charioteer, talks to him about karma yoga, i.e., doing your duty and acting without worrying about the result of your actions. The discussion forms the basis of *Bhagavadgita*, which has been analysed by numerous Indian and non-Indian authors and philosophers.

The *Mahabharata* was serialized on television by the noted Indian filmmaker B. R. Chopra and his son Ravi Chopra for the state-owned Indian television channel, Doordarshan. This followed the huge success of *Ramayana*, which had been adapted into a television serial for the same channel a few years earlier by another noted Hindi filmmaker, Ramanand Sagar, and his sons.

Mitra (1993) argues that the feature film industry provided television not only with producers and directors, but also with guidelines for the development of the soap opera text. The *Mahabharata* as serialized on television represented a variety of social and religious practices without necessarily distinguishing between the two. This brought together central social concerns and the practice of Hindu rituals. Models of social conduct were ascribed to the *Mahabharata*. Mitra, while articulating his views on the depiction of the *Mahabharata* as a television serial, defines culture as a commodity belonging to an elite group of society, which is obviously keen to guard such events as authentic Indian culture. Conceptualized around specific stages in Indian history, religion, and language, culture plays at the heart of Indian visual media, television in this instance. Ninan (1995) highlights that Indian television's gift to a still largely poor Indian society has been to promote consumerism. Indian television has also affected theatre and cinema audiences. The growth of television and its materials has run parallel to the march of history since Independence. The telecast of both the *Ramayana* and *Mahabharata* led to an increase in the acquisition of television sets around the country.

The *Ramayana* is the story of a family whose head is Lord Dashrath. By his three wives, he has four sons: Rama, Lakshman, Bharat, and Shatrughan. Rama is the eldest son, born of the first wife. The third wife asks her husband to banish Rama from the kingdom so that her son, Bharat, can become the King of Ayodhya. Much against the wishes of Lord Dashrath, Rama agrees to go into exile. Rama's wife, Sita, and brother, Lakshman, decide to accompany him to the forest. One day, the demon-king from Lanka, Ravana, kidnaps Sita and holds her hostage. Rama has to raise an army to win her back. With the help of Hanuman, the king of the monkeys, and his army, he defeats Ravana and brings Sita back. While the festival of Dussehra celebrates the slaying of Ravana, another festival, Diwali, celebrates Rama's return to Ayodhya.

The impact of both these stories on the Hindu psyche is immeasurable. From early childhood, these stories are inculcated into the minds of children, who grow up enacting the Ram Leela. When these serials were being shown on television, weddings were delayed and meetings postponed for the sake of watching these teledramas as they were being broadcast. The daily poojas, rituals, and storytelling speak of the devotion of the middle classes to these stories. Hindi cinema has been hugely influenced by these two stories on multiple levels. The depiction of love and feuds within the family in these form significant sources of storytelling. The practices of swayamvar (choosing one's groom oneself) and gandharva vivah (love marriage) are described in these stories, and have had an important influence on the storylines of Hindi films.

MIDDLE CLASS AND CINEMA

For a short while, the middle class saw cinema as an exclusive activity that was a challenge for their minds. This changed with the arrival of the era of Hindi musical films, especially in the 1960s and early 1970s. Part of the change was due to a decline in the standard of music as well as to a shift in the political and social climate. In addition, there was a shift in the content of literature, which became a major source for Indian cinema. Prasad (1998) makes the suggestion that in the early 1970s, when the country was in the midst of a national crisis, the cultural economy of cinema underwent a transformation. During this period there emerged a new type of film in which the law was no longer a mere supplement, but the most important stake in the conflict and resolution of the narrative (Prasad, 2000). Criminal characters in films were disinherited, marginalized, and brought under the purview of the law and the state, a focus that cinema audiences liked and continued to enjoy. Although these films did not eliminate the feudal family romance entirely, it was somehow subjugated to identify a sense of help-lessness, alienation, and being an underdog. This then responded to the protagonist working full time to avenge an act, often without the help of the police, who had to play a role but would always arrive just a bit late, e.g., by the time the hero had overpowered the villain.

Exclusivity came to the fore again with the emergence in the mid-1970s of art cinema or parallel cinema, which targeted the urban middle class. The 1970s saw the rise of parallel cinema. The political and economic background within which parallel cinema emerged is detailed later on in this book. Suffice it to say here that the aspirations of the middle class grew, as did their sense of privacy and exclusivity.

The advent of video films in the 1980s allowed people to watch films in the privacy of their homes. As a result, the number of cinema halls showing Hindi films dropped considerably. The simultaneous growth of urbaniza-tion was a key factor reinforcing perceptions of exclusivity. In addition, the 1980s saw a phenomenal increase in television channels showing soap operas. From then on, television became an element of the exclusive image of the middle class and has continued to be so.

LITERATURE AND MIDDLE-CLASS CINEMA

Some of the significant components of plays written in Sanskrit in the third and fourth centuries were song, dance, and music as Bowers (1956) suggests; no separate terms existed for drama and dance. The notion of drama as a separate entity, independent of the other elements, is still strange and disconcerting to many Indians.

Sanskrit theatre eventually entered a period of long decline and virtually died after 1000 AD. Its downfall was hastened by waves of Muslim inva-sions that swept over large parts of northern India during the following centuries. As Muslims had no theatrical heritage and considered drama a sacrilegious activity, drama no longer received court patronage (Barnouw & Krishnaswamy, 1980), although this was not a universal phenomenon. Under the British, Indian drama did reappear around the 1830s, but flour-ished only in the form of private family theatres maintained in the homes of large, educated joint families, especially in Calcutta. Public theatres emerged in the 1870s and the impact of Victorian theatre has already been mentioned. Although Barnouw and Krishnaswamy argue that the new Indian drama started out by adapting and imitating European models, there was an immediate reversion to the ancient notion of drama, with song and dance as inseparable elements.

Bowers (1956) proposes that Indian drama itself originally developed from dances performed at religious festivals, and that folk drama emerged with the addition of dialogue and narrative.

In Bengal, the jatra, a form of folk drama, was performed at festivals; songs were its central features. Whereas Sanskrit drama was meant for the courts, the jatra was a source of pleasure, entertainment and education for the common people. Travelling artistes took the jatra (which did not need a stage) from place to place, and the tradition lives on. These dramas had no written scripts and tended to be improvised. They had a powerful hold on the viewing public. The jatra also became an instrument of religious and social reform at times. Hindi filmmakers have used songs and stories from jatras. Other states had their own corresponding traditions. For example, Punjab had swang, Kerala had kathakali, and Orissa had kuchupudi. These forms of folk drama exerted an immediate influence on folk theatre, as also on "talkies" a century later (Barnouw & Krishnaswamy, 1980). Films and the touring talkies made a great impression on the public, which led to a decline in folk theatre. Music worked in a different way in the film and the film absorbed music in a different way. There was a change in the traditional role of music in the narrative. The presence of music and song in the Hindi film reflect these traditions.

At the time when silent films were being made and shown in India, the threat of Hollywood constantly loomed large on the horizon. However, this threat disappeared when the talkies arrived because the Indian traditions of song, music, and folk gave Hindi films a distinctive look and identity.

The development of cinema as a tradition in any society depends on many factors, the chief among these being social and financial factors, cultural roots, and social stability. For example, Mayer (1972) argues that the false autonomy of economism led to the destruction of the universal theatre of the Elizabethan epoch (in Britain, at least), and what remained was a distinctive class theatre.

Theatrical art and drama declined in ancient Greece and Rome when these states became imperial, a situation not dissimilar to that in Mughal India. Cinema has always been an open medium, something which is borne out by the way its very form has changed according to changes in the social structure of our cities over the past five decades (Karnad, 1982).

The financial accessibility of modern cinema compared to the universal theatre that preceded it has had a bearing on the latter's growth and its acceptance by the public. Modern cinema also serves as a potent channel of information and influences the attitudes of the society it sets out to entertain.

F. Kazmi (1999, pp. 56–57) makes the distinction that conventional cinema, which is spectacular, focuses on heroic characters, has a clear beginning and a clear end, restates in an intense form values and attitudes that are already known, and stresses the repetition or performance of something that is already known rather than the creation of something new. This guarantees that what is experienced in one film is not very different from what has been experienced in most others. It has by definition a number of conventions: the role of women, the role of the long-suffering wife, the brave hero, death of the villain, twists and turns in the story due to fate, bad Karma, and punishment. But everything comes together in the end. Kazmi argues that within these conventions, the classical narration is influenced by tight narration, psychological motivation, goal-oriented characters, and careful spatial continuity. The audience recognizes these conventions and knows and relies upon the fact that everything will come right in the end. The characters are black and white, and the films within such conventions are not the same. These will include variations on how songs are picturized, how the story develops, and how the denouement is reached. The distinction between conventional and innovative cinema is important. Conventional cinema is also concerned with the values, attitudes, and beliefs of the subordinate classes, therefore the portrayal of mental illnesses in the conventional cinema has to be influenced by these.

It is worth emphasizing that, although my focus here is on commercial Hindi cinema, such cinema in itself is heterogeneous. The middle cinema of Hrishikesh Mukherjee, Bimal Roy, and Gulzar on the one hand, and the popcorn masala (commercial, populist, successful) of Manmohan Desai on the other, do target different audiences. However, sometimes there is a crossover and masala films become hits because they appeal to a major audience group. New or parallel or arts cinema gradually disappeared in the 1990s and beyond. As Pendakar (1990) emphasizes, this is because the cost of production quadrupled between 1975 and 1985, and the salaries of the technical teams increased. Also, the increasingly abundant supply of films necessarily spelt doom for a large number of films. Pendakar observes that the downfall of parallel cinema was also related to the fact that it lacked a coherently expressed ideology.

It is difficult to make a film that caters to all tastes, as attitudes vary from place to place, such as from village to city. Director Karan Johar, who produced and directed a couple of major hit films in the late 1990s, notes, "in a village a woman is a wife, a woman is a mother, a woman is a sister, but a woman as a friend? No way. That's their belief" (Kabir, 2001, p. 17). This means that the films made for sophisticated urban audiences may well not appeal to rural audiences.

Karanjia (1990, p. 23) points out that another limiting factor in the success of films in the 1990s was the whimsical likes and dislikes of the public. Filmmakers tended to emphasize the lowest common denominator in audience taste, to the extent that when the rare, discriminating critic found fault with a picture the producer flaunted the film's tremendous box office returns in response. In presenting the challenges of the 1990s, Karanjia (p. 137) notes that cinema or the failure of cinema depends upon its ability to recall and recapture the past, when significant films and films that were truly Indian were made. The success of *Lagaan*, which has echoes of *Mother India*, is an example. Both films were nominated for Oscar awards for Best Foreign Film.

Given the virtually institutionalized formulaic elements found in Hindi commercial films, one might say that to see a handful of them is to see them all (Hood, 2000). Hood notes that the arguments that the producers give the masses what they want and that formula is a success on the box office are spurious and hackneyed. He observes that these arguments speak of an underlying capitalist strategy, in which clever marketing enhances the "sales". The marketing is aimed at convincing the masses that they must see the film, whether for the sake of seminudity, songs, or the reputation of the hero or heroine, or because the film highlights the relationship between the hero and heroine in real life. As they say, any publicity is good publicity. A conclusion of this approach is that the portrayal of madness has to be terrifying for people to see the film. The trend outlined by Hood has become much more important recently for several reasons; more films are failing than before at the box office, and the profusion of television channels need more fodder, which is supplied by clippings of song-and-dance sequences and romantic interludes. The money invested is proportionately much greater, thus making commensurate returns essential for survival. A similar development is that producers are now making films of the same genre, so viewers knows what to expect once they know the name of the production house.

Hindi commercial films often juggle several genres. Kabir (2001) notes that the average Hindi film does not pretend to offer a unique storyline. Benegal (cited in Raha, 1982, p. 132; also see Datta, 2003) makes a similar plea:

> We have no infrastructure to show our films to specialized audiences and, therefore, the only thing we can do is to take them to the masses. All films need an audience and there is no use in us behaving as if they do not need an audience. And unfortunately since all films are in one bag and there is no other bag, this audience must of necessity be the general mass audience.

The roles and portrayals of heroes and heroines have changed over the years. The trends of each decade have influenced the clichés and stereotypes of film scenes and dialogues. Kabir (2001) argues that the only thing that really changes in the story of the Hindi film is the way songs and dances are developed and integrated into the story.

ROLE OF MUSIC AND SONG IN CINEMA

Since the introduction of sound in the cinema, songs have formed an integral part of the story. The number of songs in a film varies from two or three to as many as seven. Premchand (2003, p. 11) estimates that there were about 36,000 songs in approximately 4334 Hindi films made between the years 1930 and 1970. There have been changes in the type of songs and music used in films. Premchand attributes the deterioration in the quality of the music to the dying down of the post-Independence euphoria; the music reflects the current "chalta hai" (anything goes) attitude towards work and life. With the change in the shape of romance in the 1960s, when love was symbolized by energy (Somaaya, 2004), music turned into a metaphor for romance. A picture without songs is unheard of and no film can be popular at the box office without good music (Shah, 1950/1980, p. 97). Therefore, the producer has to include a generous sprinkling of songs. The music is either oriental or occidental. Sometimes, a preoccupation with western music influences the film's musical output. Shah (p. 98) regrets that film music has ruined great Indian musical traditions, and that classical music has been falsified to create film music that is cheap, hybrid, and vulgar. The songs are accompanied by dances that are equally hybrid and, often, cheap and vulgar.

In its early days, Hindi cinema used the *mushaira* tradition, the *qawwali*, and the *mujra* to a large extent. *Mushaira* is a gathering of poets who recite their poetry in accordance with a specific, scrupulous tradition of behaviour. The *qawwali* is a form in which many singers sing in tandem creating waves upon waves. It is a mode of praying, and is meant to take the singers and listeners into *wajd* (ecstasy, or a heightened state of mental and emotional abandon). The *mujra* is a form of dance usually performed by dancing girls to the accompaniment of *ghazals* (semiclassical songs). It is derived from the kathak school. All these, together with the use of certain musical instruments, highlight the Muslim culture. Hindi films continue to use these forms today, though to a much lesser degree.

Initially, Hindi films were influenced by the Parsi theatre, which held sway from Calcutta to Bombay. The language used in Parsi theatre was elegant and flowery, and its narrative was interspersed with ghazals, naat, and marsiya, all different forms of Urdu poetry, accompanied by music. In fact, Hindi as a language (together with its various dialects) was associated with rural folk theatre, and Urdu with urban theatre. Hence, the Hindu elite in north India and Bengal used Urdu in their social intercourse, whereas Hindi remained confined to the schools.

Mainstream Hindi cinema has had very few films with no songs whatsoever. Songs, and the dances often associated with them, indicate the unconscious, the unsayable, the unsaid, or the unwritten. Dance may also represent an extension of a religious ritual. Associated with a song, it often communicates love to the loved one and to the public at large. Film songs are symbolic events; for example, they speak the language of the heart. The audience yearns for them, responds to them, sings along with them, and envelopes itself in the sentiment of joy or sorrow associated with the song. Songs represent coordinates of emotional development besides giving vocal and spatial narratives. They fill a void and establish a link that cannot be achieved in any other way. They provide a context within which the emotional needs and aesthetic demands of a situation may be grouped.

The success of a film does not solely depend on the popularity of the songs it has, though by and large songs do play a major role in its success. The cassettes and CDs of film songs are generally released 6 weeks to 6 months before the cinema release of the film, in an attempt to encourage the audience to look forward to the film. Though these songs may be hits, they cannot always work wonders for the film.

Why is it considered essential for Hindi films to have songs? Other than the fact that they express hidden feelings and emotions, songs provide the film and the audience with the natural break that they need. It is worth considering whether the need for songs can be attributed to the possibility that individuals cannot communicate adequately within their culture and hence take to alternative modes of communication. The intensive use of songs cannot be explained away by the fact that folk songs were very popular, as Barnouw and Krishnaswamy (1980) have argued. Instead, according to Ranade (1980), the real causes lie in the actual context of the films themselves. As it was vocal music that predominated in India rather than instrumental, it was inevitable that this would be reflected in films. In the early phase of Hindi films, classical music was predominant, which probably reflected the nature of the musical traditions current at the time (Hindustani and Carnatic). Ranade suggests that as, initially, the two main centres of film production were Calcutta and Bombay, Hindustani music was bound to be predominant then.

Nayyar (1960, p. 39), a well-known music director in his own right, observed that

> if we music directors are to march with the times, we must have our hand on the pulse of the public . . . And it is imperative that in our compositions we set a pace that conforms with the spirit of the age.

Taking uninformed criticism (maybe critics) as a target, Nayyar challenges them to prove that our ancient cultural heritage is being destroyed by the musical fare in our films. Some 40 plus years after his observations, things have indeed moved on and changed. Nayyar (p. 39) notes that

> the scenes in our film are frequently set in such places [which reverberate with jazz and other forms of western music and cabaret] and since films are expected to mirror life as it is lived, filmmakers depict this fact of life in their pictures.

He emphasizes that tunes needed to have a flourish to indicate the spirit of the age. The magic hold of music in films on the young and old alike was attributable to the fact that it is a harmonious blend of the music of the east and the west, which gives listeners a musical experience and pleasure not normally available to them.

Chatterjee (1995a) asserts that the Hindustani film song is a twentieth-century musical phenomenon. No other modern musical form from any part of the globe can boast of such diversity, inclusiveness, subtlety and reach. Chatterjee argues that the reason for so much emphasis on song in Hindi films lies in the historical development of music. Poetry of saints and folk music contributed to it. It is interesting to note that Chatterjee saw Lata Mangeshkar's singing for film heroines as counterpoint to the anxious desires of the actress involved. This myth of the purity and virginity of the heroine in most of the films was made necessary by people who had lived through (and in many cases participated in) the carnage of Partition and therefore needed all the hope to face life again and seek acceptance for their real and imagined sins.

The song contains the hidden message: the true intentions of the director. Chatterjee (1995a) highlights that, since the stories are all the same, the director needs songs to demonstrate his élan, elegance, and sophistication. A lot of attention is paid to the lyrics, the tune, and, finally, the presentation, so that the song becomes a film within a film, a testimony to the filmmakers' artistic credo. Songs are the vehicles for multilayered thoughts and feelings. Lyrics contain vital information and are interpreted with care.

Chatterjee (1995b) notes that the act of the song picturization is unique to Indian cinema. In the 1940s and 1950s directors used songs written in the film to pass on the real intent of their scripts through telegraphic audio-visual signs to the viewer. Men and women danced together in rural areas at special festivals but this stopped because of urbanization. Cinema, on the other hand, with its ability to go forwards and backwards in time, revived these social customs in stories. In early films, dances were rudimentary but gradually became more sophisticated. The film song had started to mirror life and the fantasy that grew out of it.

From the time of Independence to 20 years later, melody was king in the film song. Cherished values of filial piety and selfless friendship began to disappear quickly and alongside jingoism, hypocrisy in personal and professional life slowly but surely took over. These negative values and developments, according to Chatterjee (1995b), led to visual dance and banal dialogue, and dance took over one of the functions of the song. It is difficult to think of a memorable film without thinking of its songs. The songs and all its components can contribute significantly to the commercial success of the film. The visual expression thus becomes crucial not only in establishing artistic credibility but also to commercial success.

Nair (2001) also notes that songs are an expression of inner conflict, an element of dramatic narration, a celebration of life, a means to comment and allow the characters to move from the particular to the general, and a medium of poetic exchange of feelings.

Speculating on the sociopolitical nature of the song in Hindi films, Aziz (2003) hypothesizes that song may be associated with vulnerability, weakness, and femininity. A song is a "musicalized" speech in an emotionally charged language. Aziz articulates that a song is information in many forms, such as emotional, psychological, and abstract. He argues that the development of the song and the use of female singers in particular after Indian Independence are very clearly linked with the position of the women in the society. He concluded that wittingly or unwittingly the male creators (music directors, lyricists, producers, directors) have participated in thwarting women's progress and, ironically, they have employed female voices to achieve their aim.

Art, music, and mythology appeared to have come together. Ranade (1980) draws the distinction between the verse-in-time phase of Indian film music and the plot and song dichotomy. In the former is the crystallization of the narrative function. The songs, although a part of the film plot and story, also have to be able to stand alone and out of context of the film itself in order to sell records. Film music often gains more popularity than the film itself. The changes in the style of film music, from classical to folk to western, reflect not only changing political, social, and economic scenarios, but also exposure to wider global influences and the targeting of large overseas audiences. From singing actors to playback singers, the film song has come a long way. The song is seen as the brainchild of the music director, who fuses the voice, instruments, and words into a creation, which may well have a life of its own and bear the stamp of his personality (Sharma, 1980). The lyricists have the expertise to find words for different situations. The film song is meant to be effective for the situation for which it is written.

If we assume that songs are a form of communicating desire, a method for expressing the inexpressible, and a means of indicating what lies ahead, then it becomes important to have knowledge of the way the members of the larger community and society communicate. For someone unaware of the opera styles, watching *La Bohème* or *The Ring Cycle* may evoke surprise over why overweight women and men are dying of tuberculosis, and the singing may not make aesthetic sense. The roles of gender, social, and class factors, besides that of patriarchal hierarchy, dictate how songs are used in Indian society. The pining hero and heroine who are miles apart will sing from the same hymn sheet (as it were). The erotic nature of the communication may be conveyed through the vamp or the cabaret artiste—though over the last quarter of the twentieth century, this trend has changed. Until recently, the eroticism of a relationship could not be shown directly, but only through images of, say, two flowers entwined, waves breaking on the shore, or a train entering a tunnel. However, there has been a distinct change, as illustrated by the recent film, *Raaz*, in which the second lead is shown licking the hero's nipple. The process of sublimation earlier indicated mostly through songs is now shown much more blatantly. The reasons for this lie in the changing social mores. The fact that the character played by Amitabh Bachchan in *Hum* could sing, "*Jumma, chumma de de* (kiss me . . .)" and the heroine in *Khalnayak* could be asked, "What is under your blouse?" reflects the social shift towards a more open acknowledgement of sexual desire and erotic thoughts. However, until recently these were confined to female sexuality, but they are now beginning to influence male sexuality.

Ray (2001) argues that erotic emotions can be repressed according to the ethos of the caste system. He says the shaping of a specific ethos arising from this particular combination of repression and sublimation determined the course of Indian civilization and influenced its modern transformation. The patriarchal hierarchy and the caste system, according to Ray, were so designed as to inhibit and undermine the process of voluntary repression and sublimation at the lowest and most oppressed level of society. Sexual relations are exposed to the anarchy of exploitation, which is often the case where a pretty village girl is raped, exploited, or abused by the zamindar (landowner), the moneylender or the villain. Psychoanalysts would argue that the infantile psyche will be universal; therefore, what is reflected in the cinema—the historical and social context—cannot be left alone and needs to be understood.

Songs can be used as a political device to highlight patriotism or a hidden meaning sought to be conveyed to the audience. The songs advance the narrative, but also tend to follow it at times. Film music today makes use of traditional Indian musical instruments. As Thoraval (2000, p. 65) notes, more than playing a role in the film, music, song, and dance are vital elements of enjoying the film. The inclusion of songs, according to Thoraval, is aimed at preventing too direct a realism on the screen. Songs turn fact into fiction and fiction into fantasy, allowing the unsaid to be said. Song and dance can also play a purely lyrical role by indicating an ambience, a state of mind, or an emotion. They can also contribute to political, social, or religious sentiments and can make such statements.

The songs in Hindi cinema have been broadly divided into the following categories: (1) love songs, in which one or both of the protagonists declare their undying love for each other; (2) songs of celebration and accolade, which are usually sung to the members of the family, a group, a party, a platoon, or colleagues; (3) songs of separation, which may be sung during an occasion, such as a birthday or a festival, and in which one or both protagonists express their desperation and sorrow; and (4) special songs, such as bhajans (in which the character prays or asks for something from the gods), lullabies, comedy songs, and soliloquies.

The picturization of the songs reflects the views and skills of the director. Celebrated and successful directors have developed and used a characteristic style when it comes to using songs to indicate a turning point in the narrative. Also, they have worked closely with certain music directors to develop what has become known as their hallmark music.

The appearance of a song in the narrative of the film signifies one of the following aspects:

(1) *Turning point in the narrative*: The appearance of a song in the story sometimes represents a key turning point in the narrative. It allows the story to progress. Yet, the convention in Hindi cinema has led the audience to expect that songs will appear at regular intervals. When a song is badly placed or badly written, there is a mass exodus from the cinema hall, with the audience taking the opportunity to stretch their legs or go for a smoke. It is similar to the way people watching a video might fast-forward a song if they did not like it.

(2) *Hidden meanings*: The songs can express love and pining, or emotions that are not publicly acceptable. The language they use may be too flowery to be incorporated in the dialogue. A significant majority of the lyricists in Hindi cinema have been poets in their own right, and have written in Urdu, Hindi, or both. The style of poetry and the use of language allow the protagonists to express their emotions in a way that their partner (who may also be represented by the viewer) may not be able to. The songs are also an extension of the dialogue and bring out the character in a particular way.

(3) *Fantasy locales*: The unusualness and inaccessibility of the locales at which most songs are picturized indirectly tell the viewer that the song is unique, besides bringing out certain sociodemographic characteristics of the character. Recently there has been a remarkable shift to overseas locales stretching around the globe.

In the 1950s, the genre of romantic films was at its peak. This genre represented a post-Independence national idealism and purity, and the films were popularly known as "socials". In the 1960s, romantic films continued to stir the public imagination and became extremely popular. In the 1970s and 1980s, action films began to dominate, and they relied less on music or song and more on action sequences. The switch to the new romanticism of the late 1980s and 1990s saw a resurgence of musical films, though the nature of romance portrayed was different. This trend also reflected the emergence of a new middle class, which had come into being as a result of economic, social, and cultural changes. Liberalization and globalization meant a new kind of consumer emerged. The present younger generation is confident and assertive about its style, and the lifestyle of the middle class is not dissimilar to that in the west. The songs are more likely to be written in, set to the music of, and picturized in the western operatic style, with huge sets and casts of hundreds.

Shah (1950/1980, p. 92) notes that Hindi films dwell on stereotyped subjects. Most producers believe that the audiences expect the same stories. The stories lack realism, as do the amorous episodes, often making Indian films ridiculous. Hindi films try to camouflage romantic episodes to the point of unconvincing artificiality. However, over the past 50 years or so, the portrayal of romance has changed somewhat, though the portrayal of romanticism has not. Shah (p. 94) feels this is because of unimaginative directors, who are often unable to handle such scenes successfully. Further, romantic scenes are often shot with an awareness of the possibility that they may be censored, so expressions may be used in order to bypass the censorial eye.

From the 1960s onwards, with the introduction and easy availability of films in colour, cinema became the premier form of entertainment for the Indian masses. However, Thoraval (2000, p. 117) notes that Indian culture, which mixes up film characters, mythological actions, and the problems of contemporary daily life, is founded on a very strong social, artistic, moral, and religious tissue, which has not yet been dislodged by postindustrial modernity. Popular cinema itself, therefore, functions like a myth, and the identification of the public with the characters is a way to escape from the harsh realities of life. In addition, as the story creates the voyeur or the viewer, the film plays up to this faux character.

The beginning of a film and the way it is structured creates certain expectations among the audience. These may be subsumed in the genre to which the work of the director or the actors belongs. Thus, the audience expects different things from a film starring Tom Cruise or Amitabh Bachchan, or from the films of John Woo, David Lean, or Hrishikesh Mukherjee. The initial 10 minutes or so can lay the roadmap of the film. At the end of the film, the audience leaves the cinema with clear memories, closure, and retrospective comprehension of the structure. The endings, too, are determined by various factors such as the genre of the film, the auteur's style, and the persona of the star. Directors are known sometimes to change the ending of the story: They rewrite the scene either after the film has been completed or after it has been shown to select, invited audiences for their opinions.

The emotions experienced by individual members of society and portrayed by the actors in films have to be understood as universal representations. There is little doubt that films tend to universalize the sentiments of their characters, thereby creating stereotypes: The villain wears loud clothes and speaks loudly; the comedy is physical. The sexual, psychological, and cultural differences between the characters portrayed in most films represent an extreme position that is, however, rooted in some kind of reality. Ray (2001) argues that the emotional history of a culture is the history of the particular process of sublimation in that society, beneath which lies repression. However, my argument is that suppression and the denial of desire and opportunity also influence sublimation and repression in the case of song and music.

The impact of social, political and economic changes was evident in the music industry as well. As Sharma (1980) points out, many national tragedies befell India in the 1960s. The war with China, though short in duration, shattered India's economy and reputation. Two prime ministers (Nehru and Shastri) passed away. Further, the war with Pakistan adversely influenced the country's morale and economy. According to Sharma, the world did not take India as seriously as before, and Indian behaviour showed that this view was justified. This was reflected in the music of Hindi films, with the music director and singer giving little importance to the lyrics. In the 1980s, the combination of songs and violent movies led to an exercise in extroversion.

CONCLUSIONS

The role of the cinema and its sociological importance for the audience, be they from the middle class or the working class, is important. In addition, key factors in Hindu personality influence films that are also affected by the impact of Hindu scriptures on drama, theatre, and literature. The use of songs is virtually mandatory in Hindi films for a number of reasons. The songs not only are employed to convey the feelings and emotions which cannot be conveyed otherwise, but also form a significant part of income generation. The music directors, lyricists, and playback singers are stars in their own right and are revered as such. The emotions in films are a reflection of the genre of the film and the directional style of celebrated directors.

CHAPTER SIX

History of Hindi cinema

Hindi cinema became much more its own master and creator after the advent of sound, but it also had to struggle with the development of a new language of cinema and a new language that could be understood across the nation. This chapter highlights only some of the major landmarks.

BACKGROUND AND HISTORICAL DEVELOPMENT

It is now well recognized that the very first performance of moving images in India occurred in 1896. On 7 July in Bombay, Lumière shorts were shown at Watson's Hotel. The Lumière envoys circled the globe with their machines and film reels, with instructions that they were not to share their secrets with anyone. They were also to photograph key events in the countries that they were touring and to send these back to Paris. Barnouw and Krishnaswamy (1980) suggest that the French exhibitor did not succeed in getting good-quality pictures from India. Hence, in spite of the country's exotic locales and colourful festivities, no film from India figures in the first Lumière catalogues. However, the next couple of years saw a change, with films using Indian scenery and culture coming into circulation.

Despite its slow start, film exhibition gradually gathered momentum and the number of shows continued to grow. As noted in the previous chapter, by the end of July 1896, reserved boxes were made available for ladies following the purdah system and a broad scale of prices was introduced. Barnouw and Krishnaswamy (1980) suggest that in spite of the four anna (quarter of a rupee) seats and the special provision for the ladies in purdah, the early shows attracted mainly British residents, along with a few Indians of the educated classes, especially those who identified their interests with those of the British.

The impact of these shows on the Indian population was crucial. A Bombay photographer, Bhatvadekar, became the first Indian to order a movie camera from London. He filmed a wrestling match, an item on circus monkeys and the return of a Cambridge graduate to India. He also started exhibiting imported films in tents. In 1903, the Durbar celebration of the coronation of Edward VII, with all its oriental and occidental splendour, was recorded on film and exhibited.

Madan (1856–1923) in Calcutta and Esoofally (1884–1957) in Bombay were early pioneers of the exhibition and making of films. However, the most significant contribution of the era came from Dhundiraj Govind Phalke (affectionately known as Dadasaheb Phalke). Born in 1870, he studied art in Bombay and received training in Germany. When he saw the film *Life of Christ*, he considered the possibility of making a similar film on the life of Krishna. He visited England and returned with a camera but instead decided to make *Raja Harishchandra*, based on a story from the *Mahabharata*. The film was completed in 1912. Its heroine was a man dressed in female attire. The overwhelming success of the film inspired a range of mythological films based on the Hindu scriptures. These included *Lanka Dahn*, *Savitri*, *Krishnajanam*, and *Bhasmasur Mohini*.

A key factor contributing to the success of these films was their typically Indian outlook and relationship to Hinduism. As they brought to life the heroic figures of long-told stories, their impact on the audiences was overwhelming. When Rama or Krishna appeared on the screen, members of the audience prostrated themselves before the screen, as they did before the actors playing these characters in television serials as late as the mid-1980s.

Phalke also turned into an exhibitor and toured the country with his projector, screen, and films. In 1915, the first south Indian feature film—again based on the story of Krishna—was released. Phalke's success between 1918 and 1919 laid the foundation of the Bombay film industry. However, his studios were in Nasik and the members of his production team remained close to the studios, virtually as part of a joint family system. Phalke was also instrumental in encouraging women to start participating in filmmaking. His daughter played the role of Krishna and he persuaded a Maharashtrian woman to play the lead in his second production.

From the 1920s, historical and social films started being made in India. In 1918, the British rulers introduced a Cinematograph Act, modelled on the one in Britain, to censor cinema in the postwar scenario. In 1919, D. N. Sampat established the Kohinoor Film Company. A Gujarati mill owner,

Sampat turned this company into one of the most significant producers of the films of the silent era. Suchet Singh established another company, the Oriental Film Company; however, it lasted only 2 years because of his sudden death in a car crash.

Parallel developments were occurring in a number of spheres. In Bombay, up to 1910, films were shown in tents. Subsequently, however, cinema halls became semipermanent places, although it took another 10 years for more permanent cinema halls to emerge. As noted earlier, in the beginning there were only two classes of audience; this increased to five classes later on. The films of the Phalke era were mythological, and were also made and released with religious festivals and holidays in mind. By 1923, the number of Indian films had risen remarkably. Most of the cinemas being built were in urban areas with civilian populations. By 1925, the length of films had started to increase. Between 1923 and 1925 Bombay had three cinema halls which exhibited Bombay films all year round.

The first film magazine that covered Bombay cinema extensively was established in 1924. This was also the year that saw the great success of the Kohinoor Film Company. Three of the company's films succeeded in establishing the social film as a genre, and one of its oriental fantasies proved a great success at the box office. The company created multiple stages for its studio. Soon it had set up an all-India distribution business.

Around the first three decades of the twentieth century, social films and costume dramas, including stories about saints, folk tales, and appropriate dances and costumes, targeted the western and westernized audience. This could be attributed to purely economic reasons, but the maximum number of copies made of each such film was still only five. The oriental fantasy emerged in the 1930s, together with the urban thriller. The latter had some political content, but it was often very subtle. In reality, princely state life was seen as adventurous with intrigue in courts, encounters, dacoits, bandits, etc. Thus, these films were not as far removed from the social films as one assumes. During this period, different studios started to specialize in different genres of films. By now the film industry was also seeking a sense of respectability. It tried to engage the middle classes as its audience. These classes were also willing and able to pay more.

The other developments around this period included the emergence of female superstars, with a very clear emphasis on female sexuality. Sulochana established herself as a superstar in Bombay. In 1925, Himanshu Rai, a film director, started to collaborate with German technicians. The first female-run production company was established and, at the same time, a film industry was set up in Lahore, Punjab. Ardeshir Irani launched his own film company, specializing in the fantasy genre, and most of the stars and directors of the Kohinoor company moved across to work with him. Irani was the producer of the first Indian talkie, *Alam Ara*, the impact of which was astonishing. The Majestic cinema, where it was being shown, was besieged with black market tickets being sold at up to 20 times their normal price. Changes and developments were taking place in Calcutta and Madras as well. In 1927, Indian Cinema Arts—a precursor of New Theatres in Calcutta—was established.

The outbreak of the First World War had made the import of films from Great Britain quite difficult, and raw stock was becoming very difficult to obtain. The pressure from the American markets created another complication for the Indian film industry in the 1920s. In some cases, theatre chains were buying studios and in others film studios were buying theatre chains in order to expand their base. As large American studios became more secure in their home markets and were amply supported by their foreign markets, American films overseas came to represent pure profit. In the 1930s and beyond, in India, this meant that these films could always be offered at prices lower than those of most other films, including Indian films (Barnouw & Krishnaswamy, 1980).

In 1927, Britain passed the Cinematograph Films Act to restrict blind booking and advance booking of cinematograph films and to secure the renting and exhibition of a certain proportion of British films and for purposes connected therewith. The Government of India announced the setting up of a committee of enquiry, the Indian Cinematograph Committee. Its brief was to deal with censorship of American films, which "degrade the white women in the eyes of the Indians". Another of its tasks was to examine the possibility of exhibiting more Empire films, including the Indian films. On the matter of Empire films, the Committee felt that if cinema were to have any impact on Indians, it would be difficult for the average Indian to distinguish between American and British films, habits, and social milieu. It felt that the important thing was to nurture the Indian film. Consisting of three Indians and three Britons, the Committee reported on a number of key issues afflicting the infant Indian film industry. The need for censorship was stressed for several reasons, such as degradation of western values. The political aspect of films was not addressed at all. Nearly 50 years later, the Tamil film industry used subtle hints in dialogue and images, as well as discourses by crazy or mad people, to criticize the ruling Congress Party and support the Dravida Munetra Kazgham party and, especially, its leader, Annadurai. After Independence, the emphasis in Hindi cinema was on the construction of the country. There was a glimmer of hope and nationalist virtues were advocated. The trend of freelancing by directors and artistes became more pronounced. After the Second World War, black money poured into the Indian film industry.

Smith (1998) asserts that, following the breakdown of the studio system, the narrative structure of the Hollywood cinema changed, and that such a breakdown was not complete. Various components that contributed to the stability of the system still continue to exist. Many critics, Smith notes, have argued that Hollywood filmmaking has crossed the threshold into a new epoch. Such a scenario can equally be applied to Hindi cinema. From the disintegration of its studio system to changes in the genre, it was inevitable that the Bombay studio system would exist in parallel to the Hollywood studio system. Different studios were known for their different genres and, with the dissolution of the studio system, even though some production houses continued to produce similar types of films, the new Hindi cinema in the 1970s created new/art or parallel cinema. Gradually this was absorbed in the mainstream, creating a variation of middle cinema. In the past decade or so the younger generations of filmmakers have created a new genre targeting nonresident Indians and the second generation of migrants/Indian Diaspora around the world, some of whom are very well off, with an affluent lifestyle.

Thoraval (2000, p. 48) notes that the fall of the studio system and the strengthening of the star system were related to the entry of black money into the industry. Dyer (1986) places stars as individuals who anticipate the ideas of personhood in relation to capitalism, sell their labour, express opinions, and get themselves heard. This may also reflect why and how Indian film stars get attracted to politics. Barker (2003) outlines several stages of stardom, including how the public became interested in the offscreen antics of film actors. Agents and agencies are also said to contribute to this by packaging scripts, directors, stars, and financing together. Agents and agencies do not play a significant role in Hindi films, although some secretaries and personal assistants of stars yield considerable power by virtue of the fact that they hold the star's diary dates, and they have gone on to become producers themselves. Shah (1950/1980, p. 141) observes that the primary aim of the star system is monetary gain. While discussing the golden age of popular Hindi cinema, Thoraval (2000, p. 49) insists that the rules of the game changed gradually after the break-up of the studio system. From the 1960s onwards, Hindi cinema continued to make formula films targeting the urban poor, the labour force and the lumpen elements, and played a unifying role in this "new" urban society. These films are like fairy tales with a moral, which remains a profoundly Indian concept. They dwell on the evil nature of money, moneylenders, and the urban elite (typified by the urban rich), and the poor are seen to espouse a virtuous life in spite of being poor. Thoraval (p. 50) argues that these films centre more on expressing a story than coherently developing a plot. (This makes the films seem disjointed in the eyes of westerners.) This tendency diffuses the sense of rebellion, and sublimates the dissatisfaction and conflicts related to socioeconomic disparity.

The first 10 years after Independence were hard for Hindi cinema. The Second Film Enquiry Committee (1949–1951) was set up with wide terms of reference. Its report led to the establishment of the Film Institute of

India (1960), now known as the Film and Television Institute of India; the National Film Awards (1953); the Children's Film Society (1955); the University Film Council (1956); the Federation of Film Societies of India (1959); the Film Finance Corporation (1960); the Indian Motion Picture Export Corporation (1963); the Hindustan Film Manufacturing (1964); and the National Film Archives (1964). India's governmental network dealing with films thus has become the largest in the world.

Mishra (2002) identifies three concepts as the key legacies of the epic precursor texts: epic genealogy, the persistence of dharmik codes, and the power of the renouncer. He feels these components are essential for Hindi films, even if their proportions vary in each film. He believes that the renouncer and the mother are two important, basic character types in Hindi films. According to him, many leading roles conform to the role of the renouncer. The role of the mother and its significance in the Hindu psyche, in addition to the Indian Oedipal complex, are discussed elsewhere in this book. It is sufficient to say here that often the characters of the joker, villain, heroine, and the double of the hero or heroine are equally important. For example, the concept of the double, good versus evil twins, which portrays the splitting of the individual psyche and the difficulties in bringing them together, is also worth bearing in mind. The split represented by Nargis' character in *Raat aur Din* is concerned with sexual freedom and sexual desire, but also with repressing the western, "evil" half and upholding the traditional self.

Socially it was clear that immediately after Independence, the people of the country saw themselves as primarily Indian. Subsequently, however, with the rise of regional political parties, regional identity became important. As a reflection of this, the heroes and heroines started to use their surnames. Virtually all the surnames used were north Indian, perhaps to highlight the importance of Hindi as a language and also the "dominance" of the north. The Mandal Commission's recommendations in the 1980s split the country in a way that no other event had done by subconsciously urging people to don their caste labels for perceived or real advantages in the political and social arenas.

Hindi cinema has undergone several mutations. First, in the pre-Independence era and immediately afterwards, its focus shifted to the dilemma of the individual at home at a time of sociocultural interchange. The films of that era reduced the larger struggle to a family melodrama, which took a superficial form in Bombay, a literary one in Calcutta, and a theatrical one in Madras. Films that pitted the individual against contemporary trends, such as social inequality, religious strife, and caste restrictions, represented the second mutation. The traumas of the Second World War, the Partition of India, the assassination of Mahatma Gandhi, and communal strife had their own influence on the storyline of films.

Another mutation concerned the interior landscape—a personal hell in the life of the urban man. This, together with the personal obsession with materialism and possession, led to a wave of psychopathic characters. The failure of the individual to remain an individual and find peace led to further mutation. The focus shifted back to romance and the bosom of the family, accompanied by the peaceful coexistence of tradition and modernity.

The mutations in Hindi cinema saw changes in its music and songs, too. Originally, the artists used to sing their own songs. The live music director replaced the Indian soloist tradition by incorporating different instruments for better effect. Light film music became a passion and the continuous influence of western pop music lent it a hybrid form peculiarly its own. The songs and dances employed descended from different folk forms, such as lavani, tamasha, lori, bhajan, kirtan, bol, ghazal, and mujra. For a long time, song-and-dance sequences were an imposition on the film's structure. However, they heightened the emotional appeal of the film, and intensified audience response and participation. Mahmood (1974, p. 36) notes that as late as 1955, members of the audience in the front rows (i.e., the cheap seats) would appreciatively throw money at the screen as a dancer finished her dance.

In addition to music, the language of written cinema also changed. As cinema springs from and reflects the society in its visual aspects, it brings forth the symbols of the culture concerned. In its aural aspect, the dialogue, dialect, and the songs and lyrics, all reflect the society. In concept, Hindi film has hybridized itself from Hollywood, folk theatre, Russian film traditions, and the influence of Muslim culture and tradition. Urdu as a spoken language dates back several centuries and the two major languages used under Muslim rule were Persian (used in the court) and spoken Urdu. It was, therefore, inevitable that Urdu would be accepted in the film medium (except that it was called Hindustani). The Urdu speech patterns and its poetic traditions were both critical factors in the early days of Hindi cinema. The changes in cinema's visual and aural language are a result of influences of directors and producers. For example, after Independence, with the mass migration of Punjabis into India, the Punjabis managed to liberate the Hindi film from the clutches of theatre. They placed it firmly within a purely literary framework of written dialogue and story. Urdu poetry was used before Independence as a covert means of indicting the British rule. The songs in films were also used to give anti-Imperial messages.

After Independence, a vast majority of lyricists were Urdu poets in their own right, and the elegance, rhythm, richness of meaning, and charm of the lyrics made Hindi films what they were. In north India, music remained the monopoly of the courts and *kothas*. The only music available to the masses was the devotional music of the temples—*katha, kirtan*, and *bhajan*, or the Muslim public performances of *qawwalis, mushairas*, and so on.

In an interview with Mahmood (1974, p. 184), Ritwik Ghatak, a famous film director, said "Indians are epic-minded people. Every year thousands of Indians flock to see *Ramilila*. They know every word spoken in the scenes. It is not to see *what* is presented that they go there: It is to see *how* it is presented." Another celebrated Indian film director, Chetan Anand, said in an interview with Mahmood (1974, p. 188) that "Until recently, dancing and music were . . . regarded as the arts of *mirasis* and courtesans . . . Sanskrit storytelling began in verse form." He suggested that the integration of songs in the story gave the latter an emotional thrust and could also be symbolic. The songs become an adjunct to the drama; some songs have an integral role, while others have a suggestive or illustrative significance. The language of songs also reflects the prevalent societal influences. From Urdu poetry in the 1950s and 1960s to more sanskritized and Punjabi songs in the 1990s, songs remain the backbone of successful films, even though their style, contents, and music continue to change and evolve.

South Indian cinema contributed three types of films to the nation: the spiritual travelogue, in which the story takes the character on a pilgrimage; the authentic devotional film; and the family or social film, which not only absorbs the current social trends but also reflects them. The story of the family film unfolds within a given moral premise. Many of these films succeed at the box office because they present a view of culture and Indianness which is both acceptable and enjoyable.

The emergence of the social film as a rival to the mythological and the devotional film was the highlight of the 1960s. For the first time, the Indian film became conscious of its ecology (Mahmood, 1974, p. 41). The reformist hangover of the nineteenth century and the anti-British nationalist fervour of the early twentieth century provided the inspiration. The Hindu mind had responded to the challenge of western culture in a paradoxical manner, a phenomenon that continues to this date. Though there was a perceived need for rebellion against obscurantism, there was an unwillingness to embrace a total change over to the western way of life or style. The reformist sentiments gave rise to films that dramatized the tragic consequences of child marriage, dowry, untouchability, and other social evils, such as the tyranny of the mother-in-law. At the same time, the sentiment of revolt inspired films that highlighted the national heritage through the social and devotional milieus as represented by the lives of saints and reformers. The tenor of these films was perceived by the viewer as overly sentimental and moralistic. These films championed the cause of freedom, though this had to be done in such a way as to avoid any censorship problems from the British government. Some films decried the aping of western values, giving a clear message that nationalist values were the best.

Mahmood (p. 41) describes the cinema of the time as a cinema of lofty ideals, nationalistic, and with revivalist flavours.

Several factors played a key role in the shift of content of films. In the 1950s and 1960s, several Muslim socials (as films with Muslim stories and characters were often called) of the time represented the zenith of that culture in Hindi cinema. After the initial shock of the Partition, these films were placed very much in the Islamic context, and they exploited the culture of a bygone and much mourned era. The use of Urdu poetry and Ghazal music reflected the influence of the Persian tradition. In the late 1960s, this tradition started to disappear, as did the use of Urdu in Hindi cinema generally. The films reflected great love tragedies, and the general despondency of the Urdu poets and writers working in films at that time led to writing influenced by the universal context of pain and suffering on the one hand, and hopefulness on the other. This may well be attributed to two major conflicts in the 1960s; the optimism of socialist triumph was dashed when India went to war with China in 1962, and then Pakistan in 1965. These conditions produced some of the most moving poetry in Hindi cinema, dealing with suppressed grief and the loss of not only the loved one, but of idealism and hope as well. Songs of grief and lost love became very popular, marking the lyric writers' anxieties, loneliness, desperation, and despondency. The preponderance of producers and directors from north India ensured that conventional morality was upheld, in spite of, or maybe because of, their pretensions to modernity. Artistically, during the first two decades after Partition, this group of directors carried a streak of revivalism that allowed them to reflect what was going on in society, rather than to influence it. The Hindi film portrayed love affairs that had society or circumstances as hurdles to their union, and villains who were not the same as in the earlier decades.

Hindi films may often be called formulaic because they follow the pattern of boy meets girl, loses girl and then finds her, with some villainy and comedy thrown in. The villain or the vamp may be evil or simply bad but, until recently, not beyond redemption. The villain or the vamp could be redeemed by repenting, by sacrifice of their love or love by their family, or by meekly accepting what is coming to them. The vamp is generally portrayed as being alone, sometimes even lonely. She unwillingly and often unwittingly falls into the clutches of the villain, or he happens to be the only person who is willing to support her. She usually comes from a poor background, and is portrayed as a materialistic moneygrabber who wants the comforts of life. Her badness is the extreme antithesis of the good heroine. She dresses in miniskirts and mixes with men, drinks alcohol, and smokes, in contrast to the heroine, who is generally demure, wears traditional Indian clothes, and behaves in a traditional way. This changed in the 1980s and 1990s, when the heroine, too, became more modern and started donning western clothes and revealing dresses.

The villain and vamp add spice to the film. They represent the demon as personified by Ravana in the *Ramayana* and symbolize the badness of society. Certainly until 1976 or so, they were redeemable. They were able to repent and recover their and their family's good name. The problem with villains and heroes, or vamps and heroines, in the formulaic Hindi film has been that they represent one extreme or the other (good or bad), and never a mixture of the two. This extremist philosophy has its roots in the Hindu psyche. Those who have been dealt a bad hand by fate are looked upon with great sympathy by the audience.

The role and perception of the villain has changed dramatically over the last three decades. During the days of Nehruvian socialism, the villains were either feudal landlords, mill owners, or their sons. However, with the growth of economic liberalism and capitalism, it was the smugglers or antisocial elements who became the villains.

The changing role of the villain in Hindi cinema over the last 40 years or so reflects the sociopolitical reality of the country. When the villain was the smuggler, the hero managed to trounce him; but when the smuggler became the hero, the establishment became the villain (this heralded the arrival of the angry young man). The days when the hero and villain had clearly defined roles were characterized by a clarity regarding the sociopolitical dos and don'ts. Once this clarity started to erode in the mid-1970s, and more so in the mid-1980s, the roles of the heroes and villains became very confused and often merged.

F. Kazmi (1999, p. 152) argues that this led to a clear psychological need in the 1970s to identify the villain(s) responsible for the wrongs in society. As the structural defects of the system became abstract and the relatively new had unforeseen and unknown consequences, it was essential that "the other" thus identified was clear. Villains had always existed in Hindi films, but until then their role had been to keep the hero and heroine apart. The new villains, on the other hand, were businessmen: smugglers, dacoits, politicians and corrupt policemen, terrorists, and what the politicians of the day had euphemistically started calling the "phoren [sic, meaning foreign] hand or agents".

THE 1960s

The 1960s are sometimes considered the golden age of Hindi cinema. Several spectacular films were released, including *Mughal-e-Azam* (1960), recently re-released after black and white portions were colourized, *Ganga Jamuna* (1961), and Muslim socials such as *Chaudhvin Ka Chand, Mere Mehboob, Nur Jehan, Ghazal*, and *Bahu Begum*, all of which were extremely successful at the box office.

The films reflected the political climate of the time. The country's first Prime Minister, Pandit Jawaharlal Nehru, with his vision of Nehruvian socialism, believed in industrialization together with building government-owned dams and factories. Five-year plans were drawn up along Soviet lines. India's highest paid actor, Dilip Kumar, was once offered five million rupees to play a role, but he declined and advised the financier to invest the amount in five-year plans instead.

The box office success of *Mother India* (1957) also reflected post-Independence sentiments. The film revolves around the story of a single woman bringing up her children after her husband is injured in an accident and, ashamed of his disability and resulting loss of manhood, he had abandoned his family. While bringing up her children, the woman deals with various natural catastrophes and a greedy village moneylender who wants to exploit her. *Mother India* is based on an earlier film, *Aurat*, by the same director. *Aurat*, too, was a mega-hit and reflected society's concerns about the role of women in the reconstruction of post-Independence India, which could be seen as a screaming infant left (or abandoned) by its rulers. The romanticism of the 1960s was also evident in the gentle melodies, good lyrics, and storylines, which reflected a nation settling down to be at peace with itself. The decade has been termed the golden age of Hindi cinema both because of the music and the quality of the films. The films were essentially family socials or melodramas, and could be watched by the entire family. Even though India fought three wars with two of its neighbours (with China in 1962, and with Pakistan in 1965 and 1971), the fallout of these wars on the films and society became evident only in the next decade. The 1960s were also the decade during which film stars became well established, so much so that films could sell on their names alone. Another feature of the films of this era was the romantic triangle formula.

Film journalism in India is as old as the talkies (Masud, 1997), but has always lacked a degree of legitimacy. From *Filmindia* in the 1940s and beyond, several Hindi film magazines as well as Times of India Group's publication *Filmfare* reached their peak in the 1960s. Masud regrets that film criticism, which is different from film journalism, has remained relatively undeveloped in India, compared with foreign countries. Film criticism became well established only after the 1970s. It helped people see cinema as a craft. This may also have been a result of the coming of age of the Film Institute of India and other organizations.

THE 1970s

In 1974, Prime Minister Indira Gandhi declared the Emergency, imprisoned a large number of opposition leaders, and virtually took control of the media, including the newspapers. Indian filmmakers woke up with a jolt.

The censors initially banned two films satirizing the politicians and the political system and the print of one was destroyed by the then heir apparent, Sanjay Gandhi, the Prime Minister's younger son.

The highlight of the 1970s was a curry western, *Sholay*, which proved to be one of the biggest box office grossers in the history of Hindi cinema. It is the story of a police inspector who loses his entire family to a villain, then hires two petty thieves to take revenge and protect the village from the villain. Soon after *Sholay* came *Deewar*, which tells the story of a single mother bringing up two sons. One son is a labourer who goes on to become a smuggler, while the other becomes a police officer. The ending of the film is similar to that of *Mother India*, in which the mother ultimately shoots her younger son. In *Deewar*, she allows her younger son to shoot his older brother. *Zanjeer* came close on the heels of *Deewar*. In this film, a lonely police officer seeks revenge on a smuggler/villain who had murdered his parents when he was a child. All three films starred Amitabh Bachchan, whose arrival on the scene was hailed; he seemed to personify the "angry young man" following *Zanjeer* and *Deewar*. These films spoke of the state of society at that time, a society in which an individual had to stand up to a corrupt and controlling system. Gokulsingh and Dissanayake (1998, p. 46) are not the only ones to attribute the success of these Bachchan films to the deep crisis afflicting urban India. With the rise in urban crime, spiralling inflation, and corrupt and sectarian politics, the romanticism of the late 1960s went out of the window.

The success of these films heralded the arrival of a new formula, which consisted of high-pitched melodrama, sex, and violence. *Sholay* made violence a highly marketable commodity (Garga, 1996, p.184). This streak continued from the 1970s into the next two decades or so.

The social upheaval in society in the 1970s is worth noting. Masud (1997) highlights the problem of the middle class/intelligentsia at the time of the Emergency. He notes that the intelligentsia had started to dislike Indira Gandhi's increasingly manipulative and fascistic way of securing personal power. Being the income-tax commissioner of Bombay, Masud observed that poets with leftist leanings had "sold out". The corrupt side of the Emergency came into evidence only after the initial first few months. He also illustrates the expedient use of television during the Emergency, giving the example of how a prominent Congress Party leader, Rajni Patel, was sacked live on television. Masud notes that the fascism of the Emergency was an Indian kind of fascism because its success depended on the voluntary subservience of the people. He calls the defeat of Indira Gandhi in the 1977 elections India's second day of independence. These changes also influenced how films responded by changing from romantic to violence-based dramas.

A side-effect of the increased portrayal of violence and the more dramatic storylines of the films of the 1970s was that the music and songs started to take a backseat in the film. Not only did the number of songs drop to three or four per film, but these were also extrinsic to the film. Paradoxically, Bachchan, with his limited musical ability, sang some of his songs himself rather than relying on playback singers (Gokulsingh & Dissanayake, 1998, pp. 105–106).

The hero-based formula films of the 1970s also whittled down the role of the heroine. The 1970s no longer adored women, and openly asserted the right to treat them as insignificant possessions. Associated with this was an increase in the number of cases of molestation, rape, and the burning of women for dowry, all of which were done with greater impunity than ever before (Das Gupta, 1991, p. 238). With the arrival of the angry young man, the roles of women became secondary and simply decorative. The woman was "ill treated by society, seduced, raped and widowed in violent action to build up the macho image of the hero" (Rao, 1989, p. 25). Until the 1970s, rape on the screen was not central to the film, but was implicit. However, this changed dramatically over the next two decades.

The 1970s did have a few hit romantic films that featured women in key roles, such as *Bobby* and *Kabhi-Kabhie*, but these were the exception rather than the rule.

By the 1970s, the euphoria of Independence had disappeared and the contradictions of the socialist path of development that India had adopted had sharpened and become quite evident (F. Kazmi, 1999, p. 168). It is as if the childhood of the republic was over and the angst-ridden, rebellious teen years were upsetting the parents. The romantic twenties of the youth would emerge later.

In this era, the protagonist is shown as a marginalized individual and the audience identifies with him as "one of us". He does what we would like to do, but are unable to because of social mores and our own private morals. He is much wronged and exploited, and has suffered physically, emotionally, and psychologically. These themes continued in the next decade, and their portrayal became more prominent, aggressive and violent.

THE 1980s

Basu (2000) notes that India's fiscal deficit had become unmanageable by the end of the 1980s and its international debt had become too large for comfort. The crisis blew over only by the beginning of 1993 when the economy started to pick up following major policy changes. The Indian economy had a growth rate of over 6% per annum between 1993 and 2000 (Basu, 2000). In the 1990s, the literacy rate grew (especially among females) from 52% to 62% and Basu observes that by now, the many institutes of technology and higher education—most of which were conceived in the Nehruvian era and caused unemployment and frustration in the 1960s and

1970s—had started to yield results, perhaps because of globalization. The romanticism of the 1960s gave way to violence in the 1970s and 1980s, and to idealism of joint family films in the 1990s.

Thapar (2000) argues that upper caste nationalism gave way to middle class chauvinistic nationalism, which is now being confronted with the demands of the underprivileged, partly as a result of the Mandalization of politics. There was appropriate representation of the marginalized individual in the 1970s and 1980s blockbusters.

While discussing the influence of Tamil films on the urban poor in Tamil Nadu, Dickey (1993) notes that one of the major Tamil actors, M. G. Ramachandran (often referred to as MGR), took advantage of his fan following, turning it into a political tool. However, the melodrama the audience were watching on and off the screen brought suppressed fears and devices into public realm, but intriguingly suggested personal solutions. While giving concrete form to the anxieties caused by shared socioeconomic circumstances, the melodrama rarely advocated collective solutions, especially in the 1970s and 1980s. The blurring of the boundaries between reality and cinema is reflected in many ways where former heroes from films became real life leaders and yet real life leaders stopped being heroes.

The 1980s were a stressful period for Indian society in general, and for Hindi cinema in particular. This was the decade when Indira Gandhi was re-elected and separatist movements took root in many states including Punjab, Kashmir, and Assam. Indian society was in turmoil, and the post-Independence idealism rapidly gave way to parochialism. Another factor that caused crucial damage to the film industry, not only in India but worldwide, was the advent of video recorders. In India, the indigenously built machines were sold as video players, which did not record programmes or films at all. The easy access of the middle class to these machines and their increased emphasis on privacy, coupled with the threat of violence in public places, meant that cinema-going dropped dramatically.

In the early 1980s, some of the themes of the previous decade continued. However, another strand emerged during this decade following the success of *Insaaf Ka Tarazu*. This was the first movie focusing on the rape of the heroine, who gets no judicial recompense. When her sister, too, is raped by the same person she decides to take revenge. As is usually the case, the success of this film spawned a large number of films imitating the same theme: the woman avenging her physical and sexual humiliation by taking the law into her own hands because she knows that she will not get any justice from the establishment. These women have to look after themselves because, paradoxically, their men are becoming impotent and less supportive. In Hindi films, women are often portrayed as goddesses, especially Durga or Kali, to show that revenge is divine or justified. By locating the protagonist within the subordinate classes (in social, economic, caste, or work-related terms), and by focusing on how such an individual is exploited, oppressed, and wronged, the film is able to directly interpellate and involve the audience. The process of interpellation is furthered by linking the fortunes of the protagonist with those of the entire society. Thus, any attack on the protagonist is an attack on society. The villain is simply the enemy of society. Such viewer identification is related to the narrative authority of the film (F. Kazmi, 1999, pp. 170–171).

Two of the surprise big hits of the 1980s were the romantic films *Qayamat se Qayamat Tak* and *Maine Pyaar Kiya*. These had new younger heroes who were not confined within the angry young man image. Around this time the proliferation of cable and satellite channels for television began to influence the state-owned television channels, which started marketing extremely successful serials (mostly mythological), such as *Ramayana* and *Mahabharata*. The winds of change that were to sweep across the political system and economic system (liberalization, to be precise) changed the face of Hindi cinema yet again.

THE 1990s

Inden (1999) classifies the late 1980s and early 1990s as a distinct, new period for the Indian film business. Two of the reasons for such classification are the explosive growth of television and the "demise" of the Bachchan character over this period. Also, in the 1990s, Kashmir and other locations became no-go areas for shooting fantasy scenes and producers/ directors started to look further afield. According to Inden, a brutal dystopia of crime and rape had displaced the mediocre familial utopias by the 1980s. Furthermore, economic liberalization led to a sense of global belonging so that the middle classes were attempting to reclaim cinema as a vehicle for representing themselves, not only to themselves, but also to the nation and the world. The heroes of the films of the 1990s were icons of the transitional class. Inden concludes that the ensemble of characters in Hindi films can be seen as complex, shifting icons of the people, of their leaders and enemies, of the elites and masses but represented as middle class, or as urban or rural poor.

In the 1990s, two different strands emerged in Hindi cinema. The first was characterized by the continuation of the angry young man, but now this anger was not directed at society. Rather it was as a symbol of love. The roles of Shah Rukh Khan as the love-obsessed stalker in films like *Deewana*, *Darr*, *Baazigar*, and *Anjaam* heralded the arrival of a psychopath who feels no remorse or guilt. In a nasty, narcissistic, and egocentric way, he also fails to understand why he cannot have the woman he loves and why she does not respond to his overtures. His underlying feeling is that his possessive love should be enough for the object of love to reciprocate this.

The second strand was of a new romanticism, which, interestingly, was again personified by Shah Rukh Khan in films such as *Dilwale Dulhaniya Le Jayenge* and *Dil to Pagal Hai*. Both of these were smash hits in India and abroad.

There are two threads to this new romanticism. First, the romance involves young (teenaged) people with high aspirations of good jobs and money. The young ones either live abroad or in India, but carry the traditional Indian values in their hearts. Even if they live in India, their dress, setting, music, and environment are modern. This explains why these films were also big hits with (or perhaps because of) the Indian Diaspora, the members of the younger generation who could identify with these values. This feature of the new romanticism reflects the impact of global-ization and economic liberalization. Second, these films revived the role of music and songs in film. Music, song, and dance returned to the screen with a vengeance. This was accompanied by a trend of using very long titles, based on the romantic songs of the 1960s and early 1970s. These choices may reflect a need to revert to gentler, romantic times. Great success attended the release of three family-oriented films, which represent the overwhelming victory of family values, even though the protagonists are modern: *Maine Pyar Kiya*, *Hum Aapke Hain Kaun*, and *Hum Saath Saath Hain*. *Hum Saath Saath Hain* was financially less successful than *Hum Aapke Hain Kaun*, which was reported to have been the biggest ever box office success in the history of Hindi cinema. F. Kazmi (1999) has provided a very interesting critique of this film, and of special note is the way it is linked with the rise of the Hindu nationalist party. Power relations related to religion were apparent in the politics of the country and then started to be reflected in modern Hindi cinema.

Other successful films, like *Kaho Na Pyar Hai* and *Hum Dil De Chuke Sanam*, herald the arrival of the younger generation of actors and directors whose parents and grandparents had been in the film business. Though they appear more modernized, their ideas of romance are not dissimilar to those portrayed by their parents. This peaceful coexistence of modernity and traditional values is of great interest. And yet a sense of pessimism, too, is evident in the films of the 1990s. Some of these show female psychopaths keen to assert themselves, not for revenge but for love, as in *Gupt*, and for no reason at all in *Kaun*.

CONCLUSIONS

The history of Hindi cinema is influenced by the prevalent social factors, including the political climate and the entry of different types of individual and financial resource, which have built studio systems, destroyed studio systems and changed the medium by the introduction of colour, Urdu poetry, and Punjabi folk dance. In each decade after Independence there has been a different aspect of growth of Hindi cinema. For example, the romanticism of the 1950s and 1960s was reflected in social films where the hero and/or heroine were engineers or doctors attempting to rebuild the nation; the 1970s and 1980s reflected the angry young man's solitary stand against bureaucracy and political and police corruption; in the 1990s, an idealistic Hindu joint family became the preferred norm and the role of villain and vamp underwent a further transformation, leading to an increase in the portrayal of psychopathy.

CHAPTER SEVEN

Indian personality, villainy, and history

There is no doubt that in the twentieth century the Hindu personality emerged from and was influenced by a sense of inferiority as a result of historical events, such as the Mughal invasion and the British Raj (Narain, 1957). According to Narain, the salient traits of the Indian character include an absence of commitment, a particular identification with the mother, a peculiar attitude towards authority, along with other contradictions. He observes that when the Muslims subjugated the Hindus, a feeling of inferiority set in among the latter. Several Muslim rulers pursued policies of active discrimination and persecution against the Hindus. These policies were (by and large) passively endured, with a feeling of helplessness in the absence of political strength. The problem was further compounded by British rule; Hindus had to accept British supremacy and, interestingly, looked up to it initially, perhaps as a relief from the Muslim rule. The structural changes introduced by the British in the spheres of the economy, education, and transport further contributed to a sense of inferiority and inadequacy. Narain believes that these feelings have contributed to certain traits found in the Indian character even today, such as sensitivity, vanity, and arrogance. Narain defines the absence of commitment in the contemporary Indian character as an absence of the total involvement that enables one to carry a task from start to finish through all trials and difficulties. This may also be due to the Hindu philosophy that urges individuals to be in this world but not of this world. There is, of course, a problem in equating Hindu personality with Indian personality.

Narain (1957) explicates that, at the individual level, promises are freely made, but are either not kept or are incompletely kept. There is a great amount of initial enthusiasm, which gets dissipated very rapidly. At a collective level, faith in objectives is proclaimed but the requisite amount of sustained effort is not forthcoming. Even in fantasy, loved objects are given up or surrendered when difficulties crop up.

In situations involving a love triangle in the Hindi cinema of the 1950s and 1960s, the theme of the helpless or even voluntary surrender of the beloved to a rival was extremely popular (though this passivity gave way to psychopathy in the 1980s and 1990s, perhaps as a reaction). In such voluntary surrender, the individual can transfer his or her love from one object to another, say, from lover before marriage to husband after marriage.

Narain (1957) argues that the Indian character lacks definiteness, resulting in a capacity to show forthrightness, determination, and doggedness. There is great patience, but little perseverance. Although it is impossible to accept that such character traits are universally found among all Indians, such a generalization can, nonetheless, explain some of the actions of the crowd. The paradox between western values and the Indian tradition pulls the individual in two opposing directions. This ambivalence is also reflective of the depersonalizing factors faced by Indians during childhood, when, even in nuclear families, children are seen as communal beings. Several adults may exercise many parental functions in common for a particular group of children and vice versa. Thus, there is a tendency not to fix affection on single individuals (Taylor, 1948).

Another factor that induces a sense of resignation among Indians is the rigidity of the caste system, even though the caste system may also provide an anchor for some individuals. As for the Indian male, his identity is whittled down and his sense of masculinity denuded by his close identification with the mother. The Hindu ethos itself may be seen as passive, characterized by an attitude of "let it be". Narain (1957) attributes this sense of acceptance and submission to foreign rule, which engendered an attitude of dependence on authority as well as on the Indian family environment (which is contrary to the growth of personal autonomy). The family environment does not prepare children to predict the kind of reaction they are likely to get in response to specific actions. The dependence on and distrust of authority runs very deep. However, it is possible that the culture of dependence antedates foreign rule. The feudal landlord was seen as *mai–baap*, "mother–father"; and was expected to support, nurture, or protect the person (while the landlord, in turn, relied on the gods).

The Indian character is also regarded as being fragmented, unintegrated, and even contradictory. These features give rise to internal compartmentalization so that the psyche can cope with the jumble of paradoxical and confusing characteristics. The gap between the ideal and the actual may well represent the lust for materialism while looking for spirituality. Individuals may lust after material possessions as they see them all around them, but the religious teachings focus on spiritual growth. Thus the individual's hankering and aspirations do not match what he or she ought to be doing. Such a paradox feeds into a feeling of dissonance in wanting to be comfortable materially but expecting to be ascetic, and produces a sense of frustration. These paradoxes also make Indians experience intense feelings of aggression and anxiety. These feelings are considered too threatening to be consciously permissible, but when they are unleashed their expression is chaotic and leads to an utter loss of control. Usually, immediate confrontation is avoided and the guiding principle is that what can be done tomorrow does not need to be done today. In Hindi cinema, these feelings and emotions are then projected onto the villain on the screen, who represents extremes of evils with which the audience can identify, without getting their hands dirty. This identification with the chief protagonists against the villain then becomes a key to the success of the film.

As a psychoanalyst, Spratt (1966) argues that the Hindu personality is narcissistic. Spratt goes on to hint that the Hindu male invests a lot in the semen, and the desire to conserve it turns into a fear of loss. This does not reflect a castration anxiety, but a narcissistic attempt to preserve something that reflects the ego-ideal. Like Narain (1957), Spratt points out that although the aggressive component of the Hindu conscience is weak, and although the typical Hindu is strongly attached to his family and caste, it does not follow that educated Hindus have ill-developed personalities or lack individuality. The conscience and the personality which forms around it are well developed in other ways; the personality trait may be submissive to the father and thus dependent on the authority figures. Spratt (pp. 12–13) compares the Ayurvedic model of *satvik*, *rajasik*, and *tamasik* characteristics to the narcissistic, punitive, and impulsive personality types.

The higher or the best *satvik* types are inspired by a love of the good and have a strong sense of morals. People belonging to the lower levels of the *satvik* type are inactive, self-satisfied, self-indulgent, and self-centred, the classic narcissistic type. Narcissistic personalities are of two types: those belonging to the first type are aware of the danger of vanity and their deliberate efforts at self-control do not allow it to get out of hand. They cherish an altruistic moral ideal and their very narcissism accentuates it. Yudhishtir, the eldest Pandava, fits this profile. The other type consists of egoists and egotists, who have more or less adapted to conventional standards, but are apt to succumb to vanity and temptation. The higher level *rajasiks* are self-controlled, tense, active, and moral, but are liable to indulge in unconscious aggression; the lower level *rajasiks*, on the other hand, are less moral, less aggressive, and less active. Cinema, too, portrays these types of personality.

Borrowing from the themes of the *Mahabharata*, Hindi cinema often portrays the hero as an idealist in the narcissistic mould. Sometimes, though, the hero is modelled after the second type of narcissist.

As a result of narcissistic development and the consequent weakness of repression, a high place is given in Hindu culture to the physical body, its attractiveness, and beauty. Physical handicaps were a disqualification for kingship. This tendency to look down upon those with physical handicaps allows individuals to laugh at such people. This is reflected in Hindi films, which often rely on physical comedy with a strong emphasis on the physical characteristics of the comedian rather than the situation. The portrayal of the characters is often influenced by these personality types. The development of Hindu personality is of significant interest in understanding how people deal with family and society.

The narcissistic personality is the product of an upbringing in which the father does little to provoke the son's hostility, and the positive Oedipal complex (i.e., hostility) in the Greek sense is not strongly developed in India. The negative Oedipal complex (i.e., fear of castration by the father, the passive homosexual attitudes towards him) derives from a strong maternal attachment to and identification with the mother. Spratt (1966, p. 57) views the last two phases of Hindu life, *vanprastha* and *sanyasa*, as self-castration in preparation for returning to the womb. The close relationship with the mother is a reflection of the style of mothering.

Spratt (1966) suggests that among Hindus the worship of goddesses, and more particularly of the mother goddess, is to be attributed to the mother fixation. He points out that most village deities in south India are female (but this is true of large parts of north India as well), and the wives of male gods are also worshipped, sometimes together with their husbands and sometimes by themselves. In addition, he observes that the most sacred room in the temples (from which the image is never removed) is dark and small, with only one entrance, and is called the *garbhagriha*, "womb house".

In Indian art forms and sculptures, the female is often portrayed as a virgin. Her breasts are noticeable and literature contains numerous allusions to their weight and size. This speaks of the mother fixation, which is also evident in the veneration accorded to the cow, rivers, and lakes (the latter representing amniotic fluid). Spratt (1966) also points out that the narcissistic tendency to retreat into safety is an unconscious desire to return to the mother's womb. Furthermore, the emphasis placed on milk, dairy products and sweets also reflects a mother fixation, though Carstairs (1957) holds that these substances are identified with semen. The personality traits and the development of the personality are a reflection of child rearing patterns, influences of peers, and cultural and social factors. Cultures determine and define what is deviant and what is abnormal, as well as how deviant and deviance are defined and developed. Cultures also determine how abnormal or deviant behaviour is dealt with (Bhugra, 1993b). Bearing in mind that features such as mother fixation are too ingrained, the response of the culture to any kind of villainy will be influenced by prevalent norms and attitudes towards deviance.

The thin line between the villain and the social construction of the psychopath suggests that given the right (or wrong) circumstances, most individuals have the potential to become villainous. The line between clinical cases of psychopathy, as discussed earlier, and the psychopaths depicted in literature and cinema is not marked either. There is a spectrum of psychopathic or antisocial behaviour that demonizes such individuals and their acts. The difference between one end of the spectrum and the other lies in the purpose of the act and the end gain. For example, the success of the villain in vying for huge material gains gives a clear message to the viewer regarding (1) the immorality of the act, and (2) whether these acts and the individuals performing these acts are redeemable or not. For example, if a child is shown to be deprived of material goods when growing up and then steals, the audience may feel sympathy, because an under-standing of the underlying causes vindicates the theft. On the other hand, if the child has been brought up in lavish surroundings with parental love, the act of theft on the part of such an individual will raise a different set of responses from the audience.

Whether the hero turns into the villain or vice versa is essentially linked with the individual protagonists and the viewer's perceptions of the acts and the morality underlying them. Using demons as examples, and struc-tures and strictures implied by or imposed upon these demons within the scriptures, means that the viewer sees these representations on the one hand as extremely alien yet on the other as totally and completely understand-able, thereby feeding into holding paradoxical and compartmentalized views. The collapse of various structures and certainties in the society can only add to the prevailing confusion, and when a man or woman emerges as a superhero this success is often guaranteed. This was highlighted by the enormous success of *Mr India*, directed by Shekhar Kapur. When wearing a pair of special glasses, the hero becomes invisible; he goes on to use this technology to beat the villains and obtain the heroine. Although completely impossible hokum, this meets with great favour by audiences around the country. When the invisible hero beats the villains, who are quite befuddled, cheers can be heard in the auditoria.

Indians have followed stories from the scriptures in various forms, and villains have always had a major role in these stories. The key purpose of the villain is to keep the hero and heroine from marrying or, if they are married, to use every possible opportunity to destroy their happiness. The villains are romantic fools who, because of their habits, greed, or lust, cannot obtain the heroine. They are also family members: either the *chacha* "paternal uncle" who, in spite of the brotherly love, does not hesitate to interfere with the smooth functioning of the family, or the *mama* "maternal uncle", who does the same. Both these stereotypes are derived from the *Mahabharata* and the *Ramayana*. The villain can also be a cousin of the hero (again a shade of the *Mahabharata*), or an outside demonic representation (the *Ramayana*).

Hindi cinema of the 1950s and 1960s was laden with romance. The stories were generally simple. For example, the hero might be a doctor or an engineer trying to do the best; he would fall in love with a girl; the villain would poke his nose in to separate the couple; and, following some intervention, divine or otherwise, the couple would get back together again. If they got married, as in the south Indian social films, at least the mother-in-law or older sister-in-law would make their lives very difficult. They would suffer, but would struggle on for the sake of the honour of the family. Ultimately, their selflessness would bring the errant mother-in-law or sister-in-law round and they would live happily ever after.

In the age of optimism in the 1960s, the villain often wanted to marry the heroine in order to get her father's money, or to blackmail her or the hero's family. His motive was largely personal gain. In the end, the villain would be eliminated, generally by the police or the hero. He would redeem himself by bringing the hero and heroine together, asking for their forgiveness and that of the elders, and apologizing for his wrongdoings. Thus, in the era of optimism, even the villain remained optimistic for redemption. Later, the villain took on a new shape: The hero became the villain and the villain was fêted as a hero. Certain organizations became the symbol of villainy and the hero (as a villain) had to stand up to them. In the process, the villains became psychopaths. The extension of villainy to a level devoid of shame or guilt reflected the direction the country and society were taking.

Popular cinema has always preserved and propagated society's ethical and political norms, and its role as a pacifier has invariably become magnified during times of distress. N. Kazmi (1996, p. 24) notes that popular cinema has attempted national well-being, the enemy of the nation being shown mostly as an individual (foreign or native), and never the political system or the institution of governance. The success myth is perpetuated, with glory and failure being linked to individual effort rather than infrastructural pressures. It has also glorified lack of opportunity and the like. However, we can safely say that sometimes the villain has been accorded an equal degree of glorification. Even in *Ramayana*, Ravana, despite being the demon king, was an acknowledged scholar who had prayed for long periods of time to the gods for redemption.

Villainy in the new context has taken a different shape and a frightening form. The psychopath is shameless, guiltless, and not only irresponsible or irritable, but also manipulative and impulsive. This makes him an ideal storybook/comic book character. The switch to the new types of villain is quite an interesting phenomenon, which is explored further later. The villain provides a counterpoint to the love story because there has to be a demon in every story.

The phases of villainy can be seen as parallel to periods of post-Independence India. Morris-Jones (1979) divides the political events in India into three periods. The first five years after Independence were the years of construction, when the Constitution was drawn up and democracy started to take root. The Partition was followed by a period of self-discovery and assessment, the primary task being to hold things together, ensure survival, and get accustomed to the feel of being on the water and keeping the vessels afloat (p. 72). The mood was upbeat and cinema responded to the optimism in the air. During the second period, between 1952 and 1964, the system started to operationalize its voyage. This period has been described as "a period for achievement or containment" but, at the same time, long-term disunities appeared (p. 73). Even though the periods outlined by Morris-Jones make sense, I believe that the period of optimism lasted until the time when the Chinese invaded India. This war marked the end of the Nehruvian dream, disproving Nehru's view that the Indians and Chinese could be brothers. The Chinese attack brought the childhood years of the nascent democracy to an abrupt end. The country was forced to grow up very rapidly and, although it had reached its teenage years going by the calendar, it had not reached the requisite level of maturity when the Indo-Pakistan war of 1969 broke out. The aftermath of the war saw a massive exercise in soul-searching and, by the time the next Indo-Pakistan war broke out (in 1971), India was beginning to struggle with teenage angst.

Mehta (1993) gives a poignant account of the Nehruvian childhood of the country. India and China were engaged in a continuing quarrel over territories along the Sino-Indian border through the 1950s and 1960s. Both China and India tried to establish their claims to these two territories by appealing to place names, to old maps, to old treaties, and more generally to religious and racial affinities. The Sino-Indian discussions that began in the 1950s were so vague in their early stages that it was difficult to grasp exactly what areas were being disputed (p. 169).

In 1954, China consolidated her political hold on Tibet and concluded with India an Agreement for Trade and Cultural Intercourse. The spirit of this was set forth in the Panch Sheel Agreement, with five principles suggesting that the two powers would refrain from interfering in each other's internal affairs, would respect each other's territory and sovereignty, would work towards each other's benefit, would forswear aggression, and would adhere to the ideal of peaceful coexistence. However, within months China had occupied parts of the disputed territory; then gradually the Chinese demands increased and the Dalai Lama escaped to India in

1959. Nehru was attacked in the Parliament for allowing himself to be duped by the Chinese for 5 years into a one-sided observance of the Panch Sheel Agreement. Nehru remained publicly unconcerned, as did his Defence Minister V. K. Krishna Menon (Mehta, 1993, pp. 170–171). In the summer of 1962 the Chinese made their strongest border incursion. Both the Prime Minister and the Defence Minister dismissed these as mere jostling. They continued to believe that the main enemy was Pakistan. On 8 September 1962, the Chinese Army crossed the McMahon Line and on 20 October invaded India. India had no alternative but to defend herself. The two most populous countries of the world were at war. The Indian Army had not only become weakened by a deficiency of funding and training officers by bureaucratic, financial, and economic problems; but it also was a victim of religious, racial, linguistic, and regional schisms besetting the country at large. The motives for this attack were many and Mehta (p. 173) outlines these.

The Chinese withdrew and struck again, making it obvious that the Indian Army and India's government were at their mercy and were unable to hold the onslaught. The country rose in support of Nehru but the damage to his reputation and governance had already been done. Nehru acknowledged that India had not been prepared for the war. This failure and its consequences on the Indian economy hit Nehru and his Congress Party very hard indeed. The Indian economy in 1959–1960—the last year of the second 5-year plan—had shown a 7.10% increase in national income, 10.5% increase in industrial output, and 8.1% increase in agricultural output, but this dropped to 2.2%, 4.3%, and 1.6% respectively in 1961–1962 (Chandra, Mukherjee, & Mukherjee, 2000). This, combined with the Chinese invasion, ended the era of optimism.

The death of Nehru in May 1964 brought about a change in the political landscape of India. Shastri was elected Prime Minister. During his reign of less than 2 years India was invaded again, this time by Pakistan. Shastri "didn't have a modern mind. He was an orthodox Hindu and full of superstition" said Indira Gandhi in an interview with Ved Mehta (Mehta, 1993, p. 500). The second era, when romanticism and optimism gave way to aggression, violence, and disaffection, especially on religious, ethnic, and linguistic grounds, began after the election of Indira Gandhi as Prime Minister. The period during which optimism gave way to pessimism and helplessness had set in.

After the second war with Pakistan and the creation (or some would call liberation) of Bangladesh, the country was still not at rest with itself. The middle class, instead of being able to rise to a higher economic status, was reduced to the penury of the little man, which could be blamed on rising inflation, the spiralling cost of living and growing corruption at all levels of social and national bureaucracy. Indira Gandhi's response to the Allahabad

High Court decision that her election as an MP was unlawful was to declare an Emergency and arrest opposition leaders. As the tensions and contradictions of the Indian political scene increased and the consensus politics collapsed, it was obvious that the days of *mai–baap* ("mother–father") looking after the children and their needs were over.

The population's rebellion against the mother (personified by Indira Gandhi) reached its peak in 1974. The imposition of Emergency led to the country's rebellion (akin to that of teenagers), and at the subsequent elections the Congress government was thrown out in favour of the paternalistic government of Morarji Desai. This government, however, also caused disillusionment among the electorate. In turn, the country forgave the mother, who rode triumphantly back to power. The teenage rebellion continued off and on into the next decade or so. This period was marked by many changes and traumas related to the political state of the country. The teenage years ended with economic liberalization and with the young "grown-ups" looking to settle down by getting married.

All these phases were reflected in the kinds of film being made in Bombay and in the success or failure of different films. I would describe the three periods of Hindi cinema as the era of optimism, the era of new villainy, and the era of new romanticism. These roughly tally with the period of Nehru's prime ministership, that of Indira Gandhi's prime ministership, and the post-Indira Gandhi period up till the present. The preoccupation during the era of optimism was with reconstruction and restructuring. The era of new villainy was characterized by a sense of bewilderment, helplessness, and loss, while the period of new romanticism highlights the new and younger generations' dreams about globalization, westernization, and modernity.

The personalities of characters portrayed by the top three heroes are worth noting. The trio of actors at the top in the 1950s and 1960s comprised Raj Kapoor, Dilip Kumar, and Dev Anand. Each had his own style and favourite actress for the heroine's role. Each catered to specific sections of the audience and played certain types of character. Kapoor played Chaplinesque characters: naive but good-hearted men let loose in the big bad city. Kumar was the tragedy king par excellence. Anand was identified with romances, and his dialogue delivery never changed from character to character. The cinema of the 1960s had two brothers of Raj Kapoor, Shammi and Shashi, playing different and certain kinds of roles. Another actor, Rajendra Kumar, played doctors whose souls were tortured in one way or another, yet the romance was light and fluffy. The actor most famous for playing the villain, which he did in innumerable films, was Pran, who is reported to have said that people consequently stopped naming their sons Pran. Among the others who played villains were Prem Chopra, Prem Nath, and K. N. Singh.

Desai (2004) argues that the most important aspect of a male lead Indian actor is that the notion of manhood, of male identity, is not rigidly fixed in the Indian imagination. The mad people are equally men and women in the way they are seen on the screen. Desai's hypothesis is that there is a tremendous premium in the Indian imagination for the person who is above action and inaction. Such an individual renounces worldly goods and shows no interest in worldly life or results of actions as highlighted in the *Bhagavadgita*.

The heroines of the 1950s and 1960s included Nargis, Meena Kumari, Waheeda Rehman, Vaijayanthimala, Madhubala, and Mala Sinha. Each actress too played a specific type of role and had a particular kind of fan following. Several actresses started off with light romantic roles, then went on to gradually build their careers and reputations. Among the actresses playing the vamp were Shyama, Helen, and Nadira. Seven to eight well-known music directors provided music in the romantic era, with a similar number of lyricists. Due to the formulaic nature of cinema, the viewer knew exactly what to expect merely by knowing the faces and names of the stars. In both their form and content, the films were predictable and the viewer could rely on the directors, actors and the studio to be consistent in their style.

In the late 1960s, Rajesh Khanna, a new romantic actor, arrived with *Raaz*. The peak of romance till then was represented by Rajendra Kumar, who was referred to as Jubilee Kumar since he had been instrumental in numerous silver and golden jubilee hits. In this surcharged atmosphere, the romanticism of the 1960s gradually died down. Rajesh Khanna, who became the romantic superstar replacing the early trio of Raj Kapoor, Dev Anand, and Dilip Kumar, lasted at the top for barely 4 years. Khanna was a real superstar in the sense that a number of females married his photograph, or threatened to kill themselves; he was hounded in the streets and he generated a wave of enthusiasm in the country. He was followed by Amitabh Bachchan in the 1970s and Anil Kapoor, Shah Rukh Khan, and others in the 1980s.

CONCLUSIONS

Hindi films emerging at that time dealt with ideological tensions in society and, happily or otherwise, incorporated its contradictions. The economic, social, and political climate and expectations dictated the portrayal of protagonists and the storylines followed a formula that on the whole was reasonably successful, although it had to evolve and change in response to changing circumstances. The films reflected the state of society but in turn also influenced the society through fashion, style, and emphasis on social responsibility. The events in the history of the country, both external (such as wars) and internal (such as declarations of Emergency), influenced public attitudes, responsibilities, and expectations, and it was inevitable that these would be reflected in the literature, drama, and films of the time.

CHAPTER EIGHT

1950s fun, *Funtoosh*, and Kishore Kumar

From the day of Independence, the nation stood for secularism. In spite of the Partition, the riots that followed it, and Mahatma Gandhi's assassination, the country remained loyal to the secular vision of its founding fathers. Independent India's foreign policy of nonaggression, the five principles of Panch Sheel from which arose the Non-Aligned Movement, along with Nehru's stature, helped India gain international recognition and a sense of national pride.

As noted earlier, the years between 1951 and 1964 have been defined as years of hope and achievement (Chandra et al., 2000). Nehru (1947–1964) himself noted in his letters that, in spite of the multitude of problems and difficulties, the atmosphere was one of hope and faith in the nation's future and in the basic principles of Panch Sheel. As Chandra et al. observe, these were also the years when India was, politically, more or less stable. The country's political system acquired its distinct form and there was progress in all directions, including massive reconstruction of the polity and the economy. Chandra et al. note that people were beginning to experience and advance towards the basic objectives of democracy, civil liberties, secularism, a scientific and international outlook, and economic development and planning with socialism as the ultimate ideal. The films of this period reflected this hope and exploited the sense of stability. The identification of "the other" in defining one's own existence shifted from the colonialist ruler to the moneylender or landowner. The fact that it was the latter who was seen as standing in the way of progress meant that mentally ill individuals

107

who could have been considered "the other" were still cared for within the framework of the family. This is evident in *Funtoosh*, *Raat aur Din*, *Karorpati*, and *Half Ticket*.

In the 1950s and up to 1964, there was a degree of discontent among the intelligentsia especially regarding the slow nature of the progress towards a socialist ideal. The biggest shift was in the area of social change. Social liberation of the backward and suppressed sections of society, abolishing untouchability, and introducing equal rights to men and women under the Hindu Code Bill all led to a genuine sense of freedom.

As noted in the previous chapter, India's relationship with its neighbours was relatively cordial until 1962, when China attached and dislodged Indian troops in September, followed by a massive attack in October. Not only a feeling of panic ensued, but also a feeling of being let down, and Nehru really never recovered from the blow. This ended the period of hope and India's claims for leadership of the Non-Aligned movement. The failure of the policy and the Armed Forces Command played a large role in the sense of general demoralization of the country and its population. The architect of the peaceful coexistence was shattered. It was only in the second Indo-Pakistani war that Indian pride reemerged. However, such a massive let down changed the way the society saw itself and this too was reflected in the portrayal of characters in Hindi films.

Chandra et al. (2000), among others, call Nehru the architect of modern India. The Nehru era is looked back upon with nostalgia even though it was full of misery and poverty. Chandra et al. call him a veritable Renaissance man besides being a product of the Enlightenment, with his commitment to rationality, humanity, respect for the individual, independence of spirit, and secularism. His commitment to democracy and civil liberties was total.

To Nehru, socialism meant several things: a greater equality of opportunity; social justice; more equitable distribution of high incomes, generated through the application of modern science and technology to the process of production; the ending of the acute social and economic disparities generated by feudalism and capitalism; and the application of a scientific approach to the problems of society (Chandra et al., 2000). The socialist transformation was a process and not an event.

Cinema was the only form of mass entertainment that was widely available in the 1950s and 1960s. Although bound by caste and religion, the members of Indian society allowed cinema to permeate their daily lives. Cinema halls were referred to as temples with seats. Within this space, the boundaries of caste and religion disappeared, both on and off the screen. The love stories being shown allowed the young audience (bound by tradition and arranged marriage) to dream and to lose their inhibitions, albeit for a short while. Because of the social approach of the songs and films, cinema outings were akin to picnics. In the world of films, both on and off the screen "normal" people went mad, escaping from their failures, whether in love, business, or other significant life events.

After declaring itself a sovereign democratic republic, the ruling Congress Party won the first election and different states were established. In the 1950s, the country's first Prime Minister announced certain socialist principles for taking the country forward through the Soviet-inspired 5-year plans. The first communist ministry was formed in Kerala. Steel mills and dams were inaugurated. The romantic ideal was alive and reflected in what has been called the Golden Age of Indian popular cinema (Gokulsingh & Dissanyake, 1998). Cinema was firmly established as an art form, as Satyajit Ray won international acclaim and recognition for his films, some of which had been funded by the Bengal state government. State-owned television and radio controlled the output. Thus, Indian films started making their mark in the international market and at film festivals.

It is worth speculating that in Nehru's India, the lessons of the *Bhagavadgita*—principally the virtue of being above all worldly things—were taken more seriously. Desai (2004) argues that the undercurrent of dynamism and social uplift was evident in Dilip Kumar's films during this period. The splitting of the nation at the time of Independence did lead to bloodshed, but the enthusiasm and energy of the leaders helped the population come to terms with the loss of land and power. The changes in public response to certain kinds of films reflected this.

Das Gupta (2002) observes that the 1950s remain true to the spirit of the times and shared the modernist progressive outlook of a new India; disillusionment had not yet set in and this upbeat mood dominated the 1950s. Film directors like Guru Dutt, Raj Kapoor, and Bimal Roy gave expression to a passionate desire for justice, the rehabilitation of the neglected, and the recognition of an individual's worth.

One of the earliest films portraying madness in Hindi films in the 1950s was *Funtoosh*, made under the Navketan banner. Two brothers, Chetan Anand (a director) and Dev Anand (a star), started the Navketan Film Company in Bombay. This was one of the independent producers of films through which members of the Indian People's Theatre Association found their way into the film industry. Chetan Anand, who won international recognition for his film *Neecha Nagar* in 1946, has been likened to Frank Capra (Rajadhyaksha & Willemen, 1999) and, certainly, there are traces of the latter's realism in the film *Funtoosh*.

Having worked with the lyricist Sahir and music director S. D. Burman, the two brothers previously made *Afsar*, *Aandhiyan*, and *Taxi Driver* before making *Funtoosh*. For its time, *Funtoosh* was a daring film. It starred the evergreen actor, Dev Anand, who was well known for his romantic melodramas. In *Funtoosh*, he plays the role of a mad individual.

The film opens with Ram Lal Funtoosh (Dev Anand) being released from the International Lunatic Asylum. The asylum is full of various stereotypes of patients: people laughing manically, performing repetitive actions, and so on; one patient keeps saluting another, two Africans keep dancing, while three patients from eastern Asia dance in a circle. Someone asks, "Where is Funtoosh?" and Funtoosh appears, behaving in a manic fashion. Before Funtoosh is released from the asylum, a panel of experts discuss his case. A doctor says he has improved as much as he can, and that staying with mad people would only worsen his condition. Another doctor responds that Funtoosh will probably get better automatically upon facing some struggles in life. A person who appears to be the senior doctor agrees with these observations. Funtoosh is garlanded by his fellow patients because he is being discharged: An American patient gives him a hat, a Chinese patient gives him a stole, and an African gives him a pair of dark glasses, telling him that the glasses will show him the world in its true colours to which Funtoosh replies, "It is black". He is also given a ring, a fountain pen, paper, and a pipe. A sense of optimism appears to prevail and, oddly enough, there is no sadness and not a single depressed patient. Funtoosh finally leaves the asylum singing and in a happy state, riding in a rickshaw and garbed in odd clothes. He is garlanded with his recent gifts and is holding a pipe. Jaunty music from Laurel and Hardy films accompanies him into the outside world. However, within a few hours, he has lost his gifts and the world outside has denuded him of all his dignity.

He meets a character, played by Krishna Dhawan, and together they laugh at the greed of those around them. Dhawan remarks that since God has given Funtoosh a body, He will give him money as well. Suddenly, somebody who was shaking Funtoosh's hand runs away with his ring. At one point, he runs after his hat, singing and asking it to come back to him, and people follow him, smiling at him benignly. At another point, he runs after a lady to return some money she has dropped, but she misunderstands him and he is beaten up. In the process, he breaks his glasses and somebody makes off with his money.

Funtoosh uses his pen to write to his friends in the asylum. Another character (who is his brother in real life, Vijay Anand) encourages him to do this; Vijay Anand's character claims to be a writer who will write Funtoosh's story. Funtoosh wonders what he should write; his attempt is analogous with the newly liberated India establishing links with its international friends. Funtoosh says that life has two parts: one is the question and the other is the answer. The innocent babe in the wood Funtoosh is then surrounded by four gang leaders who discover he has no money.

Dhawan runs into Funtoosh again and on hearing his sad tales about everyone being selfish, says that the world has no place in it for good men. The silence, death, and desolation of madness in the world is broken by "a scream". Dhawan cites the saint Kabir, and Funtoosh takes up the refrain, "O, my heart! Listen to me. Do not stay where there is no peace or contentment."

Funtoosh's illusions about surviving in the real world are now smashed, and the sadness in the scenes accompanying the song is self-evident. In these, rich men walk past young children and women begging on the streets. In the song, Funtoosh grieves that there is no one to listen to the pain in his heart and no one to whom he can talk; he is in a strange country with strange people. Leaving the asylum represented a change towards freedom, a change that should have been welcome, but the loneliness and harshness of the streets (representing urbanization) create another problem for the hero. On seeing beggars seeking alms without success, he continues, "You may outstretch your hands, but the world will not give you anything and your tears will not melt stony hearts." These lyrics reflect the poet Sahir's roots and his personal disillusionment with Nehruvian socialism, although these were still early days after Independence.

Funtoosh accidentally steps in front of a car being driven by the villain, Seth Karori Mal (played by K. N. Singh), whose immediate reaction is to yell that if Funtoosh wants to kill himself, he should drown himself in the ocean or jump from a building. We next see Funtoosh on the roof of a high building waiting to jump and a crowd has gathered below. Some of the crowd are encouraging him to jump, while others try to persuade him to come down. One man is selling the option of viewing the fall when it happens. Funtoosh sighs, "They don't let me live or die." Intriguingly, the shop Seth Karori Mal drives past is called Hindustan Fabrics shop. The films title indicates that it may be a comedy and, indeed, there are some comic moments. However, the film's message, that the world can drive an individual to madness, is a black one.

Seth Karori Mal (K. N. Singh) appears again and convinces Funtoosh to come down with a plan that he should commit suicide a week later. Meanwhile, he has decided to have Funtoosh insured for 100,000 rupees, making himself the beneficiary of the insurance plan. For this purpose, Funtoosh is taken to Karori Lal's house. Lal gets Funtoosh to sign the insurance policy, and it is only after he has signed the papers that he asks what they are about. Karori Lal tells him that the insurance policy will make him richer. If the film were realistic and Funtoosh was portrayed as truly mad, his signature and consent would be questionable unless it was medically certified that he was fully aware of what he was doing. However, these technical details just get in the way of a good yarn. There follow a couple of scenes highlighting Funtoosh's lack of sophistication. Karori Lal recognizes that Funtoosh is poor, but greed for money leads to him ask his niece to look after the guest (Funtoosh) because he is hoping to do business with him. On first seeing Funtoosh, Karori Lal's niece, Neelu (played by

Sheila Ramani), who lives in the household exclaims, "What is this thing?" Funtoosh tries to "prove" his madness by behaving oddly—his walk is funny, he eats spaghetti with his hands, and drinks water directly from the jug. However, in a couple of songs, he demonstrates his multilingual and multicultural skills by singing in different languages and dancing in different styles. This special gift makes him attractive to Neelu, although a poet is wooing her.

At a party, Karori Lal tells the guests that Funtoosh is funny and very rich. Funtoosh behaves "madly" and sings songs, radiating a sense of fun and involving all the guests, making them enjoy the party. All the styles used by Funtoosh are faux, but that does not appear to bother anyone. In a moment of philosophical revelation, he criticizes God for giving sweets to donkeys and blankets to buffaloes. He talks of good people being punished and evil people rewarded. During this party, Funtoosh falls for Neelu. The next morning, the butler asks Funtoosh, "Are you a congenital idiot, or are you simply pretending to be so?!" The butler is puzzled because he wonders how a madman picked up from the streets is now lording it over him, and leaves the employment. Funtoosh's odd behaviour could pass off as the eccentricity of a rich man.

In a little aside, Funtoosh asks Neelu to teach him to dance and drive, and says he could get rid of the poet who has been pestering her. Some stereotypical encounters follow. There is a song sequence reminiscent of a situation in another Dev Anand film, *Nau do Gyarah*, involving the hero, heroine, and her lover, but the dialogue between the heroine and hero bypasses the lover altogether. It is at this point that the audience discovers that the poet is engaged to Neelu. He objects to her performing a western dance with Funtoosh and would rather have her perform Indian classical dances. This implies that Indian values are superior to western ones, at least in the eyes of the poet.

When the week is up, Karori Mal reminds Funtoosh that it is time to execute his plan of committing suicide. As a gift, Singh takes Funtoosh to a cabaret on his last night on this earth. Karori Mal tells Funtoosh that everyone is mortal and, when he dies, he will be remembered by him. In a rather lengthy scene, Funtoosh is encouraged to place his head on the railway line, waiting for the train to come. Intercutting editing and loud music are employed as he is told that dying is easy and living is difficult, so it is better if he lays his head on the tracks. Meanwhile, Funtoosh puffs continuously on his cigarette, which reminds us of the puffing of a steam engine. It transpires that the train was passing on another line, and Lal asks why Funtoosh cheated. Funtoosh appears to be hyperventilating. Initially, Singh tells him that another train will pass by in 10 minutes, but later they reach the compromise that Funtoosh can live for another month.

After the month has passed, Karori Lal reminds Funtoosh about committing suicide. Funtoosh asks, "Is it necessary to die?" A very popular tune from another Navketan and Dev Anand film, *Taxi Driver*, plays in the background (its words are: "Where shall I go from here? Who will listen to my story?"). We find out that four creditors—a Marwari, a south Indian, a Bania, and a Sindhi—are demanding their money back from Karori Lal and that Karori Mal plans to have Funtoosh killed in order to collect the insurance money. Funtoosh runs to Neelu, asking to marry her. However, Karori Lal takes Funtoosh to a hilltop under duress and tells him to jump. Funtoosh lands in a truck full of cotton which is being driven by the butler, who asks Funtoosh, "Have you gone mad?" Funtoosh pretends to be mad, acting as if he is in water rather than on a pile of cotton. He is then taken back to Karori Lal's home, where he continues to utter chants, and speaks in an odd voice. Karori Lal tells Neelu that Funtoosh had jumped from the hilltop of his own accord. He avoids calling a doctor since the doctor is bound to send Funtoosh to the lunatic asylum. Neelu believes that Funtoosh jumped for her sake, and even when he tries to explain that her uncle was behind it, she refuses to believe him. Funtoosh finally escapes from the house but is beaten up, losing consciousness for nearly 24 hours, resulting in a loss of memory.

An old friend of Funtoosh's, Jaggi, recognizes him and reminds him that they had been colleagues. Jaggi tells Neelu that he and Funtoosh had known each other for years and that Funtoosh had gone mad as a result of his promotion at work, that soon after his mother and sister died in a fire, and that he subsequently spent 5 years in the lunatic asylum. Funtoosh is unable to remember that his mother and sister had died, and Neelu is worried that he would not remember that he was in love with her either. Both Neelu and Jaggi help to remind him of his past, and he slowly begins to remember. Dhawan also returns and sings a sad version of the song "O my sad heart", which Funtoosh used to sing; this brings back memories of the period when he was mad. He eventually recovers his full memory and he and Neelu decide to get married.

When Neelu tells her uncle that they wish to get married, he refuses to give his consent but then throws an engagement party for them. He then takes Funtoosh out on a drive and when they reach a boating area they have the classic hero–villain struggle, after which Funtoosh is presumed drowned. When the uncle returns home, however, he discovers that Funtoosh is still alive. It is now Karori Lal's turn to go mad, and he is admitted to the same asylum in which the film began. Karori Lal is later discharged with a hat and feather and garlands and sheets, and leaves the asylum on a tricycle. The background music is jaunty, again reminiscent of Laurel and Hardy films.

The film therefore completes a full circle, conveying that madness is all-pervasive and exists in different forms in different individuals—from the very rich to the very poor.

The portrayal of madness is superficial. The madness, therefore, is of two types: the good kind, in which the hero suffers as a result of a traumatic event; and the bad kind, which afflicts the villain as a natural punishment for all the sins he has committed. The natural justice demands that the free country has to lock up its villains in the institutional sense and indicates that there are deserved and undeserved types of madness. The impact of the mad individual's condition on those around him is shown as being variable. Towards the end, when Karori Lal goes mad, the look of fear on Neelu's face is telling. However, there is no hint of any long-term implications as in the very next scene she seems to be well settled with Funtoosh.

This film has several unusual aspects. First, the international nature of the asylum places its inhabitants, and the country, in a cultural context that is truly international. The modern nature of the heroine's life is emphasized by the fact that the guests at the party that evening include many foreigners. Also, one song sung by Funtoosh says that "When God gives/He gives in abundance", emphasizing equality and saying that God gives to all those in need, whatever their race. Funtoosh goes on to sing in various styles— Chinese, African, Russian, and Spanish—demonstrating that he has an international awareness. This may be seen as a parallel to India's independence from the alien cultures of colonialism. Next, Funtoosh's loss of innocence as he is forced to confront the cruel realities of the world is somewhat reflective of how India had to deal with problematic situations after Independence. Also, the problem that insurance companies do not pay up in cases of suicide (the act of suicide remains illegal in India), and the underlying hint that human lives can be bought and sold in the true capitalist mode of production, cannot be ignored.

Funtoosh had a couple of memorable songs: When Funtoosh has lost all the gifts he mournfully sings, "Dukhi man mere sun mera kehna" ("O my sad heart, listen to me"). Another song is "Aey meri topi palat ke aaa" ("Oh my hat, return to me"), reflecting an unexpected volition of the hat, which keeps darting about in the air. Valicha (1988b) notes that *Funtoosh*, a successful film, reflected the mood of the 1950s when the new and emerging middle classes were seeking comfort and solace in soft lingering and breezy cinematic romances that help to keep the hard reality at bay. We have already mentioned this phenomenon during the golden age of Hindi cinema, following the break-up of the studio system. A few stars, such as Dev Anand, influenced every branch of filmmaking. As Valicha points out, scripts were written with the stars' images in mind and the image was considered the perfect idol. Any strong deviation from a star's image was punished by the audience, which ensured that such films flopped. In the viewers' eyes, it was self-evident that Dev Anand would remain Dev Anand and act as such. Thus, the madness portrayed by him (in *Funtoosh*) also has a star-like quality. It seems impressive and shining but, in the end, is very vacuous. This is because the screen image of the romantic hero had to remain romantic and pure, and since madness would make it impure it remained secondary to the entire film.

The review of *Funtoosh* in *Filmfare* noted that though pleasing and entertaining, the picture suffered from a confused story, deals with ill-defined characters and was utterly contrived and over-drawn. A lack of logical sequences in the film also infects the film with a touch of fantastic unreality. The reviewer points out that the entire comedy and humour in the picture are drawn from the actions and utterances of a hero who is a semilunatic (sic) for most of the time in the film, and it is doubtful if any adult cinema-goer can laugh at or with a person suffering from lunacy, which is a major calamity for any human being.

Dev Anand's zany acting as neither sane nor insane individual was seen to please the groundlings in his attempts at clowning and comedy. The direction, with the exception of his character, was seen as excellent in the handling of the actors and the film's presentation of the individual sequences. The heroine was praised as an accomplished mature natural artist. Other artists were praised as well, but the music was noted to be the chief asset of the film, and the production values as good with photography as excellent.

Another film dealing with so-called madness, *Karorpati* ("Multimillion-aire"), was released in the same decade. It starred Kishore Kumar and Shashikala. In that decade, Kishore Kumar played the hero in several comedy films, such as *Half Ticket*, *Dilli ka Thug*, *Chalti ka Naam Gadi* and *Aasha*. *Karorpati* is the story of a very rich Rai Bahadur who, in his dying moments, asks his lawyer to read out his will to all his relatives. The lawyer persuades the heroine, Rupa (Shashikala), to stay on for the reading of the will even though she acknowledges that she was adopted and was an orphan and should therefore leave. Dharam Dass, the guardian of Rai Bahadur's grandson Ram (Kishore Kumar), who had been banished because he was said to be mad, is invited as well and asked to bring the grandson along. At this point, it becomes clear that Ram has been dead for 15 years and Dass (allegedly under pressure from his wife) not only failed to inform the grandfather about this, but also continued to receive and accept the monthly stipend sent as payment to look after Ram. The husband and wife then plot that he should catch hold of someone resembling the dead grandson; as Ram had been sent away at the age of 10, and would now have been 25, no one in his family was likely to recognize the substitute.

Dass goes to the Junior Cine Artistes' Association office in Bombay to find a suitable substitute. After looking through the album, he chooses Kishan (Kishore Kumar), who is acting as a stunt double for a film star (played by his real-life brother, Ashok Kumar). Kishan initially refuses to cheat anyone, but changes his mind after being offered a hefty sum of money. He is briefed on the background and asked to impersonate a mad person. He is told that Ram committed suicide at the age of 20, and the fact that the family had not seen Ram for a long time is to Kishan's advantage. Kishan asks Dass how he is supposed to impersonate a mad person when he has never seen one. Dass responds that there is nothing to being mad but two things: one, to look into people's ears and two, to make faces at people. Thus, it is clear that the film focuses on the comic potential of madness, rather than realistically portraying the condition. Kishan is cautioned to beware of "his" Uncle, Dewan Hakumat Rai (K. N. Singh again), who is accompanied by his son, Himmat Rai (played by Anoop Kumar, another brother of Kishore Kumar).

It is clear that the large extended family is no longer considered very desirable, even though a relative comments, "If a sparrow takes a drop, it does not diminish the ocean." It is self-evident in the film that the new regime is in place.

Kishan is brought in, acting as Ram. He is dressed in Scottish garb, plays the bagpipes, and does Highland flings. Kishan behaves like a child, as if he has a low IQ. The uncle decides that he should be sent to a lunatic asylum. When Ram/Kishan tells Dharam Dass (the name means "slave of dharma") that he is worried about the prospect of being sent off to a lunatic asylum, he is assured that no one can declare a sane person mad. Dewan Hakumat Rai (which means "ruler") says that one should not be afraid of mad people and, instead, they should be dealt with firmly. Rupa points out that "Ram" talks like a child, where upon Dharam Dass says children and mad people are alike.

Ram/Kishan continues to act mad when the will is being read out. After opening three boxes in the style of Russian dolls, the lawyer announces that, although the property should (ideally) go to Hakumat Rai (the uncle), then on to Himmat Rai (the uncle's son), all relatives have been set aside as beneficiaries and that the will states that the property should be equally divided between Rupa and Ram/Kishan. Also, because of the latter's mental condition, Rupa should look after the property, which she will inherit only after her marriage. There is a scene in which Hakumat Rai tries to indicate to the lawyer that Ram/Kishan's behaviour is abnormal, by pointing to his own head, but the lawyer interrupts with "Oh, he is mad" (this is said in English). Hakumat Rai assures Rupa that he will help her look after the property and he also persuades Ram/Kishan to stay back. Dharam Dass wants to leave, but Rupa tries to persuade him to stay by saying that Ram/Kishan will need him in order to settle down in new surroundings. Dass then makes the observation that "mad people settle down very easily", and says that Ram/Kishan's madness has now become a habit.

Ram/Kishan's mad behaviour includes yodelling, sliding down banisters, and making people eat while sitting on the floor. To demonstrate the westernized middle class the family eats at the dining table and to revert to eating while sitting on the ground indicates at one level the traditional view and at another Brahminical (superior) behaviour. The perceptions of madness include using philosophical questions. Once, Hakumat Rai slaps Ram/Kishan while Rupa and Dass are out of the room and in a "fit of madness", Ram/Kishan slaps Hakumat Rai back. In another scene, there is an argument about which came first, the chicken or the egg, and Ram/Kishan calls the others mad.

At the instigation of Hakumat Rai, Himmat tries to get Rupa to fall in love with him. Ram/Kishan hears of this plot, as he was hiding in the back seat of the car when it was being discussed. On several occasions, Ram/Kishan disrupts the meetings between Himmat and Rupa. Himmat complains to his father that he is unable to understand this type of madness. Subsequently, Ram/Kishan and Dass are locked up to enable Himmat to seduce Rupa. Himmat's observations on mad people include, "Who shouldn't be afraid of mad people . . . these people are very wise in some ways."

Ram/Kishan falls and "hurts" himself, as a result of which he "recovers" from his madness. The doctor pronounces him cured of his madness and emphasizes that this sort of recovery is quite common; with Ram/Kishan having broken his arm, his mind has been set right. Ram/Kishan claims that he does not believe he was ever mad, and the doctor gleefully informs everyone that Ram/Kishan will no longer remember anything about his past. Ram/Kishan and Rupa gradually fall in love.

In another ploy, Hakumat Rai gets a girl, Meena, to pretend that Ram/Kishan had been in love with her. He chides Ram/Kishan for pursuing Rupa, at which point Ram/Kishan decides to tell Rupa the reality. Himmat overhears this and soon Ram/Kishan and Dass discover that their secret is out. Hakumat Rai confronts Ram/Kishan, telling him he knows that he is Kishan and that the real Ram is dead. He blackmails the two, asking Kishan to tell Rupa that his love for her is untrue so that Himmat can marry her. Kishan is worried but agrees under duress; he pretends to be in love with Meena, and Rupa gets a glimpse of this. He then tells Rupa that he was mad earlier, but in contrast the whole household was mad for money. Next, he is kidnapped by Hakumat Rai's goons and locked up.

Hakumat Rai proposes that Rupa marry Himmat. When Hakumat is talking about the climax of his plot, i.e., killing Rupa, the old nanny overhears him. She informs Kishan, who escapes and saves Rupa. The police inspector comes into the picture and, finally, announces that Kishan is actually the real Ram, who had survived the suicide attempt and lost his memory as a result (which had apparently cured him of his madness). The film relies on the comic potential of its hero, Kishore Kumar, who acts mischievous and naughty, rather than focusing on madness *per se*.

The third film I will discuss in this chapter is *Pagla Kahin Ka*, directed by Shakti Samanta. Many people call the hero, Sujit (Shammi Kapoor), "crazy"; he works as a musician in a hotel and is in love with Jenny (played by Helen), a cabaret dancer there. He lives with his friend Sham (Prem Chopra). Once, when Jenny asks him what will happen if one day she changes and forgets him, he says (in a song) that she will remember him whenever she hears his songs. He accepts that people call him mad because he believes he is in love with a woman who is like the moon (thereby linking the moon with madness). At one point, he say that he dances like a madman at gatherings, at which point he also makes funny faces with rolling eyes.

At the New Year's Eve party, the owner of the hotel tries to get Jenny drunk and it is obvious that he is worried about losing his cabaret dancer to Sujit. After the party there is an argument and the manager is killed by Sham. However, since Sujit is a true friend of Sham's, he takes the blame while Sham and Jenny run away. As the basis of his defence, the lawyer decides to use the fact that everyone thinks Sujit is mad. He says that Sujit will have to be certified mad if he is to escape being hanged. As Sujit stands in the court with a "mad" face, the lawyer informs the court that Sujit has an abnormal personality. He states that his expression and talk clearly indicate that he is mad. The prosecutor challenges this, at which point the defence lawyer presents a witness who was the warden of an orphanage to which Sujit had been admitted after his mother died. Sujit, he says, was only 6 when his father went mad after the loss and was confined to a ward for dangerous lunatics. The warden states that, as a child, Sujit was serious, quiet, and hard-working. When he was taken to see his father in the lunatic asylum, the father did not recognize him and then lost his temper. Thereafter, Sujit's personality appeared to change. He became almost mischievous and, as a result, was beaten by the warden. Sujit, in turn, attacked the warden with a knife. According to the warden's evidence, his mental condition continued to deteriorate after that day. At this point, Sujit starts to babble. In his evidence, Sham states that the defendant suffers from fits of madness. When asked why he shared his rooms with him, given the circumstances, Sham replies that he wanted to support him. Sham testifies that Sujit hit the hotel owner on the head. Sujit intervenes to say that the owner lost his head and hit himself with the bottle! In her evidence, Jenny says that she is not mad, so how could she love a mad person. Sujit continues to behave "oddly" and yet maintains that he is sane, although others around him do not agree. The court decides that he should be sent to a psychiatric hospital (they call it a lunatic asylum), and stay there till he is cured.

Thus, the film tries to raise the topic of madness that is hereditary, and precipitated by stress/death/loss/bereavement (in this case, the loss of both parents at a young age). However, the personality of the patient is "abnormal" and portrayed comically. The film uses madness as a peg for the story to introduce the notions of lost love, lost friendship, and social isolation starting in the lunatic asylum. Interestingly, in the court scene, Jenny is dressed in a white sari, indicating widowhood, even though she is not married.

The unrealistic portrayal of madness continues as Sujit is taken to the asylum. Before going in, he tells a policeman that he is there to buy a bungalow and the psychiatrist plays along with this. A patient even tells him that it is a madhouse, which is followed by loud laughter all around. The scene includes a patient dressed in shabby clothes and with leaves in his hair, and others patients who are dancing. Sujit runs away and ends up in the female psychiatrist's quarters. The senior psychiatrist comes along and tells her to close all the doors and windows. The junior doctor appears frightened, even though she is a psychiatrist, and is hurt in the ensuing scuffle to run away. The senior psychiatrist tells her that he arrived at the right time, otherwise Sujit might have killed her (with no evidence to justify this at all!).

As in *Khamoshi*, the senior psychiatrist chairs a meeting with at least 10 other psychiatrists to decide whether Sujit is insane or not. They take turns in asking questions to assess his mental state. One psychiatrist asks him his name and he gives not only his name, but the names of his father, grandfather, and great-grandfather as well. Another psychiatrist (unusually) asks Sujit to keep his answers short while asking him what he did for a living. The interview is more like an inquisition with rapid-fire questioning. Sujit keeps saying he is not mad. On being asked if he would murder someone if he did not like their face, he talks nonsense for a while. He is then sent away and put under "observation". Everyone except the female psychiatrist Shalu (Asha Parekh) immediately declares that Sujit is mad and has committed murder. Shalu, on the other hand, wants to study him further.

There is a scene where one of the patients talks to Sujit about the daughter he has lost. However, this tinge of seriousness is erased in the very next scene, which is suddenly comical. The bed next to Sujit's is occupied by a patient who claims that he is a film hero; the inmates crack a few jokes about various stars. They burst into song out of the blue. A "comedy actor" pretends to be the buffalo of another patient. Sujit buys the buffalo, but the previous owner hits it and all the patients sing, "Why did you hit my buffalo with stick, she was grazing in the field. How has she harmed your father?" The purpose here is to identify that the world of buffaloes and mad men is the real one in that the buffalo climbs trees, eats sweet meats, and sings! The question of reality and whose reality is paramount in psychiatric assessments. Towards the end of the song, singing patients surround Shalu. Clutching her stethoscope (the symbol of her power: her sceptre), she looks scared and walks away.

Meanwhile, Sham tells Jenny that Sujit has been declared insane by the doctors and he will have to stay in the asylum for a year or two. Jenny expresses dismay that Sujit will definitely go mad if he has to stay with mad people for so long. Sujit writes to Jenny, "All the mad people are sleeping as I write to you. I have met a lovely girl, Shalu, who is trying to cure my madness. But hopefully, she will go mad herself." This also reflects on the possibility that falling in love is a madness itself.

Shalu tries to express her doubts to the head psychiatrist (her senior). "Every mad person always follows the same action or same thought [assuming all patients have obsessive compulsive traits]. This person sings and dances and does other things. I note an artificiality in his madness", she says. Another doctor (possibly a psychiatrist) counters that there is no doubt that Sujit is mad, because the research committee said so. Thereupon, the senior psychiatrist (played by the veteran actor/director, Manmohan Krishna) says, "In such medico-legal cases, fake madness can appear." They agree that Shalu should feel free to treat him as she deems fit since she has the patient's full confidence. When Shalu enters Sujit's room, he says that he is imprisoned and will try to escape. She promises to take him on a picnic the next day. Wardens accompany the inmates to the picnic. Sujit pretends to strangle Shalu. At this point, she says she is convinced that he is faking his madness. He then acknowledges that he is neither mad nor is he the murderer, but that he had to pretend. Shalu says that, as a doctor, it is her duty to report it. He then tries to impress upon her that had she known the power of love, she would have known why he behaved the way he did. He blames the act on his love for Jenny. He tells Shalu that she knows nothing about him (which actually is an astonishing statement, since a psychiatrist is supposed to get the patient's background or history). By hinting about a deprived childhood Sujit is perhaps trying to gain further sympathy from the heroine. Shalu then talks about a patient who has gone mad because his loved one married someone else.

Between all the fluff about love and its permanence, Sujit says, "I wonder how you don't go mad working with all these mad people." He then sings the song he had sung to Jenny ("You won't forget me . . ..").

Meanwhile, Sham rapes Jenny after admitting that he loves her. Shalu tells Sujit off for giving false hopes to another patient and yet she does the same things. She explains to him that "everyone who comes here does so because of sorrow". One day, Shalu invites Sujit to her place for dinner. It is obvious that she is in love with him, but he is still in love with Jenny. She tries to tell him that she loves him. Soon, he is discharged from the asylum. Before leaving, he tells Shalu that he will always remember the sympathy she gave him. She asks, "Only sympathy?"

On reaching his place, Sujit discovers that Sham has married Jenny. He goes to a hotel where a cabaret is in progress. The cabaret depicts a love triangle reminiscent of Jenny, Sujit, and Sham. Sujit then, almost as expected, goes mad. In a scene showing the onset of his madness, Sujit gets angry, plays the violin, saxophone, and piano in turn, and the loud music reaches a crescendo. His eyes go wild and he is seen sweating. He is then taken back to the asylum. The warden tells Shalu that Sujit has returned, that he is different and refuses to recognize anyone. Shalu hears a scream, "Leave me alone!", and she runs to the electroconvulsive therapy (ECT) room, where Sujit is about to be given ECT (in a sitting position!). Sujit mumbles that they wanted to kill him. He fails to recognize Shalu. In a situation similar to that in *Khamoshi*, Shalu goes to meet Jenny. Unlike any decent doctor, Shalu initially treats Jenny shabbily to say the least, and blames her for Sujit's mental state. She refuses to allow Jenny to meet Sujit. Jenny then describes the rape; Shalu gets on her high horse and says that she should have killed Sham, in which case Sujit might have forgiven her. All of Shalu's statements are, of course, completely implausible coming from a psychiatrist. Jenny holds herself responsible. She tells Sham that he acted selfishly, in spite of the fact that Sujit had taken the responsibility for the murder on himself.

On one occasion when Sujit calls out Jenny's name in wistful, romantic tones, Shalu reminds him that Jenny is married. She also tells him that she likes him, and sings the same song he used to sing for Jenny. In the middle of the night she closes the door and there follows a scene in which she acts maternal, but also seductive. Later, she is unable to sleep and worries that she might go mad if she does not take care of herself.

In another scene, one of the nurses appears at the window of Sujit's room and calls out to him. In his mind, the nurse transmogrifies into Jenny. She acts as if she is actually Jenny and tries to tell him that she does not love him. Sujit attempts to strangle her. In the ensuring scuffle, he is held back by the wardens and ends up slapping Shalu. At one level, this violence represents the madness of the Indian male, for whom the female is a passive receptacle who can be slapped and raped without compunction. Later, the nurse says it was for Shalu's sake that she took such a risk (knowing what Sujit meant to her). In the next scene, Shalu is in Sujit's arms, counter-transference of the highest order.

Sujit helps one of the inmates escape, but the man falls down the stairs and dies. Sujit promptly bursts into song, talking about difficulties of the heart's loneliness and craziness called love. Shalu is obviously overinvolved, has no other patients to look after (so it seems) and again takes him out on a picnic. She tells him that love is the chain that binds two hearts together. She also reminds him of their previous visit to the spot, but he is struggling to remember. She then reminds him of the song he used to sing. At this point, Sujit joins in and happens to remember their previous outing. They go on to declare love for each other. Shalu bursts into tears, saying that she has been waiting for him. Next, she tries to tell him about what Sham has done, but Sujit is in no mood to listen.

Shalu goes to visit Jenny, but runs into Sham instead. He refuses to acknowledge that he is a friend of Sujit's. Shalu tells him that she knows about the murder and blackmails him, telling him to accompany her to the hospital. Sham defends himself by wondering how Shalu can believe a mad person's ramblings despite the fact that she is a doctor. On the way to the hospital, Sham tries to murder her. It becomes clear that this situation was set up and that Sujit and the chief psychiatrist are witnessing it. Sujit thus discovers the "real" Sham. In the struggle that follows, Sham kills Jenny and is arrested.

The chief psychiatrist tells Shalu that she should now end the act of being in love with Sujit. In response, she admits that she is in love and it is not just an act. "But you are a doctor", he says. "But I'm a woman also", is her response. The chief psychiatrist tells Sujit he knows all about their romance, but that Shalu is bound to act in accordance with the treatment plans of patients. In an effort to follow her line of duty, Shalu tells Sujit that he has misunderstood her. She says, "You can give sympathy to your patients, but not your heart." In the end, however, she gives up her job and leaves with him.

Of the three films discussed, *Pagla Kahin Ka* is the most commercial film and, perhaps, also the least successful in box office terms. The portrayal of madness is appalling. Those with mental illness are clowns, feeble and weak. Those treating them are caricatures, all in white coats and, absurdly enough, they get the hero to face the truth by setting up situations, as a detective might. At the same time, the film portrays some of the nurses as having a genuine empathy towards those with mental illnesses. It also depicts the nurses' loyalty to the doctors and the patients' loyalty to each other. The patients appear to form a closer network and, to their minds, "the other" is obviously the hierarchy and the establishment. It is possible that the caricature of those with mental illness and a sense of loss of reality are such that the comic conclusion is the only possible solution. It is also possible that mental illness ends up being caricatured because of the lack of knowledge of the phenomena mentally ill people experience. Further, there is no doubt that, as with producers in Hollywood, Hindi film producers are keen to make money, rather than concern themselves with accurate portrayals of mental illness.

Pagla Kahin Ka was identified as a good film by the reviewer in *Filmfare*. Shammi Kapoor was noted to show his real mettle as an artiste, earnestly putting across the character he acts. However, there are scenes where he plays to the gallery when he fakes madness to draw a favourable verdict from the doctors (none of them professionally competent with the exception of a lady doctor, who is obviously the leading lady of the film) in order to free himself from the charge of murder. The reviewer praised the acting of Asha Parekh, Helen, and Prem Chopra but noted that there are many flaws too, most of them resulting from a somewhat half-hearted commitment to the subject and mixed intentions on the part of the makers, who apparently set out to make a seriously emotional film but lost courage and decided on a compromise.

While this is understandable, there is, however, considerable scope to make the portrayal relatively more realistic. For example, in films like *Funtoosh*, the portrayal is perhaps more gentle and soft, compared to *Karorpati* and *Pagla Kahin Ka*. In the former, mental illness is depicted as comical; in the latter it is used as a ploy or a device to turn the story on its head. By faking madness, the hero tries to be empathetic with other patients. It is when he really becomes mentally ill that the emphasis on his treatment shifts. It is to be noted that in all three films it is the love of a woman that cures the "patients". The female, through nurturing, caring, or playing the doctor, is like a mother to the errant son (who has become mentally ill, which represents his deviance). The woman brings him in line with a combination of nursing, love and affection.

In *Funtoosh*, as in *Pagla Kahin Ka* (even in the subplot) and other films like *Pyar Ka Mausam*, *Caravan*, *Hera Pheri*, *Lal Patthar*, *Shukriya*, and others, the madness is precipitated by a significant loss. The portrayal of mental illness is not classic and cannot be fitted into any clinical diagnostic category. It is simple, superficial, amusing at times, and distressing or frightening at others. A major reason for this must be that the viewers perceive of and fear madness in such a way that very few films dealing with mental illness have been successful at the box office. Hysterical conversion symptoms were also caused by sudden loss, for example hysterical aphonia in *Ghazal*. In *Woh Kaun Thi* the villain uses the heroine to drive the hero mad so that he can inherit the estate.

Baharon ki Manzil is the story of a young woman who wakes up one morning and does not recognize anyone around her. She thinks it is her wedding day but she is told that she is already married with a teenage daughter. She recognizes her "husband" as her brother-in-law. The "husband" gets perplexed and calls a psychiatrist who suggests that she be admitted to his hospital and investigated. Meanwhile, she is getting increasingly suspicious; she discovers a body in her wardrobe, although when she gets others to see it the body has disappeared. She goes to Bombay to trace her fiancé and finds that he is already married and has a family. The psychiatrist starts to believe in her and by carrying out some detective work he finally solves the mystery.

The reviewer in *Filmfare* saw this film as a diverting show with considerable artistry. The writer was noted to have exploited the various possibilities to explain this peculiar situation and made them credible in the eyes of the spectator. The reviewer noted that Meena Kumari as the heroine and Rehman as her husband played the two most intricate characters of the film (if not of their careers). Rehman was seen as doing full justice to his job, but Meena Kumari looked alienated from her role at times. The reviewer lay the blame squarely on the director. Dharmendra, playing the psychiatrist, gets acknowledged as playing the role with quiet dignity. However, the reviewer laments that with story material such as this, the film could have been much more absorbing than it is, and various incidents could have been made more effective if the director had brought to his work the finesse it demanded. Using the scene of the heroine's visit to her fiancé, the reviewer calls it flat because of the haphazard manner in which it was treated and the wooden portrayal by the male actor.

The psychiatrist is smart and suave and has an EEG machine, which helps him make the diagnosis, notwithstanding the fact that EEG is used to diagnose epilepsy primarily and, although epilepsy and mental illness are associated, one cannot diagnose mental illness from EEG alone. Perhaps tongue in cheek, he is called Dr Rajesh Khanna (a hero who was at the top of his powers as a box office draw around the period this film was released).

In another review, *Baharon ki Manzil* was seen as a fair film but the opening scenes as shaky and unconvincing. The process of gradually halting psychiatric sessions is suggested rather than actually shown. There is no last minute confession, and unravelling (though incomplete) is left to scattered scenes along the way. Some specific scenes were singled out for commendation, but the weakest link identified was the characterization. Meena Kumari as the heroine was noted to have a realistic role as the amnesia victim contemptuous of the man who calls himself her husband; and in spite of the amnesia, or perhaps because of it, she is willing to risk an extramarital affair. Neither of the male leads has sharply defined roles. Yet the film was seen to leave a clean taste and no hangover.

A degree of romanticism still existed in the beginning of the 1960s but, as the decade wore on, a macho outlook emerged, possibly as a result of disillusionment. Films about bandits and dacoits made their appearance. Das Gupta (2002) suggests that the failure of the popular film of the 1960s to find a suitable formula indicated the uncertainties and fears of the post-Nehru era and had to contend with developments of art or parallel cinema around the world. In *Aya Saawan Jhoom ke*, one of the minor characters plays a madman who kills his cabaret dancer girlfriend. The portrayal of violence was hidden behind the wholesome family drama where even the vamp is seen as deserving to die because she is planning to be independent. Das Gupta (2002) sees the replacement of patriotic faith by a mafia set of values leading to hiding behind family values, and the enthusiasm for modern energy and independence was becoming shaky. The cynical age of the 1970s prepared for the arrival of the extremes of violence to achieve its aims. The faults of development led to the appearance of indigenous consumer goods which were not generally available to everyone, so the hero had to grab them. On the other hand, the 1970s also defined motherhood as the sole destiny of the woman; the only free women were cabaret dancers or courtesans, even though they yearned for manly and maternal love. Sexual love and the superficial acceptance of modernity and sexuality in women became dominant in the 1980s. Das Gupta emphasizes that an interesting anomaly exists between the new freedom in film and the absence of it in real life. Marriage is a family affair where money plays an important part in that the families marry into each other. The love enacted between unmarried people is thus fantasizing of freedom before marriage, so limited afterwards by familial pressures.

Anuradha is the story of the eponymous heroine, who gives up her singing career after marrying an idealist doctor and moving to a village. After feeling neglected by her husband she starts to feel lethargic, withdrawn, and dysphoric, without reaching depression. With the encouragement of her male friend she is about to leave her husband when circumstances change and she decides to resume her career of looking after

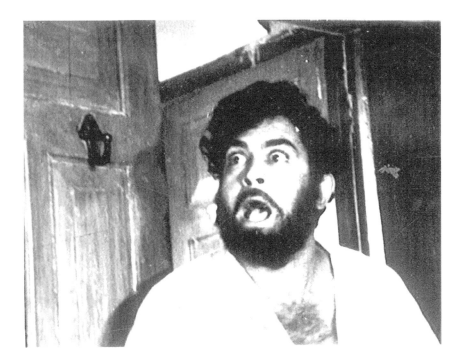

Figure 8.1 Scene from *Anhonee* (courtesy of National Film Archive of India)

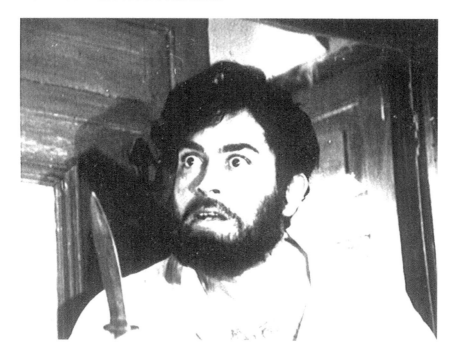

Figure 8.2 Scene from *Anhonee* (courtesy of National Film Archive of India)

her husband and daughter. The film's director, Hrishikesh Mukherjee, in an interview with Prabhu (2001, p. 36) pointed out that, "In life you might achieve something, sometimes you might be *instrumental* in others achieving something. My question is, which one gives more satisfaction, more completion? A mother sacrifices her life to rear her children." Undoubtedly, Mukherjee is reflecting the patriarchal society and also the prevalent norms of the 1960s when doctors were idealistic, worked in rural areas and felt defeated (or threatened) by the likelihood that wives may have an independent existence.

Anhonee is the story of a police inspector who pretends to be mad—with torn clothes, dishevelled hair, unkempt beard, and inane grins—who is then admitted to a psychiatric hospital. The female psychiatrist who looks after him—in a white coat and carrying a stethoscope—falls in love with him, to the extent that she goes on to sing, "Idiot has fallen for me and I can't do anything about it." It becomes clear that there had been a murder in her family which was being investigated by the police inspector. Similarly, in *Hungama*, one of the characters pretends to be mad. A stronger storyline of someone pretending to be mentally ill appears in *Deewangee* (discussed later).

There is little doubt that characters in Hindi films, be they male or female, are portrayed in black and white. There are no grey characters who would add to the uncertainty and confusion in the minds of the viewers.

CONCLUSIONS

Although we have looked at only a small number of films from the 1960s in this chapter, common themes of madness are varying—it is often the hero who is ill and the heroine is the carer. Madness is used as comedy and villainy and as an excuse to demonstrate the suffering which is caused by loss of stress, and yet can be easily cured by believing in the mad individual and through love rather than medication. Custodial care was also demonstrated to be patchy and the professional carers, especially psychiatrists, are buffoons and not to be trusted. In at least three of the films, money plays a significant role in the causation of madness one way or another. The political climate influenced the portrayal in its international nature, multifaceted and multifunctional effects, and gentle caring professionals.

CHAPTER NINE

Psychoanalysis in the films of the 1960s

Psychoanalysis is based on the work of Sigmund Freud, who refined his thoughts over a large number of publications. Many were inspired by his theories, but some occasionally broke away and developed their own theories and ideas by mixing and matching Freudian readings with additional theories and viewpoints borrowed from newly emerging branches of psychology and philosophy, of religion and theology.

The term "psychoanalysis" in America came to be employed to describe loosely all three schools of thought which took their origin from the work of Freud. The theories of Fromm, Horney, Sullivan, and others are classified as neo-Freudian, though they really bear very little resemblance to the original (Jones, 1961, p. 1).

Cinematic psychoanalysis is an important aspect of film theory. Cinema and psychoanalysis developed broadly over the same period, generating a similar degree of enthusiasm in its auteurs. Heath (1999) points out that Freud's distrust of cinema was reaffirmed when he refused to lend his name to Pabst's 1926 film *Secrets of a Soul* (the first film to represent psychoanalysis as a treatment), arguing that cinema could not possibly represent his theory and concepts of psychoanalysis. In her introduction to her book, *Endless Night: Cinema and Psychoanalysis, Parallel Histories*, Bergstrom (1999) maintains that psychoanalysts and cinema scholars should be able to speak together productively on a whole range of issues, including comparisons and prospective histories. Léonce Perret's 1912 *Le Mystère des Roches de Kador* was described as the first psychoanalytic film at the 1995

Pordenone Silent Film Festival, at which cinema itself was hailed as a tool for psychotherapy (Bergstrom, 1999).

Bergstrom (1999) notes that Perret's film uses the medium of cinema as the primary tool to effect a (cathartic) psychoanalytic cure. It moves from darkness to light, in a parallel metaphor from catatonia to normalization, as the woman is reestablished within her social milieu. The power of psychoanalysis is thematized. Interestingly, the patient is female and the analyst male.

Heath (1999) emphasizes the need to consider how psychoanalysis and psychoanalysts are represented in the cinema but also how film functions in the analytic session, as demonstrated. The analyst's speech, associations, and memories may draw and depend upon cinema's sounds and images, and its provision of a residue of signifying traces taken up as unconscious material. It is fair to say that when we watch a film and understand its meaning consciously, what we interpret and retain may well be analysable even after a long time. The portrayal of psychoanalysis again raises a different set of questions. Similar to resistance in the process of psychoanalysis, there is resistance to aspects of cinema itself. The role of fantasy and of psychoanalysis in understanding fantasy is noteworthy. Fantasy is seen as another way of evaluating the experience of cinema, where the viewer uses experiences to interpret and make sense of what has been viewed. The viewer's identification with the characters and the actors is crucial to understanding what is shown on the screen.

Jones (1961, p. 1) suggests that the term psychoanalysis be reserved for orthodox views, and "analytic" as an innocuous generic term to cover all those psychotherapeutic methods that make use of investigation and explanation rather than suggestion. The development and rooting of analytical methods in the USA followed a large-scale exodus of analysts from Europe in the wake of the Second World War. The basic ideas of analysis were European in development, but it was the American influence of living and working in a capitalist society that influenced the modification of analytical thoughts, more so in the "I-ego" or egocentric models. This, combined with mode of production, led to the kind of thinking where the individual and their rights were seen as paramount, rather than kinship or family. In rural societies and cultures, kinship assumed a more important role and subsumed the "I-ego" in "We-ego"; the sociocentric views were retained more clearly.

Psychoanalysis developed in the context of Victorian Vienna, with Freud's own experiences of working with Charcot and dealing with hysteria. Clinical presentations and representations of hysteria are still present in developing countries such as India, whereas hysteria as a clinical condition has virtually disappeared from western Europe. Such presentations in clinics and in films are often dramatic, providing a wonderful opportunity for the actor and the director to showcase the talent and to move the narrative forward.

Hollywood mainstream and independent films have used psychoanalysis extensively, both in form and content. The role of Hollywood and analysis is discussed later. Hindi cinema has used these opportunities to a limited extent only. There are several possible reasons for this. First, the overall fantasy figures of characters are projected figures, thereby allowing the audience to develop their own imagination. Second, the use of mythological genres allows the Jungian analytical concepts of universal psyche to be used without terming them as such. Third, the basic formula is simplified to the extent that analysis itself becomes superfluous.

PSYCHOANALYSIS AND THE CINEMA

Kaplan (1991), in her introduction, laments the fact that no anthologies of cinema and psychoanalysis exist which emphasize the importance of the diversity of methods employed in such analysis.

Lacan's literary corpus led to numerous debates and the Lacanian theory became extremely influential in the study of cinema (see Metz, 1982, 1985, for example). Lacan's psychoanalytic concepts differ from the Freudian concepts in being textual and structuralist in the context of cinema and in the centrality of language, thereby making them more attractive to film studies. The Lacanian film theory is constituted from many Freudian concepts, based on Althusser, structuralism, and semiotics among others. The presence of Freud and his daughter in London, and the migration of neo-Freudians to America who then developed various schools of psycho-analysis, contributed to the discrepancy between the American and the British concepts of psychoanalysis influenced by social and cultural factors.

Kaplan (1990a, p. 11) suggests that the concepts of the "text" (as an organization of language, codes, and signifying systems generally designed to produce meanings) and its "reader" (or interpreter) are constituted by prior cultural history as well as by the act of reading in film analysis. Freudian psychoanalysis can be seen as a science, a tool for analysing literacy and anthropological material and medicine (i.e., as a cure).

Kaplan (1990a, p. 12) further states in her essay that psychoanalysis as a talking cure is based on the theory of human development and the analytic scene. It is used to explain literary relationships, actions, motives, and the very existence of the text itself. As a structural discourse, the interaction between the analysand and the analyst, and the literary use of such inter-actions, allows the viewer or the reader to understand the coda and the structure embedded within the interactional text. Psychoanalysis, besides being a narrative discourse, is also cultural and historical. Lastly, Kaplan (1990a, p. 13) sees psychoanalysis as a specific process or set of processes used as a discourse to illuminate textual processes. She argues that scholars of the humanities who compare the psychoanalytic exchange (analysand versus analyst) with the literary exchange (text versus reader) focus on processes. The film, however, adds another dimension of viewer/audience versus the story/text. The comparison between the spectator/screen situation and the child/minor situation is essential in understanding the film as a text. The film narrative is similar to the story the analysand chooses to tell the analyst, and this allows the viewer to pick up pertinent points in the same way as the analyst. Since viewers may not have the same training, views, or experiences, the interpretations among members of the same audience will be different. The film theorists and critics may well pick up the same things. The analysand and the analyst together constitute a history of the problems that need to be resolved, and the aim of the analyst is to get the patient better. Such a discourse between the auteur and the viewer does not exist unless the cinema viewer comes out with a sense of relief or happiness, which may not have been available otherwise.

Metz (1982, p. 9) argues that in the register of the imaginary (Klein's object relations) the institution depends on the good object, although bad objects are manufactured as well. He proposes that cinema is a technique of the imaginary and is representative of a historical epoch (that of capitalism) and a state of the society, that is, industrial civilization. The development of the signifier (in terms of mental illness) in Hindi cinema may well be related to industrial development through 5-year plans, which marked a decisive shift from an agrarian economy.

Cinema links the auteur with the audience through the medium of the story; the analysis of the story therefore is not direct, first-hand or even second-hand, but possibly third-hand. Metz (1982) states that Freudian psychoanalysis is a reflection of the strength it places on the Oedipal complex, which allows only one kind of psychoanalysis to study cinema. Other types include the nosographic approach (treating films as symptoms or as secondary manifestations from which one can work back), where the maker of the film is of interest rather than the film itself or the typological membership of the film. A psychoanalytic study of the film script focuses on the situations, characters, landscapes (manifest content), and the covert message. The cinema's signifier is perceptual–visual as well as auditory. The film, argues Metz (p. 45), is like a mirror where the viewer "sees" familiar household objects and perceives their significance. The viewer is not in the mirror, yet he is able to recognize "his" world without himself in it. This is what turns cinema into a symbolic medium where the individual identifies with the fictional character and situation, yet within this setting is able to recognize the "other" who is externalized. That "someone else" on the screen allows the viewer to place his or her ego in the imagination of the signifier. Any engagement with images arises from the collective unconscious; the psychoanalyst must therefore plot the dream's archetypal imagery against parallels drawn from mythology, religion, folklore, works of art, and other cultural artefacts in order to clarify the metaphorical context of the dream symbolism (Izod, 2001, p. 22). This process allows the patient and the analyst jointly to build a picture of its unknown meanings through the emphasis on personal associations (Frederickson, 1979, p. 188; Jung, 1943, p. 81). Izod (p. 22) argues that the significance of this method is that it can be reduplicated in the interpretations of screen images.

On the other hand, Kaplan (1990a, pp. 14–15) considers the role of the critic as different from that of the analyst. The analysis of the film is packaged in a series of diverse goals which range from professional enhancement to a search for the "truth" (i.e., intellectual curiosity) to aesthetic pleasure.

In this chapter, I aim to embed the concepts of psychoanalysis, as in the context of psychoanalytic theory treatment, as explored in two Hindi films made in the 1960s. I do not propose to use the Kaplan (1990c, 1991) model, but instead will look at the films in the cultural context of psychoanalysis.

This chapter uses psychoanalysis to understand two films made in Independent India by mainstream directors with stars as the main characters. The discussion is both in terms of the portrayal of the process of psychoanalysis and in the context in which the film itself is analysed in its narrative and discourse. Using Mulvey's Theory, Nair (2002) notes that in Hindi films, the heroines reflect the patriarchal society's gaze on them. Nair (2002) argues that for the male gaze, the female image in the films can be a source of anxiety (the castration complex), so the male attempts to nullify it by fetishism or overvaluation. Therefore, this ambivalence towards women, where they are either an object of desire or a threat, leads to male worship and fetishization of the woman on the one hand and to devalue, punish, and save her as a guilty object on the other hand. Thus the creation of the "other" in which patriarchal ideology cannot believe or accept. The ideology will deal with it in either of two ways: either by rejecting or annihilating it, or by rendering it safe and assimilating or converting it as far as possible into a replica of itself. The interdigitation between these two processes is not unusual in the context of Hindi cinema. *Khamoshi* portrays the stereotype of the therapist, the settings in which interdigitation takes place, and the role of woman as a carer struggling single-handedly to manage psychiatric patients. As a nurse, Radha (Waheeda Rehman) is expected to be the therapist, the training for which she received abroad.

Raat aur Din, on the other hand, is the story of a woman who is submitted to shamanic rites for "possession" as well as to medication and ECT, irrespective of her needs for a cure. The interpretation of both films is linked with the post-Independent India of the late 1960s, when these films were made and released.

Transference and countertransference remain the cornerstones of psychoanalysis. Transference describes the feelings that the analysand has towards the analyst, and countertransference describes the feelings that the analyst has towards the analysand. Freud saw transference as a disadvantage (Freud, 1950b, p. 314). He acknowledged that it was not clear why neurotic subjects under analysis develop transference so much more intensely than those not being analysed and why transference provides the strongest resistance to cure. One indispensable preliminary condition in such cases is the introversion of libido, when the unconscious turns away from reality. The resolution of transference and countertransference is the key principle in psychoanalysis. In addition, the psychoanalyst requires supervision to discuss his or her countertransference, because the therapist may either apply unnecessary interventions or deny appropriate and necessary interventions. This emotional involvement enables the therapist to examine feelings that may be generated in the significant others by the analysed as well. Both the analyst and the analysed are likely to be influenced by their personalities, previous experiences, past and childhood development, as well as by cultural factors that would need to be identified and understood.

Cultural differences in personality development and concepts of the self suggest that there are similarities and differences. Highlighting the Freudian and the Jungian theories and comparing these with Indian psychoanalysts will allow the reader to interpret the psychoanalytic models and methods used in the Hindi cinema. By necessity, the material covered here has to be brief.

In Hindi cinema the mother–son relationship and the subjugation of women is exploited to the maximum. However, maternal narcissism, that is, the projection of the mother's own unfulfilled desires on to the child or the use of the child to play out problems with the mother (or significant others), has to be seen in connection with the formation not only of male identity as Kaplan (1990b, p. 128) suggests, but of masculinity, which is more concerned with male patriarchal positions. Kaplan (p. 128) proposes that Freudian theory is employed more literally in the cinema. She argues that (certainly in Hollywood cinema) the desire to confine the mother within restricted pop-Freudian stereotypes is itself a symptom of the mother's increasing cultural threat in the post-Second World War world. Other relationship characterizations, such as sister–brother, brother–brother dyads, also need to be considered in the cultural context. It is essential that the reader/viewer approach these dyads and interactions both at the individual and social levels so that the formative sense of relationships can be understood. The role of parental authority embedded in the kinship, and changes in the latter as a result of urbanization, westernization, and globalization, impinges upon the individual's functioning as an exemplar of the ideal and further away from the threat of the other. Thus, the modification, or difference, of psychoanalysis in the Indian context and in the Indian psyche, is worth addressing. The concepts of Indian personality have already been covered in previous chapters.

INDIA AND PSYCHOANALYSIS

Girindrasekhar Bose, in the early twentieth century, established the psychoanalytical methods of treatment in India and was using these in 1909 (Vaidyanathan, 1999, p. 3). Bose was deeply rooted in Hindu spiritual and philosophical lore and, unlike Freud, found no evidence of castration anxiety. He found no evidence of penis envy and suggested that "the desire to be female is more easily unearthed in Indian male patients, than in European" (Vaidyanathan, 1999, p. 3).

Bose (1999, p. 26) suggests that when a person is struck it results in a desire to strike the offender back and, unless there is an opportunity for the satisfaction of this desire, a painful tension results. The desire for retaliation or revenge emerges. In every instance, the satisfaction of any wish leads to the development of its opposite.

In every individual there is an unconscious desire to be struck, so when this finds an involuntary satisfaction by the assault, its opposite—the desire to strike—rises in the conscious and is recognized as a desire for revenge. If opportunities for satisfaction of the opposite wish are wanting, there is an accumulation of tension in the system. In some cases, the opposite may have social sanction. The difference that Bose outlined was significant in the context of the Oedipal complex. Bose suggested an Oedipal triangle, which has child–mother craving and the repeated satisfaction of these cravings give rise to the opposite craving (in the mother) to feed a child, caress a child, etc. The child is interested in things in which the mother is interested and the mother reciprocates. The father, on the other hand, becomes a new centre of interest and is apprehended from the standpoint of the mother. The identification with the father is through the mother. This triangle needs resolution and the failure of identification with the father and the mother, with appropriate responses from them, produces complications. The Oedipal complex can only be resolved by favourable circumstances where each angle of the triangle is functioning smoothly.

The attitude of the child towards its mother depends upon their environment, passive experiences, and impressions from the mother. Repeated submission to such passive situations gives rise to active wishes of a similar nature in the mind of the child as "identity of reaction" (Bose, 1999, p. 29). The child acts like the mother because the mother is its object. It does not appear to form an important component of the Oedipus complex. The desire to be a woman is discernible in all analyses, Bose (p. 30) argues.

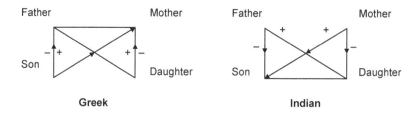

Figure 9.1   Differences between Greek and Indian myths

In the female child, the whole psychosexual constitution is in favour of the feminine attitude towards the father, where this phase of sexual development is more developed than in the male child. The castration wish is transformed into the castration dread. Bose illustrates these basic principles from his clinical work and posits that the superego must be conquered. The ability to castrate the father, converting him into a woman, is an essential requisite for the adjustment of the Oedipus wish.

The Indian Psychoanalytical Society was constituted in 1922 under the presidentship of Dr Bose. Hartnack (1999, p. 95) suggests that the Oedipal complex in India deals with the son's attitude towards the mother and altogether ignores the conflict between the father and the son. Ramanujan (1999, p. 109) found very little resemblance between the Indian mythical stories and the Greek Oedipal myth. He suggests that the Indian Oedipus pattern in father–daughter stories is similar to those of the Freudian views. These differences in the Greek and Indian myths are illustrated in Figure 9.1.

In Muslim dynasties often sons have killed their fathers, but not as often among the Hindu. Some writers point to the role of the elders in India, the general pattern of political gerontocracy, and even the long tolerance of foreign rule (as noted by Spratt, 1966), as tempting patterns. Obeyesekere (1999, p. 15) confirms that the essential components of the Indian Oedipus are the erotic-nurturant bond between the mother and the son, the patriarchal authority of the father, and the undisputed loyalty of the son.

An understanding of the Oedipal traditions (though not of the Greek variety) is essential to understand the role of the mother–son dyad and its depiction in the Hindi cinema. The role of the long-suffering woman, first as a wife and then as a mother, has previously been alluded to. Suffice it to say that the absence of the father on the screen and the presence of the widowed mother only emphasize the son–mother relationship.

As Ramanujan (1999) found in his search through Indian myths and folk tales, when a younger man kills an older one, it is the latter who teaches him a way of doing so. Is this a form of suicide? The aggressive father is sometimes replaced by aggressive villainous uncles and it is the submissive son who stands up to their cruelty and torture.

In the cinema, unconscious identificatory processes can be understood at three levels: precinematic, cinematic, and extracinematic (Friedberg, 1990). Identification with the actor and the director, or the story, is viewed in the context of how such information is obtained. Friedberg, in her description of precinematic identification, argues that the assimilative relations between the subject and the object and their interactions are the key to the identity formation. Using the Freudian concepts of displacement, primary identification (the original emotional tie with an object), secondary identification (the regressive way in which it becomes a substitute for libidinal object-tie), and tertiary identification (the perception of a common quality), the patriarchal identification allows a degree of reliance on perception. Lacan's reformulation of Freudian and post-Freudian object relations insisted on the primacy of the visual and deemphasized other channels of introjection (Friedberg, 1990, p. 39). Fenichel (1935) considers the process of ocular introjection, incorporation through the eye, in addition to oral, anal, epidermal, and respiratory introjections. Two directors of identificatory relations are identified by La Planche and Pontalis (1973, pp. 205–208): heteropathic/centripetal (the subject identifies self with other) and idiopathic/centrifugal (subject identifies other with self). The former identification is introjective and the latter is projective. The cinema plays upon introjective identification while providing the illusion of projective identification (Friedberg, 1990, p. 39).

CINEMATIC IDENTIFICATION

Primary cinematic identification differs from the Freudian primary identification. Metz (1985) defines primary cinematic identification as with the "look" of the camera and the projector. In the primary identification, the viewer constructs an imaginary notion of wholeness that does not reflect back as a mirror would.

This makes the characters on the screen transcendental subjects. Secondary identification with the star, actor or character, as defined by Metz (1985), is gendering of identification. Friedberg (1990, p. 41) critiques Metzian perceptions on the grounds that the conventions of the cinematic representations enforce a metronome of the body and wholeness is not offered here. The variables of the gendered body identification provide the next obstacle. Secondary identifications seem to be predicated on the recognition of human form, which is always available in the cinema. Extracinematic identification deals with an entire system of signifiers and as code. Friedberg (p. 43) suggests that the film star is simultaneously (acknowledged) recognized as "other" and misrecognized (disavowed) as self. She calls the film star an "institutionally sanctioned fetish". This identification allows the viewer to peel layers of the story, and understand by establishing, confirming, and learning to live with its message.

In real life, the Oedipus complex is almost never actually played out to the end by begetting children upon the mother. It remains in many states of unresolved indeterminacy, troubling the individual's mind. As the relationship is seen universally as taboo and perverse, its resolution is important for the individual's well-being and functioning. The mother becomes a symbol of long-suffering womanhood. Obsession with the mother and family is symptomatic of indifference to the good of society as a whole. Fate becomes a determinant of life. Within this misogyny, taking the woman for granted becomes an important dictum. The aspect of mother love gets subsumed into the girlfriend who should look just like mother, be traditional at home and modern outside. A man's honour is flexible, depending on his behaviour, whereas a woman's honour is more specific and rigid.

During the Golden Age of cinema in Hollywood, psychoanalysis and psychoanalysts were used to highlight the subtext: psychotic patients going on the rampage, and sympathetic friendly omnipresent therapists. Cinema has reflected the prevalent attitudes in the society to mental illness and the mentally ill as well as influenced these attitudes.

As far as mental illness and psychiatry are concerned, Hindi cinema has followed in Hollywood's footsteps, albeit rather reluctantly. There have been only a handful of Hindi films with a central character portraying mental illness, though some comedians have used it and some villains have used it to "justify" their villainy. What follows is a discussion of two early films where the protagonist is treated by psychiatrists and the narrative has expressed major components of the society's concerns. Bhugra (2002) observes that in spite of several inaccuracies the films discussed below present unusual aspects.

Khamoshi, based on a Bengali film by the same director, Asit Sen, was released in 1969, virtually after the black and white era had ended. Set in a psychiatric hospital, the story revolves around Radha, a psychiatric nurse who is asked by the head of the asylum to look after a patient using experimental treatment.

The film opens with Radha (Waheeda Rehman) looking over the balcony as Dev leaves the hospital. Significantly, the scene starts by Radha writing in her diary "Dev left today, whether he will remember how I accepted him (and made him my own), or, will he forget what I did for him. Today I hid what I was feeling from everyone. I bid goodbye to him with a smile and told him that I am a nurse after all and it is my duty to rekindle the lamps that are about to blow out." The introduction of the past relationship right at the beginning of the film reflects the process of suppression. It also indicates a lack of friendships within the social circle of the therapist, whose only confidant is a diary.

The hospital is headed by a retired colonel, who we meet presiding over a meeting to accept patients for therapy for the bed vacated by Dev's discharge. He is told by his assistant (among several others, including the matron) that the hospital had received 150 applications for one vacant bed, which included "cases of general paralysis of the insane, paranoia, schizophrenia, hysteria, manic reaction with cause not known, acute mania". The hospital chief interrupts him to ask "What did you say last? I am interested in such cases, take one of those." The matron interjects to say that they had just had a case like that. The Chief responds: "By looking after such cases, I want to prove that if *doctors* and patients form a relationship, then that relationship can be the treatment without any shock treatment. Without severe medication such relationship and trust can solve the emotional problems faced by the patient." He is reminded of the success in the case of Dev, to which he replies: "That's why I want such a case again. It is possible that Dev got better by chance. If we can cure others as well, then we can say that this cure is not coincidental." The committee agrees to admit one Arun Chaudhury. The hint at research methods of replicability of treatment and hypothesis testing are tantalizing but never referred to again.

Arun Chaudhury (Rajesh Khanna) is a young man whose rich girlfriend has jilted him. He is a poet and his family of rich landowners have also disowned him. His friend is looking after him. His psychotic experiences involve seeing the face of his ex-girlfriend Sulekha. He mistakes the dancing girl he has gone to see for Sulekha and attempts to murder her. He talks to himself: "Something strange is going on, it's all Sulekha's fault, I know." When taken to the hospital, Arun looks at the matron and asks: "Who is she?" The response "one of us" generates an even more paranoid reaction in Arun. The situation of us versus them (i.e., therapists versus patients) is clearly outlined here.

The Chief asks Radha to take the case but she is reluctant to do so, because it would mean "acting". She is told emphatically "No, no, this is not acting. This is the patient's treatment which you can do. Not everyone can." Radha refuses to accept the case and, much to his reluctance, the Colonel hands over the case to another nurse, Bina. The Chief reminds her: "You must remember about his illness. He has a girl in his heart who has deceived him and poisoned his mind. Her impression on him is very deep. You have to erase that impression and instil a new image with your love and loyalty like that of a mother." Bina questions this approach. The Chief-Psychiatrist then tells her the gist of Freudian analytical thinking: "When a child is born it is in an autoerotic stage, it becomes like looking in the mirror, narcissistic stage. The daughter develops feelings for the father and the son for the mother, which are called Electra and Oedipal. Once it is realized that these feelings are not acceptable socially, the boy starts searching for the mother in different faces. He falls in love with the face in which he finds this trust. If this trust is broken, the mental suspicion comes to the fore. Arun Choudhury has come to us in such a condition. You will have to act in such a way that his attraction for his mother and lover becomes the same. This is called establishing the rapport [sic!] with the patient, so that lost trust is regained. This was how Dev was treated and this is how you will treat Arun Chaudhury."

Arun is in a paranoid mode and the doctors decide to give him electroconvulsive therapy (ECT). Radha is drawn in despite her reluctance. Radha learns that Dev is getting married and she accepts looking after Arun, perhaps on the rebound. She visits Arun's friend to get some information on his background and discovers letters that Sulekha had written to him. Radha uses these letters to blackmail and persuade Sulekha to visit Arun, who then tries to strangle her. Sulekha gets angry and shouts at Radha, who like the therapist in *Pagla Kahin Ka* (see previous chapter) adopts a rather holier-than-thou approach. Radha encourages Arun to start writing again and uses this as therapy. Twice she mistakenly calls him Dev. Arun improves and, on a visit out, they talk and she appears happy in his arms. She refuses to see him prior to his discharge and Arun is told that Radha has gone out of town. He challenges the Chief, who tells him that Radha was only acting in order to get him better. Arun refuses to believe that Radha had been pretending to love him. He goes to her quarters and demands to see her. She is shown sitting quietly and still. The Chief says, "How did I make this mistake? I kept seeing a nurse and not the girl or woman in her—why couldn't I see that?" Radha is shown alternately laughing excessively and crying. She has become mentally ill herself.

Khamoshi is probably the first Hindi film to describe the descriptive aspect of psychoanalysis. There are several problems in its portrayal of the methods of psychoanalysis and the problems inherent in transference and countertransference.

More than once it is argued that Radha has been acting; though at the end she denies that she was ever acting. The diagnosis of acute mania is clinically inappropriate on the basis of the information given and, in modern clinical practice, psychoanalysis would be an inappropriate intervention for such a condition.

The retired Colonel who is Chief of the National Psycho-Analytical Institute uses his authority in a patrician and patriarchal manner. He is the stereotype caricature of a psychoanalyst, with grey wig and beard. His description of basic psychoanalytical principles is of much interest to the audience, and to Bina as the new nurse who is stepping in where Radha should have been. When the Colonel asks Radha to take on the case, he emphasizes the similarities with the earlier case and that there is no evidence of clinical supervision in either. Initially, he establishes Arun's sensitive

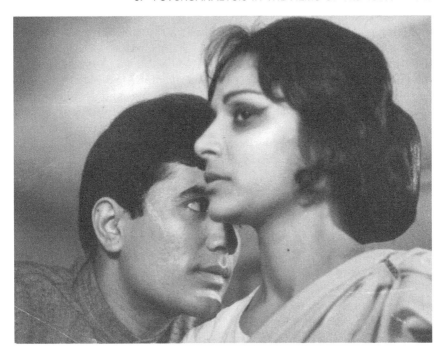

Figure 9.2   Scene from *Khamoshi* (courtesy of South Asia Cinema Foundation)

nature by telling Radha that this person is very fond of writing novels, plays, and poetry (not dissimilar to the poet in another film, *Khilona*, who also becomes insane after losing his girlfriend). At the same time he emphasizes the informality of their relationship by saying that she should stay away from writers because they are either crazy or romantic, thereby also emphasizing the close and entwined nature of madness and romance and whether both the conditions should be seen as obsessions. On her refusal, saying that she cannot act, he challenges emphatically "this is not acting. It is the patient's treatment which only *she* can carry out." At the same time, he chooses not to explain the problems associated with analysis. On one occasion he tries to blackmail her by saying that when they sent her to England she had promised that on her return she would devote herself to the service of these patients. On another occasion, the Chief asks Bina to act as if she is in love with Arun. The conflicting messages are never resolved.

Interestingly, other patients are stereotypes of alcoholics and of rocking psychotic patients, who provide comic relief to the audience. An interesting encounter between the junior psychiatrist Dr Rai and Arun's friend Bihari Babu, where they both consider each other insane, is a classic scene where the anxieties and stereotypes of the audience are confirmed, thereby providing relief. The fears that madness may be catching and that there is no possible way out of the asylum are especially evident.

The fact that Radha is shown lying on a bed embracing Dev and then on the boat embracing Arun, suggests that the therapist–patient relationship has no physical boundaries; intimacy therefore becomes much more of an issue. This may also reflect the absence of personal, private, and public space in Indian culture. Dev's mother invites her to visit their house and acknowledges, after Radha has touched her feet to greet her, "I gave him birth, but you have given him new life", thereby emphasizing the maternal/fraternal nature of Radha's relationship with Dev. Furthermore, this hint of the Oedipal complex and the way mother–son relationships work is an interesting paradox. Radha is doing exactly what she has been told, that is, to be the mother/lover. Yet her love is that of a lover, causing a conflict between her public duty and her private feelings and emotions. There is no room for her to resolve this dilemma. Although it is not true psycho-analysis, in the sense of sessions on the couch 5 days a week, it is fairly similar. Although the hospital is called the National Psycho-Analytic Clinic, they do use medication, ECT, family involvement, etc.

On trying to persuade Radha to take the case on, the Colonel begs her: "[Arun] came with trust in us and even this road will be closed to him." He reiterates his experience in the field hospital where an Army nurse had given her cloak to a dying soldier whom she did not know. She told the Colonel that he was "one of our soldiers". He emphasizes to Radha, "Since then I believe a woman can forget her own misery and take on the misery of the whole world. When Mr Dev got better, I thought, as God can't be every-where, he gives his form to the female." As one woman is responsible for turning a man mad, another is required to deal with this madness. The paradox could not be clearer. Mother and sister nurture, and lovers love, but naughty love—especially if it reflects a class divide—is poisonous, leaves an imprint, and poisons the mind to turn it mad.

Radha uses techniques of projection in getting him to write his way out of his repressed feelings, so that she can then work with him to express what love is about in a song which indicates that love is both a silence and a speech; love also listens and has no voice, and yet it is enlightening, with no barriers, and eternal. This rather moving explanation is also her expectation of life and her lover. Having been hurt once, she is still carrying on with life, and yet on the lookout for new love. She deliberately misquotes Arun and, not surprisingly, he picks up on it.

Sulekha is in Indian clothes while singing but by the time Radha con-front her; she has changed into western clothes, emphasizing her "modern" persona. Radha verbally attacks Sulekha, saying "To poison someone or poison someone's mind [obviously equitable acts] is your fault. To push him into this hell [is your fault]. Why should *we* have to suffer." When the

Colonel comes to know of this he challenges Radha. She responds "Those who are poisoning the society—you don't say anything to them, because you are experimenting and you need patients. I have a complaint against those who continue to spread the illness and we have to pay for it." Radha, as a good therapist, is taking on the role with an element of omnipotence and omniscience.

She goes beyond the call of duty, even pretending to be in love, even spending her free time with her patients, taking them on outings, and dealing with their friends and families. She is a good detective, extracting information by visiting various friends of Arun and resorting to blackmail to stage a confrontation so that Arun can forget Sulekha and move on with his life. However, in the end she, like a traditional Indian woman, is burdened with perceived obligations: The Chief has reminded her that she had been sent to England and that she had made certain promises.

Radha, as a woman and a nurse, listens to a man and a doctor with no room for negotiation or multidisciplinary consultation in this setting. Ultimately her reward is her own psychosis. That Radha, as a nurse and a therapist, is a representation of the sacrificing mother who has nurtured her son(s) in erotic-nurturant manner in the Indian Oedipal complex style is clear. She is alone and juxtaposes her professional role (there is no evidence of a personal life, of family or friends, and she confides in her diary to convey her innermost feelings) and clinical expectations in a way that makes it impossible for her to have any outcome other than what she is destined to.

Radha, in *Khamoshi*, suffers the same way courtesans and film actresses do in films and their portrayals. She falls into the trap even courtesans should not, falling in love with her clients. In the first instance her love is not reciprocated, and in the second case she's not able to reciprocate and shuts herself down, becoming psychotic. Radha belongs to no one but many depend on her. She is seen to be free, without family ties; nurses were often thought to be of loose character in Hindi cinema and Indian society. Her punishment for this freedom is her psychosis.

Chakravarty (1998) highlights the figure of the prostitute in Hindi films: "As an image of female oppression, class oppression and of psychic and moral ambivalence, [the] daunting figure of the prostitute can be a searing indictment of social hypocrisy and exploitation." This observation can be applied to Radha: She is neither a prostitute nor a courtesan, but her role and the demands made of her indicate this.

This sense of good therapy and personal sacrifice to the extent of going mad herself is interesting. Gabbard and Gabbard (1999, p. 15) suggest that movie psychiatrists may offer film students a privileged view of cinematic myth making in action. Each of their attributes can be divided into good and bad halves, producing complementary pairs of good and bad psychiatrists.

A good psychiatrist is caring, effective, omniscient, a good detective, reconciling, compassionate, human, fallible, and a healing lover. In *Khamoshi*, Radha as the therapist is all of these but in the end suffers for being too good. In *Raat aur Din*, one of the therapists has some of these attributes. Other therapists in both the films are neurotic and ridiculous. In each there is at least one character who is an exploitative lecher or libidinous clown as defined by Gabbard and Gabbard (1999).

The nurses in the asylums are female and the orderlies are male, thereby confirming the nurturing feminine role and the weak male. Even when Radha consistently refuses to take the new case, the Chief does not probe deeply to find the reasons for her refusal. The sense of isolation and desolation that engulfs Radha is palpable, as is a sense of martyrdom when she agrees to take on Arun's case. The martyrdom is like that of a mother who is willing to give herself up for her son's sake. Radha's interpretation and accusations are flung at Sulekha ("we have to pick up the pieces") and highlight the sense of martyrdom and omnipresence. Arun is a poet, therefore expected to be sensitive and removed from the real world, making him much more susceptible to madness. His hallucinations or illusions and paranoid ideations do not neatly fit into a diagnostic category, nor does the diagnosis given by the Doctor Uncle or the hospital Chief.

Radha is like a daughter of the doctor who is a patriarch. He sent her abroad to train in therapy and she is expected to treat ("marry") a patient chosen by her father figure consultant. This allows her to be rebellious for a short while, but she eventually falls into line and obeys by entering into this patient–therapist relationship; yet again the father has abandoned her. She is told off by the matron as well (taking a maternal supervisory line) when she asks for some time off in the evening, "You will do your special work elsewhere. Who will do the work here? You do what you feel like [anyway], why do you want to ask me. Do what you like." The tone implies that the matron also feels let down by Radha. Having let both "parents" down Radha, as a good daughter, has to atone for her sins; one way is to get "married" and suffer the consequences. Like other Indian marriages, her parents arrange her marriage. When Radha is due to see Dev for follow up, she is visibly excited and dresses up in a sari rather than her uniform. This preparation for her lover is obvious in her letter to Dev after she hears about his wedding: "[We] do not always get what we want. Even though I desired, I could not attend your wedding." The gesture of giving Dev a copy of *Meghdoot* (an epic poem by Kalidasa in which the heroine uses clouds as a messenger to her lover) is appropriate for a lover, but inappropriate in the patient–therapist relationship.

The reviewer of *Khamoshi* in *Screen* (11 December 1970) notes an offbeat attempt in its outward tone and set up. Being black and white, "It tries to keep away from the stock and set ingredients of our films." The reviewer feels that the film suffers from intrinsic drawback of content material and treatment, making it a sincere but a half-hearted attempt. The dialogue is seen to be long-winded and old-fashioned, but the two protagonists have done a brilliant job. Waheeda Rehman moves the audience in quite a few scenes even though the story is absurd. The reviewer notes that the scenes in the madhouse do not look realistic, with individual cases drawn in some detail, mostly for melodrama and to gain sympathy. The reviewer points with a sense of relief that they (i.e., patients) are not made ridiculous with the casting of comedians as loonies (sic!).

An important question to be asked is, "Can nurses be thus used by hospital authorities [to cure patients]?" The answer lies in the patriarchal nature of the society, where men can and do order women about.

The Oedipal complex, as described by the Doctor-in-Chief, is Freudian. It is interesting that the European model is chosen rather than Bose's (1999) model. Bose came from Bengal, as did the story writers and director for the film. Interestingly, the same director originally made the film in Bengali. This may reflect the impact of import or postcolonial experience on the story writer and whether these values were more important than the traditional Indian ones. In the setting of the psychiatric clinic there is little evidence that any other kind of psychological therapy is going on; the patients are given medication and attend a roll-call to get their medication.

When Radha is invited to attend Dev's wedding, she wants to know from Dev's relatives if Dev remembers anything. They respond by speaking highly of the hospital, doctors, and nurses, who are very good. Radha is obviously expecting that Dev misses her, but not hearing that makes her feel rejected. She deals with this rejection by reading a plaque on the wall with a quotation from Swami Vivekanand, "You are not born, you do not die, you are not destroyed, you are child of immortality—Why are you afraid?", and her cognitive dissonance disappears. As "mother" she deals with difficult patients by agreeing to their demands. For example, she gives a bottle of water (declaring it to be alcohol) to an alcoholic and soothes him, saying that she has been to his house to feed his wife and children. Freud's free association method is implicit in the story. Radha encourages Arun to write but, in a classical Freudian slip, when she reads the story, the heroine Reena becomes Radha. Her sacrifice at the altar of parental happiness and the reaction of both "parents" only emphasizes her "marriage".

Raat aur Din ("Night and Day") was effectively the last film of Nargis, the megastar of the 1950s and 1960s. Nargis started acting in films as a child and was a star at the age of 5, but became best known as Raj Kapoor's romantic lead in some of the Hindi cinema's most enduring melodramas. In *Barsaat*, *Andaz*, *Awara*, *Shri 420*, and *Anhonee*, where she played a double role, Nargis was often presented as a femme fatale doomed to destruction by her beauty. She was said to earn more from her films than her male

co-stars did (George, 1994). Like any other star, any reading or consideration of a film starring Nargis must acknowledge the contexts of her other
work and her star persona, as well as the expectations of audiences—not
only of her but also of the characters she played—as well as her public and
private life.

Raat aur Din is the story of a woman whose personality changes under
the influence of alcohol and this change gets her into trouble with her
family and friends. She goes through treatment to Dr Dey's Psycho Clinic
(sic!) and eventually recovers with the help of occasionally sympathetic and
caring psychiatrists.

In the film, Pratap's (Pardeep Kumar) car breaks down while he is on
his way to Shimla to meet a girl who was selected for marriage by his
parents. He meets Baruna (Nargis), who is alone, as her father is away.
They spend the night talking. Baruna's father returns, gets Pratap's car
repaired, and Pratap proceeds to Shimla. Against his mother's wishes he
marries Baruna. One night Pratap and his mother see Baruna dancing to
western music. Convinced that Baruna is possessed, Pratap's mother gets
a shaman. Pratap chases the shaman away. Later, at a party, Baruna's
drinks are spiked, she becomes drunk and is unable to remember anything.
Her husband Pratap and Dilip (Firoz Khan), who had been dancing with
Baruna, talk to the psychiatrists and Baruna is admitted to a nursing
home where she gains access to alcohol and again her personality changes.
She is unable to recall the psychiatrist's name and maintains that her name
is Peggy. She passes out and on waking up is embarrassed and denies
being Peggy. During the session with the psychiatrist, her mood changes
once more; she becomes flirtatious Peggy again. She makes fun of the
psychiatrist and attacks the nurse, in spite of being sedated. The psychiatrists decide to give her ECT, which has no effect, after which she
disappears. In a hotel she drinks excessively and passes out. Subsequently
she is involved in an accident.

Her father explains that his wife was rather old fashioned; he admits that
he used to gamble and drink heavily. After a fierce row they separated and
the mother took Baruna with her. The psychiatrists take Baruna to Shimla
to let her relive her childhood experiences. She recalls that in the house
opposite lived a young girl, Peggy, whose parents encouraged her to sing
and dance and attend school. Baruna's mother kept her at home because
she believed that education was a bad influence. Baruna recollects that she
used to meet Peggy, and once followed her to a Christmas Ball. Her mother
yells at her, falls down the hill, and dies. Baruna blamed herself for her
mother's death, though it had been caused by a heart attack. As a result of
this process, she starts to feel better and reconciles with her father.

Rai (1997) emphasizes that the film represents feminine binary codes and
national and cultural anxieties in postcolonial India, oscillating between

virginity/promiscuity, purity/contamination, religion/dissolution, India/the west, sanity/madness, public sphere/woman space. To this can be added wife/whore, mother/child, and stability/instability issues. These coda are for understanding the switch between different characters and the role of the explorer/ethnographer (i.e., the psychiatrist) in unveiling the unconscious motivation. The fact that the psychiatrists work as a team to bring her two disparate halves together suggests the hopes and expectations of the leaders to pull the split country together.

There is no specific psychiatric diagnosis discussed in the film. The psychiatrists initially talk about the case being "quite complex, very complicated case indeed". At one point the senior psychiatrist calls it a case of "a split personality". The senior doctor tells the new house surgeon, "The patients have no physical illness, but mental illness", thereby making a distinction between the two. Later, the psychiatrist explains to Baruna that the body is the slave of the mind. Quite rightly, they gather third party information to know more about her past and her personality. They are keen to find out how long ago this has happened and why. These "episodes" are seen to be linked with her having headaches for which she takes aspirin and goes to sleep, after which her character changes. The story may well have had some Hollywood and psychoanalytic influences in its treatment.

The husband is perplexed at the diagnosis of split personality. The senior psychiatrist explains, "It's like the myth about two souls in one body", an angle thereby bringing in the Indian concept of the soul equating life and personality. In *Raat aur Din*, despite the western clothes, smoking, and drinking, the audience appears to know that she was not an evil woman and accepts the unusual dual nature of the heroine.

The portrayal of psychiatry and the psychiatric nursing home is unusual: The patients have single rooms, the resident doctors appear to be unusually well paid, and there is no presence of others who would be working in the nursing home. Also, in only one scene is there evidence that there are other patients in the Psycho Clinic.

The split personality in *Raat aur Din* shows a good Baruna and a bad Peggy. The former is a soft-spoken dutiful housewife and the latter a woman very sexual and westernized in clothing, mannerisms, and hairstyle. These visual details reflect the unacceptable use of sexuality. Peggy is a childlike character and is flirtatious, which makes sense in the context of the denouement of the film. The explanations given to the psychiatrists make her childhood experiences clearer. Intriguingly, the character again is Anglo-Indian, confirming the stereotype in audience's mind that Anglo-Indian women are loose in character and sexually available. The awkward elements of *The Three Faces of Eve* get processed through family relationships, domesticity, and family melodrama. Within this form, attitudes towards mental illness, the use of psychoanalysis and practice, the violence and victimization of the "mad woman", and the relationship of the woman to her families is assimilated (Bisplinghoff & Slingo, 1997).

In some ways the diagnosis itself is perhaps less important than the description and representation. As Kleinman (1980) has argued, the patients are often interested in why something has gone wrong, whereas the therapist is interested in what is wrong. This explanation, which Kleinman calls Explanatory Models, is essential to the understanding of how help is sought and from where it is sought. The help sought in *Raat aur Din* is initially within the folk sector and then, either because of western beliefs or the perceived failure of the shaman, psychiatrists are consulted. There is no mention at all of the reasons why the family chooses these psychiatrists and how treatments are selected. The husband, a rich businessman, is shown to be more sophisticated than the parents, who are more traditional in their clothes and attitudes.

The aetiological factors of psychiatric conditions are often divided into precipitating, perpetuating, and predisposing factors. In Baruna's case there are several predisposing factors: The "loss" of her father before the age of 11, her parents' divorce, and a sensitive and socially withdrawn personality all play a role in the aetiology. Among the precipitating factors, marriage would be the most important. In addition to adjustment to a spouse, relationships with mothers-in-law in India are generally fraught with difficulty. No daughter-in-law is ever considered good enough for the darling son. It is likely that Baruna's upbringing may have left her vulnerable in dealing with other women. An illustrative example of this in the movie is when the mother-in-law introduces Baruna to their neighbours, till recently a common practice in rural and semi-rural India. A key function of such gatherings is to see the bride, criticize her looks, and also to assess/admire/criticize her dowry. In the scene where Baruna is brought down to meet the neighbours, two neighbours are already involved in an argument about mother-in-law and daughter-in-law relationships. These are at the core of family strife, partly to do with the son's relationship with the mother and her overinvolvement with the son, and partly to do with love-marriage where the conflict is greater, as in this case. As noted earlier, Spratt (1966) suggests that the narcissistic personality among Hindus is related to unconscious identification with the mother. Under these circumstances the individual responds in a way that is inexplicable in western terms. The Hindu personality relates to mother fixation in relation to caste, hierarchy and specific expectations. Rai (1997) points out that the film reappropriates the violence between Peggy and Baruna as a desire to kill the maternal (traditional Hindu) superego. By splitting and then "uniting" Baruna's subjectivity, the film compels a range of anxieties to recur within her. The violence imparted to mother India (portrayed remarkably by Nargis) at the time of the Partition and the ambivalence of its leader's status to make sense in the context of the film and postcolonial discourse allow the viewer to understand the role of dead mother in the genesis of splitting Baruna.

The Indian attitude to women is made up of strands of Hindu tradition where the woman is both mother goddess and represents power, is submissive and yet aggressive, nurturing and yet seductive, a combination of Madonna and the whore. Yet she is ruled by a patriarchal society. The ritual concept of the impurity of food tasted by another is extended to a woman who is, as food, to be "consumed" in a pure condition. In both these films women are made impure by their illness. In *Raat aur Din* the mother-in-law rejects the impurity of her daughter-in-law and encourages her son to marry another.

In one scene Baruna confirms what the mother-in-law dreads. The mother-in-law says in response to a query: "The girls from the hills [i.e., a cold climate] look grown up and mature. She is no older than 16/17." In reply, Baruna bursts into laughter, which is unappreciated as daughters-in-law are not expected to speak at such gatherings nor should they laugh openly. Women are also not expected to flaunt their age; Baruna says, "I was 18 a long time ago. Papa says that I am over 25." To the mother-in-law this confirms her total unsuitability for her son and she, like other traditional mothers, hides behind "I did not have your horoscope so I could just guess. I said what I thought." This self-reproach is justified because the mother-in-law has already been established as traditional and therefore backward and ignorant.

The filmmaker is making a clear distinction between the older generation and the younger, more liberated, generation. The period in which the film is set is more traditional. Post-Independence, the country is coming to terms with the aftermath of the Partition and the two wars with its neighbours, although there is no mention of these events or awareness. Pratap's modernity is mixed with tradition; he is modern enough to marry of his own volition, allows drink in the house and at parties, and believes in psychiatry. Yet his traditional views are of those of the Indian male who cannot appreciate his wife drinking or smoking and, as the owner of a coal mine, rushes to look after the injured after an accident. This contrast is even more marked with the Hindu and Christian differences. Peggy is obviously Christian with the Cross hanging prominently on the wall; the modernity of Christians is compared starkly with Baruna's life of being imprisoned in her room and not being allowed to go to school, listen to music, or mix with others.

Baruna's mother-in-law is a guardian of Hindu patriarchal tradition, argues Rai (1997), in inviting the shaman to dispel the evil spirit possessing her daughter-in-law's body with the use of a burning stick. The burning of the body is symbolic perhaps to liberate the soul but the question remains:

Whose body is being burnt, Peggy's or Baruna's? Whose scream is it? Rai proposes that the displacement of the war zone of desire (a recurrent theme in Hindu nationalist thought) may reflect gendered subjectivity, perhaps both of Baruna and more significantly of her mother-in-law. Rai suggests that the film draws on the psychoanalyst (Dr Alvarez) as the spiritual war against desire, but the violence experienced by Baruna both by herself and through Peggy reflects an ambivalence of the individual.

The family (largely the husband) identifies that Baruna needs help. The mother-in-law focuses on exorcism and believes in horoscopes, whereas the son brings her to Dr Dey's Psycho Home. The two psychiatrists interview her; they keep interrupting and the story progresses in a series of flashbacks. The nursing home appears to have at least three psychiatrists with one junior doctor who is resident, although others appear at the bedside at different times. There is only one visible nurse in uniform. Although the senior doctors are in suits, the junior wears a white coat, as does another psychiatrist later on in the film. The management includes both physical and psychological methods of treatment. Bisplinghoff and Slingo (1997) propose that in *Raat aur Din* Baruna's split personality is a personal matter and potentially a family disaster. Hence, Baruna and her family need to heal.

The interconnections between the Hindu household and psychiatric treatment emphasize to the viewer that the possession states may be the first port of call and that the "modern" view will be to use the psychiatrist and therapist as the next stop on the pathway to treatment. *Raat aur Din* assimilates the sophisticated imagery of Hollywood psychiatry, including shock treatment. Bisplinghoff and Slingo (1997) observe that the film begins with Indian alternative forms of treatment, which are rejected in favour of a more "enlightened" Freudian approach (although not labelled as such), and even this Indianized approach leads to an isolation of the heroine.

The repression can be brought out and also cured by psychoanalysis. Apparently, no traditional psychoanalytic models or techniques are employed; the strategy favoured by the psychiatrists focuses on why things had gone wrong. As part of this investigation they interview both the husband and the father, then take her back to Shimla to get her to remember her childhood and associations. However, unlike psychoanalysts, the psychiatrists are more directive in their questioning as well as in their interpretation, which may be appropriate for the film as medium. In this film the mental health professionals are psychiatrists, giving medication and ECT as well as talking therapies to both inpatients and outpatients. The stereotypes and conventions offer filmmakers the opportunities to produce fantastic dream sequences or logical explanations for the inexplicable behaviour of their characters.

Hollywood films use ECT differently off screen or on screen; beneficial or punitive, it continues to carry very strong images for the public. The

ECT is used as a dramatic device but much less in Hindi films. As mental institutions became more stark in their portrayal after the golden age of Hollywood cinema in the 1930s and 1940s, so did the portrayal of ECT.

On one occasion, medication is shown as being given where the junior doctor tells the senior one that "I have injected your recommended dose to the highest level but to no avail"; no name is given to the medication. Injections have always had a higher "perceived" therapeutic value and dramatic impact in India. There is no mention of consent, therapeutic effects, or even side-effects. The injectable antipsychotic medication was introduced in India in 1980 and here it suggests a medicalization of the condition.

In *Raat aur Din*, after medication when the psychiatrists see that "her violence is increasing", they decide to give ECT. Again, there appears to be no discussion or consent, which is representative of the doctors' patriarchal attitudes. The delivery of the ECT is very dramatic: She is tied down, a mouth gag is inserted, and a nurse presses the button. Baruna's scream is heard outside. Pratap is frightened and yells, "Stop it, stop it, Doctor, I can't see this." The psychiatrist's response is uncomprehending and patronizing: "My God! I didn't know you had such a weak heart. You go home and relax. I promise as soon as she wakes up she will be in her senses." When there is no improvement in Baruna's condition, Pratap accuses the doctors of making false promises that she will get better after the shock.

Like Hollywood, the image of ECT in Hindi films is extreme. It is seen as punitive and is used as dramatic device to highlight the cruelty of the modern psychiatry. In *Raat aur Din* it is not dissimilar to the rituals being performed by the shaman who is asked to come and exorcize Baruna, by using a burning stick to drive away the witch possessing her. In the scene, everyone apart from the shaman is female, suggesting a gender-related perception that hints that women are backward and a man is required to put them right. The weakness and backwardness of women at one level is related to their lack of education; when Baruna's mother refuses to send her to school this confirms the backwardness and yet perpetuates this myth. In the ECT suite, the female nurse is in uniform and the male doctors are holding Baruna down. In early Hollywood films, ECT is portrayed as benign, accompanied by soft music, whereas in later films it takes on a major punitive image. The psychiatrists in the ECT suite are worried, do not appear confident, and the use of the nurse and her uniform to give the ECT indicates that she is more empathic and yet authoritarian. These mixed messages appear in other Hindi films as well.

Gabbard and Gabbard (1999) include the mental institutional film as a subgenre of the prison film. With easily recognized characters and dramatic devices, the film does not allow the characters of the psychiatrists to develop and does not fill the viewer with confidence. *Raat aur Din* has nowhere near the impact of the visual horror depicted by the interpersonal conflict between the nurse, representing the institution, and the patient trying to escape, as in *One Flew Over the Cuckoo's Nest.*

Despite several inaccuracies in the story line and logical errors, this film presents an unusual story for its time. It won the President's Gold Medal for the best film of the year and Nargis won the Best Actress award. The review in *Filmfare* praised Nargis for her performance, acknowledging that, though her versatility was never in doubt, in *Raat aur Din* she put across the most difficult role of her career as if to reaffirm her histrionic talents. "It presents with unusual seriousness, and almost complete success, a complex offbeat subject with rare coherence by writer Akhtar Hussain and very ably directed by Satyen Bose", noted the reviewer. The reviewer praised all of the performers, especially the two actors playing "understanding psychiatrists" and the comedian Anoop Kumar as a house surgeon turning in a very hilarious portrayal.

It is interesting to note that the reviewer feels that, free from the box office clichés, the film offers a contrast to the screen presentations of the day, both pleasant and painful: pleasant because of what the film offers us and painful because it reminds us of what the majority of Indian films lack today.

In an interview, Nargis pointed out that, despite the film being in black and white, with outmoded costumes and no lavish sets, viewers will remember the content of the film. To prepare for the role, Nargis acknowledged that she went to the Mental Hospital in Thane, met with psychiatrists, and watched electric shock treatment being given.

Limitations in cinematic portrayal allow the dramatic concepts to take precedence over the truthful aspects. Sarris (1998) suggests that the typology of films is determined by the prevalent social mores and that most Hollywood movies were oriented towards a middle class vision of life even in the 1930s, and yet he finds these extremely truthful. This is more apparent when films started to tackle talking therapies.

Talking therapies are less dramatic on the screen than ECT, but charismatic therapists can offer their all to the suffering patients, as shown in *Ordinary People*, directed by Robert Redford. As noted in the previous chapter, Meena Kumari's character in *Baharon ki Manzil* receives counselling but there too the psychiatrist is working as a detective to explore what has gone on.

In America, by 1957, psychiatry had become a fact of life for most Americans. Consequently psychiatrists confirmed optimistic myths about how easy it is for troubled people to return to well-being. In Hindi cinema, however, no such heroes emerge, largely because the concept of personal psychotherapy is alien and the role of the family really important and marked. Hence the psychiatrists function either as ethnographers or as detectives trying to find the source of pain and resolve it. The repressed

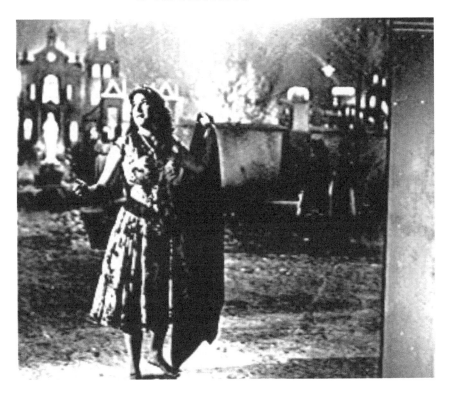

Figure 9.3 Scene from *Raat aur Din* (courtesy of National Film Archive of India)

memory is painful and either leads to a defence that protects the patient and keeps the therapist at bay or, under the right circumstances, allows it to come out.

In *Raat aur Din* the main character is a product of an unhappy parental marriage, violence leading to repression. Bisplinghoff and Slingo (1997) observe that Baruna's journey back in time is depicted as an actual trip back to her childhood home and the physical side of her trauma. In behavioural terms this could be seen as one way of dealing with her post-traumatic stress disorder by exposing her to the source of the trauma. In the Freudian context this mystery is resolved by reliving the childhood trauma, central to the core. However, what is even more fascinating is that the family is healed and both sides of the family made whole, as represented by Baruna walking into the future escorted by both her father and her husband. Bisplinghoff and Slingo comment that this is a very unusual way of depicting an Indian woman's relationship to her father even after her marriage. They interpret the scene in the Freudian way by arguing that she has been returned to both of them. However, it also reflects that even if the father and husband are distant they are important for the Indian female to survive any kind of trauma, which is a confirmation of patriarchal power.

The comparisons between *Raat aur Din* and *The Three Faces of Eve* are inevitable, although the latter was released 10 years earlier in the USA. In both films the actresses won national acting awards for their portrayal. In *The Three Faces of Eve* the psychiatrist uses hypnosis to bring together two of the heroine's personalities, Eve Black and Eve White. Eve Black is seductive and histrionic. Eve White is a depressed and withdrawn house-wife. When the psychiatrist begins to use hypnosis, a third personality, Jane, emerges as the integration of the two selves. Joanne Woodward plays Jane by adapting better posture. Through hypnosis a repressed traumatic memory of her childhood is uncovered, when her parents forced her to kiss her dead grandmother. In *Raat aur Din* there are only two selves: Peggy and Baruna, differentiated by their clothes, drinking, and smoking habits, establishing a clear distinction between the west, or Christian, and the East, or Indian, worlds. The differences are stark, as mentioned above, but Baruna represents a withdrawn, depressed (not in the clinical sense) indi-vidual who comes out of her shell after she recalls her traumatic memory. In the scene after she has disappeared from the hotel having drunk alcohol, as Peggy she is dressed in a skirt and goes around singing, "O my vagabond heart/Who knows where your destination is."

In front of the church, surrounded by the statues depicting women and motherhood, she is happily hopping and dancing to choral music, which is playing in the background. She continues to sing and she gives away her overcoat to a leper. As the camera focuses on the statue of a woman who is holding her face, Baruna (as Peggy) emotes that the night and day are two faces (of the same thing). She acknowledges that there are two facets to her personality and she does not know which is the real her. The truth experi-enced through her madness and her movements through light and shadows affect her; although aware that her heart is a vagabond over which she has no control, she is also aware of an inherent restlessness, probably a sign of her entrapment in her life and perhaps also in her in-laws' house. This is very unlike her "free" days at her father's place; which is the experience for a large number of Indian women.

This song ends with her getting drenched in the rain and being given shelter by a poor Brahmin couple. Her being drenched in the rain can also be interpreted in two ways: The rain calms her ardour as the westernized "other", and it also is a way of punishing her. ECT as "hot" treatment and rain as "cold" cure are symbolic events that indicate that she must face punitive supernatural anger from the highest father figure. The talking therapies provided by Dr Alvarez and his colleagues are mere devices in the narrative. Her discovery that she is pregnant leads Baruna to scream; she wants to kill the baby, otherwise the baby will kill her, thereby reminding the audience of the link between her childhood and mother–child relationship. It could be that she intends to punish her unborn child to avenge herself from her parents who have hurt her. As a result of the drenching, perhaps she gains some insight into her own behaviour as she realizes that as a married housewife she should not have got drenched. On her return to her in-laws she explains to her mother-in-law that she did not know what she was doing and asks for forgiveness, but the mother-in-law, who is bossy and garrulous, merely scoffs at her and throws her out, much like the banishing of Sita in the *Ramayana*.

In Shimla she recovers her traumatic memory and says, "I killed my mother." Dr Alvarez brings her a newspaper report to confirm that her mother had a heart attack prior to the fall and tells Baruna,

> It is not your fault. You held yourself responsible for your mother's death. You thought that you had committed a grave crime and hated yourself so much that you wanted to kill yourself. But there was another life where there was no regret. A life full of happiness: that of Peggy. As your mother tried to stifle you as she trampled on your wishes you were drawn more and more towards Peggy. A different personality of Peggy was etched in your mind. Body being the slave of mind, Peggy and Baruna did not recognize each other.

The cathartic recovery leads to cure in this case. The psychoanalysis of the film itself is of interest. Gabbard and Gabbard (1999) argue that the revelation of the other personality reveals a multiple personality disorder also related to multiple repetitive incidents rather than a single one.

The instant cure does not happen in real life. The diagnosis given to the heroine by the critics and Nargis herself is inaccurate. In an interview with Mohan Bawa (1980, p. 70), Nargis acknowledged that, "She was a schizophrenic character actually. A girl with a dual personality. It was one girl, not a double role. Medically it has been proved that a schizophrenic has two lives. And what are the causes, no one knows. There are two entirely different characters. Two separate entities." The actress went on to reveal in the same interview that this was one of her best performances. "The transition from one character to the other was beautifully done. Done within one shot it was very difficult, especially where the doctor is interrogating her and she is normal. Suddenly, from that normal state she is transformed into the girl who wants to smoke and take a sip of brandy. And from the 'bad girl' she comes back to the 'normal girl'." Nargis was always seen as having her charisma oscillate between the simple and the chic.

With the development of semiotics, Freudian and post-Freudian psychoanalysis became more important in Europe. For example, flashback as used in both these films more than once suggests that both philosophies of memory and psychoanalysis play a role. The story advances by bringing in flashbacks. In addition, unlike the majority of Hollywood films these films, like many Hindi films, also use song location and situation embedded in the memory. There are of course problems with flashbacks, as they give the impression that the narrator knows all. The other essential matter in this film is Baruna's recollection of her childhood and events that have influenced her character. Lacan proposes that the infant develops a dramatically ambivalent relationship with the reflected (projected) self, both loving it for being an ideal and hating it for being outside the child's body. In this context, as a child Baruna appears to have identified herself with Peggy because she is "ideal", but hates it because she is an outsider. By virtue of cinema technique, only significant and perhaps dramatic events can be illustrated. Lacan has used the imagery of the newborn child's pleasure in the sense of complete union with the mother (Oubert, 1978). The child attempts to understand his or her concept of self by a number of strategies; some of this is related to projection and hence its inability to see itself except in terms of the "other". Baruna shares her room with her mother; one window in the room is barred, whereas the other is open. This probably denotes that one route is open and the other imprisoned and claustrophobic. At another level this can also be seen as a representation of women in newly emergent and independent India; being imprisoned under the old traditions and so-called backwardness, yet westernized with a sense of independence and freedom. The emergence of Indira Gandhi as Prime Minister might have liberated women, but a majority of women in rural areas remained illiterate, oppressed, and backward. The ambivalence towards freedom and independence as a woman and being a good housewife is touched upon very briefly in *Raat aur Din* by illustrating the shopping habits and freedom attributed to Sheila, the girl whom Pratap's parents wanted him to marry. The distinct Anglo-Indian "badness" of drinking, smoking, and western dress and values represents looseness of character and is seen as a strict no-no, an extreme position to take.

Gabbard and Gabbard (1999) suggest that the Lacanian perspective in the films indicates the ability of the protagonist to identify alternatively with the exhibitionist and voyeur, the victim and the victimized. The identification of the audience with one or the other suggests that this identification allows the replication of our childhood experiences. Thus, in immediately postcolonial India, all that is western may reflect badness, although over the last 10 years or so it has changed and become more acceptable. The appeal of the cinema lies in the audience's relationship with the mirror image, confusing self with the other. There are options of watching cinema over and over, tape freezing, rewinding, and starting again, whereas in the theatre such an identification occurs rarely and the performances differ from show to show.

The cinema also reflects the relative importance of symbols. The symbolic covers the unsayable and in Hindi cinema songs and dances are used to depict and express emotions that are not openly acceptable. For example, in the opening scenes of the film Baruna/Peggy enters the club and encourages others to untie themselves (from the bindings of daily humdrum life) and celebrate by singing. She also invites the stranger (the "other" for her in this case, who assumes the guise of a potential lover) to help get rid of her helplessness. There is a not so subtle invitation to drown their sorrows in drink; in itself this is surprising but it also indicates that at some level she is very aware of the effect alcohol has, not only on her but on others. She wants to be free, and the freedom that she had experienced at her father's home after her mother's death is also inviting, although at this point the audience is not aware of this. This is further indicated to them in the flashback. When she is joined by Dilip, the undertone is that they have become united—these two free spirits, although lost in what he calls the city of dreams, have perhaps become transubstantiated into something superior. He volunteers to ask for directions (in which they want to travel as a result of their love/lust) but feels that she has not given him any indication at all. Whether this reflects her ambivalence, her innocence, or her desire to manipulate is left to the imagination of the viewer. It becomes clear as a result of the song and its setting in a club, the fact that she wears a long evening dress and uses a cigarette holder, that she is manipulating—or is she part of the manipulation (of the audience) itself? They communicate to each other and to the audience that they are aware of the consequences of their actions; although their hearts dictate them to move on forward, they are also aware of those who they may be leaving behind.

The desire here is to meet a stranger, let go of inhibitions, and look forward to leaving old traditions behind. Thus, from the beginning of the story Peggy as a character is laying the foundations for a westernized, free and available approach to life. It is also a call to new India to go forward and stop hankering after the past. The characters feel free to love, being provocative and encouraging others to be merry as well and fall in love, drink, and move ahead. Dancing a waltz also suggests the romanticism where men may lead but women have an equal stake in the pleasure.

Oubert (1978) described suture in films using the traditions of semiotics. This implies that the cinematic gaps created by cutting or editing are "sewed" so that the viewers are included to identify themselves with some aspect of the "gaze" created by the camera (Dayan, 1976). In *Raat aur Din* suture works as Pratap sees Baruna for the first time as she is singing the title song in a path lined by trees with fog emerging sporadically. This allows the character to be watched just like the audience without any sense of encroachment. There is the unique way of monitoring Baruna later when her screams caused by ECT allow the viewer to be outside the room and look at Pratap's horror intercutting with the "medical" treatment. The same is illustrated very well within the scene when the shaman is trying to rid Baruna of the possession. The symbolism of holding a skull and burning rod in the hands of the shaman as well as the use of the ECT machine suggest a strong element of simulation of burning parts of Baruna to rid her of the western values.

The similarities between shamanistic and westernized approaches indicate that both the shaman and the psychiatrist believe in their approaches even if they do not understand the mode of action of these techniques. In addition, both therapists (shaman and psychiatrist) are being used to demonize and exorcize western values, which have hurt the country in the past. The newly independent country has to find its own way to deal with crisis.

The gender and psychoanalytic theories cannot be isolated from the interpretation. An Indian female is expected to be a homemaker and her existence is not in isolation but related to kinship and society in general and family in particular. The females therefore carry the tradition and impart it to the children as well, thus the role of mother is important. Interestingly, the two key mothers, Baruna's mother and her mother-in-law, are both examples of devouring and punitive mothers. Although Baruna's mother-in-law is protective of her son, she is a strong woman who controls her thoroughly hen-pecked husband. When Baruna learns that she is pregnant and screams about killing the unborn child, it is unusual because abortion was not an acceptable option for Indian women. Her fear is of failure, and of punishing her unborn child as her mother had punished her.

The suppression and repression of her traumatic memories, leading to amnesia (which is referred to as total amnesia by the psychiatrists without any observed formal testing), is an interesting example. The use of the flashback in cinema is of particular interest to the audience (Turim, 1989). The flashback can be used to represent a dream, a fantasy, or a supernatural element, all of which are relatively common in Hindi films. The actions that seem to have the most dramatic and negative consequences are often those whereby a character intentionally or otherwise slights, insults, or injures a figure to whom veneration is due (both mother and mother-in-law are injured by Baruna in this instance). The focal amnesia may be related to such events. As Goldman (1999, p. 274) observes:

> Such an emotional climate . . . easily gives rise to a situation where the victim of abuse, encouraged to revere, even worship the abuser, can react only by an identification, coupled with severe anxiety but becomes aware of the powerful hatred aroused.

In a society where it is unthinkable to own up to one's negative feelings towards one's elders, the projection of anger, public acknowledgement, and living with the paradox are some of the solutions individuals may choose.

In *Raat aur Din* there is also the key theme of understanding the self-hood, how self is identified, and how two conflicting aspects of the self are eventually brought together. The concepts of the self in India include an inner-self (atman) and the denial of the self's reality or importance in the anatman (not-self), as well as imminent and transcendent selves. The social practices in the specific life stages provide place for a special kind of self-realization even on the margin of life in the world. Roland (1988) suggests that the Indian self comprises the person plus their extended family and caste within a "self-we" structure compared with self-regard in the west. The father–son dyad appears ruptured and the mutual esteem enhancement is missing. The film focuses on Baruna/Peggy but the men shown are generally weak, pathetic, and dysfunctional. Pratap is feeble; his father is hen-pecked and retired. The psychiatrists are ineffective and mocked by Baruna when she mimics one and calls him an old fool. This gender dichotomy along with the "split" self Baruna displays at a micro level represents the fracturing of femalehood and fracture of the motherland at macro level. As Roland has distinguished, there are two levels of hier-archical relationships in India, each corresponding to a level of self-feeling. The lower level involves response to the expectations of others, whereas the upper level is the particular self, intimately involved in self-transformation and religious activities. Baruna struggles between the two: At the "we-self" level she is lost because her mother did not allow this aspect of her to develop and her father was missing till she was 18. After marriage, her "we-self" in relationship with in-laws and husband is weak because of the behaviour attributed to her split self. The psychiatrists are struggling to work out these positive/negative values. Bisplighoff and Slingo (1997) point out that Indianization (of American things, in this case Hollywood films) is a sensitively tuned system of adaptation of the plot and structure of an alien original into the anticipated actions and familiar characters of Indian popular films, while overcoming the obstacles imposed by the Indian film censors.

The subject of *The Three Faces of Eve*, mental illness and psychoanalysis, made Indianization of the story somewhat difficult. Nargis may have been influential in the choice of the story and her iconic status allowed her to do so. George (1994) suggests that she personified the elements of 1950s cinema, which related to hope, anxiety, and social concerns of the new country.

CONCLUSIONS

Psychoanalysis and its representation in Hindi films of the 1960s indicate that the filmmakers were prepared to explore newer therapies and methods. Indigenization of Hollywood stories may have been difficult but at that point in the political, social, and film history the filmmakers appeared to be willing to take risks. Furthermore, the conflict between modernity, as represented by psychoanalysis, and traditionalism, as shown by traditional values and households (emphasis on arranged marriage), was evident though resolved somewhat by demonstrating the success of modern interventions. Psychoanalytic emphasis on gender roles, gender role expectations, and male/female and traditional/modern dyad suggest that the nation state was becoming aware of dichotomies and attempting to deal with these.

CHAPTER TEN

Arrival of the new villain

After Nehru's death and Shasti's short-lived premiership, India was still reeling from the effects of the two wars. When Indira Gandhi was elected Prime Minister, public expectations were running high. Morale was beginning to pick up after the Indo-Pak War of 1965 but the economic conditions were deteriorating. Under the circumstances, the Nehruvian dream of socialism was beginning to fade and the public's restlessness was being reflected in the restlessness of the leaders. The syndicate (the old guard in the Congress Party) had "chosen" Indira Gandhi because they saw her as a "dumb doll" and had the notion that they would be able to control her. She defeated them decisively but the early days of her premiership were traumatic for the country's pride. Indira Gandhi was elected because she was Nehru's daughter, had an all-India appeal and a progressive image, and was not identified with any one state, region, caste, or religion (Chandra et al., 2000).

Indira Gandhi's government was faced with several grave problems: political strife in the Punjab and in the North East, economic recession, poor industrial production, and the failure of monsoons to occur. A consequence of the two wars was that defence expenditure rose. The government initially vacillated by being slow in taking decisions and being tardy and ineffective in implementing them. This gave the message to the public that Indira Gandhi was in government but not in power. With the devaluation of the Indian rupee by 35.5%, the people felt abandoned and cheated, partly because they did not understand the true reasons and

161

meaning behind it; the feeling was of being generally let down and losing the value of one's hard-earned currency. The decision to devalue the currency may have been rushed through, reflecting Indira Gandhi's inexperience. However, with time she gained confidence and her subsequent populist measures such as nationalization of banks showed a sure political touch.

The year 1966 was one of continuous popular turmoil, of mass economic discontent and political agitations provoked by spiralling prices, food scarcity, growing unemployment, and, in general, deteriorating economic conditions (Chandra et al., 2000). Rising but unfulfilled expectations of the populace in general—but the middle classes in particular—contributed to an overwhelming feeling of being let down. In the Indian psyche, the uncle (Chacha Nehru) had given way to a mother who was unable to feed her children. The sense of bewilderment was palpable in the country. In addition to repeated agitations, the status of Parliament as an institution started to decline.

The fourth general elections to the Lok Sabha (Lower House or House of the People) were conducted in 1967. Large-scale disenchantment with the ruling party, increasing power of regional parties and their leaders, and factionalism within the ruling party, meant that the Congress returned to power with a marked reduction in majority from 228 to only 48. Having lost eight states, Jan Sangh (the precursor of Bharatiya Janata Party) emerged as the main opposition party in three states and another right wing party, Swatantra, did so in four states. Land reforms in the 1950s had meant that various landowners also ditched Congress and took with them some poor peasants. The 1967 elections also inaugurated the era of coalition governments in many states, which were often unstable and short-lived.

The years 1967–1969 were transitional years in Indian politics, with Indira Gandhi consolidating her position within the party and country in spite of her party's fragile majority in the Lok Sabha. With her expulsion and the subsequent split of the Congress Party in 1969, she came to lead the Congress (Requisitions) Party. Economic recession and problems continued, accompanied by a rise in corruption and black money. Restlessness and increasing discontent among students, the working class and the urban masses developed. Naxalite movements in different parts of the country and the accompanying violence and industrial unrest continued to rise. The political tensions within the ruling party increased, leading to a split between the government and the party, which meant that Indira Gandhi's position within the party was weakening. Such an intraparty struggle was inevitably accompanied by ideological differences, and handling of the economy on the one hand and mounting unrest on the other meant that Indira Gandhi had to look outside her party for support. Having adopted a nonpartisan approach initially, in 1969 with a direct attack on the syndicate over the selection of presidential candidate (she chose V. V. Giri) she sacked Morarji Desai, nationalized banks, and abolished princely privy purses; the latter two measures were enthusiastically welcomed by the masses. After the election of V. V. Giri with her tacit support she was expelled from the Congress Party, establishing a rival organization. When the nationalization of banks was declared invalid by the Supreme Court she called for elections a year ahead of time in February 1971. Chandra et al. (2000) observe that Indira Gandhi had checked the mood of despair, frustration, and cynicism and initiated a climate of hope and optimism. Campaigning on national issues of social change, democracy, socialism and secularism, she had led her party to a two-thirds majority. Working with a coalition of the poor and disadvantaged voters she ensured that the social agenda for change was highlighted and that voters were aware of it.

The 1970s, particularly after the war of 1971, were years of crisis. Politically, waves of popular unrest led to the imposition of the Emergency. Mrs Gandhi and her party lost the elections to a motley coalition of parties called Janata (People's) Party. Even after the Janata party rule, the crisis in the political-judicial-administrative axis led to the context of spiralling inflation, political uncertainty, and the increasing public perception that society and its institutions did not work. Authoritarian versus democratic models allowed the outsider–insider, weak–strong, and rich (politician)–poor (public) comparisons to emerge. Basu, Kak, and Krishen (1981) emphasized that it was Mrs Gandhi's view that social and political institutions were ineffective and ineffectual and a drag on "progress", holding up the strong untrammelled authoritarian rule as a panacea, notwithstanding the fact that it was her reign itself which was responsible for the ineffectual nature of these institutions. The Janata rebuttal, argue Basu et al., was a mere reversal of this postulate that the source of all evil was traced to Mrs Gandhi's authoritarian subversion of democracy, but the Janata argument was weakened because in office it did nothing to dispel the doubt that society and its institutions could in fact work. Basu et al. conclude that in India the 1970s provided a fertile social context in which the myth of strong versus weak was born and nourished, and to which its meanings are addressed.

Immediately after the elections, India got drawn into the civil strife between East Pakistan (Bangladesh) and West Pakistan. Large numbers of East Pakistani refugees sought shelter in India, reaching a number of 10 million. The strategy of preparing for intervention very carefully and also mobilizing international opinion meant that over the following 8 months strategies were in place to deal with the deteriorating situation. The attack by Pakistan in December 1971 gave India an opportunity to respond at both frontiers, and within a fortnight Bangladesh had been liberated. This victory had a number of consequences and the morale of the country was never higher. Some of the old idealism was back. This, coupled with the explosion of an underground nuclear device in 1974, meant that national pride was running high. However, this did not last very long. The restlessness emerged again and there was a marked deterioration in the economic situation, with rampant inflation, increasing unemployment, and scarcity of food; the burden of looking after 10 million refugees was beginning to show. Failure of the monsoons and an increase in world oil prices, coupled with a reduction in foreign-exchange reserves, meant the good feeling that followed the Bangladesh war lasted only a short while. Industrial unrest and railway strife in 1974 contributed to the closure of universities and colleges. The disillusionment of the middle class and the rich peasants further added fuel to the fire of resentment in the populace. J. P. Narayan's call for the police and the army to rebel following unrest in Bihar and Gujarat and the High Court judgement against Indira Gandhi's election further confused the situation. With increasing pressure on her to resign, she declared an Emergency on the grounds that India's stability, security, integrity, and democracy were under threat and that the economic programme was not being allowed to be implemented. The nebulousness of the J. P. Narayan philosophy and ideology and his coming together with communal organizations and parties meant that the political movement he was leading changed its colour and size (see Tandon, 2003, 2006; Deshmukh, 2004).

The agitational movement employed extra constitutional and undemocratic methods. J. P. Narayan believed in party less than democracy and sampoorna kranti (total Revolution) (Chandra et al., 2000). This meant that the rhetoric of Revolution was being encouraged and the aim was the removal of Indira Gandhi. Once again, with her back to the wall, she decided to act decisively by imposing the Emergency by claiming that in view of the extra constitutional changes she was facing she had no other option.

Chandra et al. (2000) point out that in spite of the possibility of other solutions to resolve the impasse, both sides shunned the option of elections which in a democracy are the right and appropriate vehicle for the legitimization of a political regime and for expression of the popular will. It was not surprising that with an imposition of Internal Emergency, leaders of opposition parties were arrested, newspapers were stopped and communal organizations banned. The parliament became ineffective and Sanjay Gandhi and his coterie went on a rampage, with compulsory sterilization, moving people out of their homes and the emasculation of fundamental rights. A key consequence of the Emergency was the holding of unlimited state and party power in the hands of the Prime Minister through a small group of politicians and bureaucrats (see Dhar, 2000).

The initial public response to the imposition of the Emergency was passive acquiescence and support. The general feeling was that such tough measures might help curb corruption and improve the standards of public life. In addition to some intelligentsia being against it, the Emergency started to become unpopular at the beginning of 1976. The initial bewilderment and the fear of the unknown along with curbing of the "rule" of the antisocial elements and against the extreme communal organizations may have helped. With the restoration of public order and discipline, and a reduction in strikes and crime, the universities and colleges returned to normal and a sense of calm prevailed in the country. Improvement and efficiency in government offices was visible and dramatic, and corruption was under control. The economy started to boom again. However, the public's love affair with the Emergency was short-lived.

There were many reasons for this. The government workers felt under pressure, the poor did not see any immediate dramatic change in their lives, the closure of avenues of protest and atmosphere of fear and insecurity may have all contributed to a sense of disillusionment. Trust in the media had evaporated and rumours started to circulate as the power of the police and bureaucracy increased. A denial of civil liberties and harassment on a regular basis further contributed to a sense of exasperation and bewilderment. The legitimacy of the Emergency was being questioned. Sanjay Gandhi's enforced family planning in a country where children are seen as an asset and social security for old age further contributed to a sense of feeling alienated and let down. Although slum clearance and demolition of authorized structures was confined to a few cities only, the rumour machine fed the imagination of people around the country and further contributed to a sense of fear, repression, and abuse of authority. Such a blatant abuse of authority on the part of the mother meant that the populace's resentment started to rise to the surface. The surprise in the elections held in March 1977 was the loss of power by Gandhi and her party. Chandra et al. (2000) offer three possible explanations for the decision to hold elections. First, it would reflect Indira Gandhi's commitment to liberal democracy and democratic values. Second, she was misinformed about the possibility of winning the elections. Third, her victory in elections may well be seen to legitimize her actions in imposing Emergency. Chandra et al. propose that, as the Emergency regime was being discredited, the authorization may have to be obtained by greater legitimacy and political authority acquired through the elections.

The elections led to the trouncing of the Congress Party (in north India in particular, where it acquired only two out of 234 seats in the Lok Sabha, the Lower House). The Congress performed better in the south of India, increasing its number of seats. This may have been a result of pro-poor measures, which were better implemented in the south and generally weaker implementation of the Emergency measures in that area. The new Janata government looked and behaved like the Samyukta Vidhayak Dal governments of Bihar, UP, and Madhya Iradesh during 1967–71, and Dhar (2000) observes that in some ways it was worse because of continued infighting caused by personal ambitions rather than by having any ideological vision.

In the naked grab for power, former enemies were forgotten and new unscrupulous alliances were forged. By the end of 1977 the political momentum had been lost, but the government continued until July 1979. By then the lack of confidence in its ability to govern had turned the public angry. The populace saw the infighting and the inability of the leaders to gather common cause, the lack of progress, and increasing caste tensions and violence. There were growing tensions, increased lawlessness, and violence affecting students. Having rejected the Nehruvian view of industrialization, the governing coalition failed to come up with any alternative ideology and failed to deliver on land reforms. After the first year the economy started to drift, inflation shot up to 20% and the government barely functioned. The aim of its leaders was simply to hold the fragile coalition together and hang on to power.

The Congress witnessed a further split and a revival when Indira Gandhi's faction won majority seats in two assemblies. The continuing harassment of her by the government was seen as a persecution by the population at large and their support for her started to increase. In the middle of 1979, the government fell following a split and elections were held in January 1980. Disenchantment with nongovernance, a lack of vision and incessant neutral egotistic quarrels meant that the voters once again turned to Indira Gandhi, and she returned with a two-thirds majority. Her return also demonstrated that her party could not produce an alternative leadership, thereby coming to consider herself as indispensable to both party and country (Dhar, 2000). The mother was back. The failure to focus on the problems of the country and perhaps her insecurity led her to focus on short-term gains which meant that the alliance had to be rewritten. This led to ill-fated support for Bhindrawale in Punjab which was to have horrendous consequences not only for the country but also for her at an individual level. In almost tit-for-tat on her return to power at the centre she dissolved the assemblies of nine states.

Thus, it is not surprising that the populace's attitudes towards the politicians continued to be a "plague on both your houses".

The increasing poverty and a sense of grievance resulting from high expectations and poor achievements led to alienation from the political process and the general feeling that corruption was beginning to spread among the politicians as well. Until this point there had been very little direct corruption, in that any corruption was at lower levels among bureaucrats—at least the politicians were not directly involved. This too changed with Indira Gandhi when her son Sanjay was given huge amounts of land in neighbouring Haryana, at extremely low prices, to set up his car manufacturing plant.

This potent mixture also reflected the prevalent political climate, in which Indira Gandhi, her son and her cabinet were doing what they wished. The most famous painter of the generation, M. F. Hussain (who started his career by painting film hoardings), painted Indira Gandhi as Durga, the goddess of destruction. This was meant to be a compliment and a demonstration of her strength and her intolerance towards her enemies. This "need" for a messianic leader may be construed as being related to the traditional need for a *mai–baap*, who is supposed to look after the people, as well as the need for a mother figure. The major crises that the country was experiencing (economic deprivation, exploitation, war, and so on) and the resulting sense of personal helplessness allowed people to accept a government which jeopardized their personal liberties.

SHOLAY AND BEYOND

Zanjeer and *Sholay* proved to be two key films of the 1970s. The films *Sholay* and *Deewar*, released in 1975, highlighted the thematic trend wherein the individual has to stand up against the unjust, unyielding and unforgiving system to gain justice. F. Kazmi (1998, p. 137) has argued that conventional Hindi films, unlike great works of art, become subservient to the dominant ideologies since they fail to distance themselves from such ideologies. Instead of challenging the ideological assumptions of their times, they tend to reinforce and perpetuate them.

Mishra (1985) sees films like *Baradari* and *Samrat* as the immediate antecedents of *Zanjeer* with their focus on revenge, which, in the case of *Zanjeer*, is internalized, leading to the dream text in which the importance of *ashva medha* (horse sacrifice) and the *ashvins* (the two-headed gods) in the Indian consciousness and their centrality to Indian mythology are depicted. The image of a horseman on a white horse and the importance of the horse as phallus also leads to its hero being identified with the subtext and all that is being represented. Mishra asserts that any theoretical critique of Bombay cinema must begin with a systemic analysis of the grand Indian metatext and founder of Indian discursivity, namely the *Mahabharata* and *Ramayana*.

Zanjeer is the story of a police officer called Vijay (played by Amitabh Bachchan) who, on a Diwali night, saw his parents being gunned down by the villain. All he can remember is the villain's bracelet and it is this zanjeer (chain) that he sets out to find with the help of his Pathan friend. Going beyond the legal process, he ultimately takes revenge on the villain. Bachchan's character in *Zanjeer* highlighted the frustration and anger of big-city Indian youth. The 1960s, as S. K. Jha (n.d. c) asserts, saw the emergence of a new class of vulgar rich and of a set of people who prospered from shady dealings, while the educated middle class youth struggled. Bachchan's victory over the villain resonated with and provided a catharsis for the anger of every young Indian who felt that similar real-life villains were stealing their own opportunities and future. The superb dialogue, along with Bachchan's mesmerizing performance as a serious, intense, angry young man, made the film a big hit. Banker (2001) sees *Zanjeer* as the film that changed the history of Hindi cinema. The director managed to capture the essence of the angst and seething frustration of a whole generation of young Indian men, who were caught between the dubious glamour of illicit business on the one hand, and waning fields of employment, like agriculture and government jobs, on the other. Although Banker suggests that *Zanjeer* is much less than the sum of its parts and every element of the structure has been surpassed in subsequent films, his observation that "*Zanjeer* is worth watching simply for the emergence of a persona that every Hindi film will take for granted because it traces every step of the development of Vijay, the persona that would capture the imagination of an entire nation" (p. 69), remains entirely valid.

The projection of the persona of Vijay on to Amitabh Bachchan in *Zanjeer* led to the creation of one of the biggest superstars in Hindi cinema, but perhaps more importantly, gave hope to the viewer that Vijay (victory) was somewhere out there and could be theirs too. Mishra (2002) describes the role of Bachchan in *Zanjeer* as that of a renouncer who combines revenge with his ascetic desire. This may explain the minimal role of Jaya Bhaduri, who stands at the periphery of Vijay's vision. The ruthless smuggler was taken as a fact of everyday life, but the hero's anger and violence (although related to childhood trauma) were quite out of proportion and highlighted his anger at the system's failure to deliver justice (Bakshi, 1998, p. 121).

F. Kazmi (1998, p. 138) notes that even though *Sholay* initially spent a couple of shaky weeks at the box office after its release, it went on to create history, becoming the first film ever in Hindi cinema to gross more than one crore (10 million) rupees in each territory in which it was released in its initial run (normally calculated for the first 18 months after release). In the next 15 years, another 12 films reached this milestone and of all the 12 films, 10 films centred on the theme of rebellion. Another five films were hits, even though they did not reach this mark.

Interestingly, *Sholay* is also a film that has been studied at length by filmologists and critics (see Dissanayake & Sahai, 1992; Chopra, 2001). The curry western is not a misnomer at all in this case. The film highlights not only a rural idyll disturbed by a dacoit, but also asserts the kinship and extended joint family system in a feudal setting, in which everyone knows his place and the patriarch is allowed to lord over the village.

The villain in this film is "the other", in that he is not embedded in the context. He represents pure evil; there is no guilt, no remorse and no sense of shame. His dialogue became so popular that cassettes of the film's dialogues were sold in millions. The film portrays the feudal system, but the villain, unlike previous villains, is motivated by pure greed and not by anything as complex as unrequited love or a sense of social justice. He has shades of the classic psychopath, who is not redeemable. In *Sholay*, the villain (called Gabbar Singh and played by Amjad Khan) epitomizes what I would call the "new" villain.

In their cultural reading of *Sholay*, Dissanayake and Sahai (1992) high-light, among other factors, the impact of Hollywood on Hindi cinema. *Sholay* was a curry western and not only reflected the time but was influ-enced by *The Magnificent Seven*. A feature common to all westerns is the conflict between law and lawlessness and how it is inscribed.

The story is based in a village called Ramgarh, where a retired police officer, the Thakur (a title) Baldev Singh (Sanjeev Kumar), resides with his daughter-in-law (Jaya Bhaduri) and a servant. The villain, along with his gang, keeps attacking the village in order to collect tithe. Gabbar has already been arrested and sentenced to prison in the past by the Thakur when he was a police officer, but he had managed to escape. He goes on to shoot down the entire family of the Thakur, who happen to be away at the time. His younger daughter-in-law escapes as she was at the temple.

The Thakur chases Gabbar and has his hands chopped off by the villain. In order to avenge his family and arrest the villain, he contacts his friends in the police to learn the whereabouts of two petty crooks who had impressed him in the past. They had looked after him once when was he injured and had not escaped despite having an opportunity to do so. The Thakur then invites them and agrees to pay them if they deliver Gabbar Singh alive to him. The two crooks, Jai (Amitabh Bachchan) and Veeru (Dharmendra), initially take on the responsibility so that they can escape with the Thakur's money. However, they gradually settle down, largely because Veeru falls in love with a woman, Basanti (Hema Malini), who drives a tonga (a two-wheeled carriage). Meanwhile, Jai falls in love with the widowed daughter-in-law Radha (Jaya Bhaduri) who responds, though the two always keep a distance from each other. Gabbar Singh sends his gang members to collect their dues from the villagers, but Veeru and Jai manage to chase them away.

Once they return to the hideout, Gabbar Singh shoots the gang members because of their failure to bring in the money. Gabbar Singh attacks the village during the celebration of the festival of Holi and barely manages to escape. In a dramatic scene, Jai and Veeru discover that the Thakur has no arms. Once they get to know the full story, they give their full allegiance to him and stop worrying about the payment. Enraged, they attack Gabbar, but he manages to escape. In retaliation, he kills the only son of the village Imam, who is on his way to the city. Gabbar sends the body back to the village, then demands that Jai and Veeru be handed over to him. However, following an impassioned plea by the Imam, Veeru and Jai stay on. The stage for the final confrontation and resolution of the conflict is set. Jai and Veeru kill four of Gabbar's men. Jai is killed in the shoot-out. Basanti is kidnapped by Gabbar, who, in another sadistic gesture, asks her to dance on broken glass to save Veeru's life. Veeru is winning in a hand-to-hand combat with Gabbar when the Thakur comes in, seeking his revenge. The climax comes when the Thakur hurts Gabbar and hands him over to the police.

As noted above, the imposition of the Emergency marked the start of the breakdown of consensual politics and the rise of confrontational politics. However, though this brand of confrontational politics was based heavily on repressive and coercive measures, its true nature was carefully shielded (F. Kazmi, 1999, p. 97). Kazmi goes on to argue that Indira Gandhi made a virtue of the antidemocratic act of declaring Emergency by arguing that the special powers under it were essential for her to identify the powerful "antinational" and "antisocial" elements or, put differently, the villains. If you do not have villains, you have to create them, as is done in films and literature. It was a case of real life imitating art here.

F. Kazmi (1999, pp. 98–100) puts forward the theory that the success of *Sholay* has to be seen in the context of the contemporary political climate and economic factors. Caste and class violence were projected on to the dacoits, Gabbar Singh representing one such dacoit. The establishment refused to see that the cause of this violence lay in the unjust, unjustified and unjustifiable system and, instead, projected it as a law and order problem, little realizing that the problem was created by the system itself. The definition of the psychopath in a similar way represents exactly that.

The village depicted in the film is a microcosm of society, in which the Thakur is the benevolent feudal landlord, the head of a joint family and also of the extended village family. The rich and poor coexist happily, and Hindus and Muslims live together without rancour, helping each other out. This rural idyll is disrupted by the entry of the villain, who can perhaps be considered to represent the "phoren hand" repeatedly suggested by Indira Gandhi. The next parallel is that she then uses her son Sanjay as a hero to clear up the mess. The allegory may be invidious, but the fact remains that the success of the film was astounding.

At one level, *Sholay* is a very simple film about good guys and bad guys, revenge and action. Around the dominant theme of revenge, the film weaves a number of subplots and episodes to carry the narrative forward and make it interesting (F. Kazmi, 1999, p. 97). The phenomenal success of the film was not due to its novelty value alone, but also to the dialogue. The dialogue was such a hit that it was played at weddings, social events, fairs, and festivals. Gabbar Singh was the new villain who, despite being ruthless and devoid of guilt or shame, caught the public imagination in a way that no previous villain had. This appreciation did not mean that he was not considered evil; the source of the appreciation was the fact that he represented the collective frustration of the masses. Dissanayake and Sahai (1992, p. 59) argue that his success was due to the fact that the element of spectacle predominated over that of the narrative in a way which had not been attempted in earlier Indian melodramas, and the audiences were "able to draw a distinction between the performative and constantive dimensions of the film's discourse". The audience applauded the villain in spite of his being morally depraved and despicable.

The character of Gabbar Singh represents a clinical case of psychopathy. He has no roots; we are not told what makes him the way he is and why he behaves the way he does. He is sadistic and shoots people not always in self-defence, but to teach them a lesson. He kills insects, with effort and without remorse. His violence is needless and glamorized. When he shoots down the Thakur's entire family, including a young child, the expression on his face is bland and blunt. The self-centred look in Gabbar's eyes is contrasted with the terror in the child's eyes. The subsequent chopping off of the Thakur's arms is presented in a new and startling way, unlike the images seen in previous Hindi films. Gabbar Singh is totally alone and isolated, and seen as such. The characteristics of the personality, his behaviour and his actions will reach a clinical diagnosis of psychopathy.

The violence is totally mindless and casual, not only on the psychopath's part, but on the part of the police officers and the two crooks as well. The two heroes have a casual and *laissez-faire* attitude to violence. They go about their job with a professional and detached cynicism. Jai is sullen, quiet, withdrawn, and seething with a controlled rage. Amitabh Bachchan plays the role again and these traits later became his hallmark. Death is of no consequence to Jai and Veeru, who are rootless in the same way that Gabbar is. There is no mention of their families or past, so the audience is given no idea about why they became what they did. At that level, they are not dissimilar to Gabbar because they, too, act outside the law even though the ex-police officer is their employer. They, however, have the capacity to fall in love, whereas Gabbar is shown to fancy dance girls (read: prostitutes), and this difference may make them worthy of redemption. Another difference is that they are able to demonstrate to the villagers that they are on their side. However, overall, the characteristics of the heroes and the villain are not too dissimilar. The success of this film consolidated Amitabh Bachchan's image as the angry young man.

Dissasnayake and Sahai (1992, p. 63) posit:

The lack of comforting narratives which offer the security of stable logics, the phenomenon of the social order being constantly undercut by ambiguities of meaning and the absence of human feeling and the concomitant devaluation of human life, which are dramatized in the film, work at the level of national analytics as well. This film in its own melodramatic way brings out a social thematic that has a deep relevance to Indian society as a whole.

Das Gupta (2002) emphasizes that most of the Amitabh Bachchan films of the 1970s and 1980s are inherently anticonstitutional. The hero takes the law into his hands because of the indefensible delays in the delivery of justice. Personal revenge gives greater satisfaction and the attitude is one of grab what you can, since honesty does not pay. The family is the only valid social unit. As there is no search for a means to change the system, judicial or societal, the "learned" helplessness means that an active hero or saviour is required. The growth of individualism during that period legitimized this approach. As Das Gupta says, the Bachchan figure emerges time and again among the oppressed to become the saviour. His anger is not of the rebel, but is born out of violence. However, the saviour provides a way out, even if it is only a fantasy. In the avenging woman films, the perception of the saviour is taken to its logical extreme; the avenging woman is idolized because the Hindu pantheon not only allows it, but also actively encourages it. The distinctions between male and female avenging are also related to the role of social units, e.g., family and the social expectations.

Das Gupta (2002) also raises the interesting question of why violence appeals to the lumpen (i.e., the proletariat), but more importantly why now and why here. His answer is that Bachchan provides a model of action for those who have been wronged and denied opportunities they feel are rightfully theirs, and those whose talents and abilities have been ignored by a ruthless, unfeeling world. However, the attraction to violence may have diverse roots. First, it is entirely possible that violence started gaining greater legitimacy as crime rates increased. Second, since the people were frustrated at not being able to do anything, the idea of an external marginalized individual doing the fighting for them was appealing. Third, the projection of the ill feeling of the marginal "other" is readily acceptable. As Das Gupta points out, these aspects became abundantly evident later, after Bachchan's election as an MP (which made him a part of the establishment) when he went to Assam to support his party and people threw stones at him during a rally (perhaps they felt let down by the fact that he was no longer a rebel). Thus, paradoxically, the people elected their much-worshipped rebel hero to power, yet rejected him at the personal level, besides rejecting his film persona.

Vasudev (1988) notes that, in addition to the weight of tradition for Hindu women to behave like mythological heroines and characters, the hypocrisy of the male in the Victorian mould, which still exists, leads to an expectation that women would be allowed to love but this love will be pure, all-consuming, and eternal. Even the prostitute is to subscribe to this convention. Although the male gaze expects their women to behave in an orthodox way, such an expectation is controlled not necessarily by the viewer but the creators of the film. In the past two decades or so, many female directors such as Aparna Sen, Sai Paranjpe, Kalpana Lajmi, Deepa Mehta, Mira Nair, Gurinder Chadha, Farah Kham, etc., have emerged. It will be interesting to see how, in the long run, this development may change the portrayal of the female on the screen.

Karanjia (1982) suggests that the early categorization of Indian women into heroine and vamp has transmogrified into different forms but keeps the same characteristics. The reasons for this change in cinema's attitude to women are related to a relative lack of female creators. Nandy (1981) observes that the portrayal of womanhood shows the traditional Indian's fragmented image of the woman. He highlights that continuous psychological attempts to split off the bad women and to depsychologize the problem by turning these women into an external sociological differentiation: Cantankerous mothers-in-law and cabaret dancing vamps all indicate an attempt to place such women outside the acceptable limits of bicultural living (i.e., outside the optimal mixture of tradition and modernity). Nandy identifies another social function of the Bombay film: its ability to act as an interface between the traditions of the Indian society and the disturbing modernity of western intrusions into it. Thus, the Hindi film gives cultural meaning to western structures imposed on the society, demystifies some of the culturally unacceptable structures in India, and ritually neutralizes those elements of the modern world that have to be accepted for reasons of survival. Mishra (1985) classifies the stereotypes into that of the mother, the renouncer, and the man of the world and what the parallel text indicates. Viswanath (2002) suggests that women authenticate cultural identity and the family is a significant social unit in the rhetoric of the Hindu right, hence it is the female who carries the burden. The rigid hierarchy and the personal, social, and spiritual spaces all come together in the household. Hence, all the major hits of the 1990s, *Hum Aapke Hain Kaun*, *Kuch Kuch Hota Hai*, and *Hum Dil De Chuke Sanam* portray huge houses with the family structures intact and dictating to the youngsters. The female identity is constituted within and through the family. The 1990s films have targeted the NRI (Non Resident Indian) market but have shown consistently that tradition is better than modernity and Hindutva (a political ideology with beliefs in Hindu superiority) is better than foreigners are.

The vitalizing power of the women characters is often ignored (Mathur, 2002). Mathur argues that the role of a good mother is trivialized in Indian cinema. She notes (p. 67), "This silent suffering, stoic species is so distressingly deified on celluloid that by the end of the movie you are convinced that these faces will soon be upon postage stamps." The space between a strong woman, real life and her portrayal gives paradoxical messages to the spectator.

F. Kazmi (1999, pp. 99–100) offers an interesting insight by pointing out that *Sholay* presents things from the perspective of the marginalized (the crooks), the survival sector (the villagers), and the injured and the wronged (the Thakur). The Thakur was being punished by the villain because he was doing his duty with zeal. Kazmi suggests that these two features, namely that of everyone being vulnerable to the dacoit or anyone on the wrong side of the law, and the problems involved in taking one's job too seriously, are bound to appeal to a large number of people. The moneyed feudal landlord ignores his ex-colleagues and takes charge of protecting his villagers and avenging the deaths of his family members. The two crooks, although ruthless, are shown as selfless individuals who care for others and eventually give up the idea of stealing and/or making money from their commission. Thus, their pathology is reduced. Their visions of settling down to have children and a family give them a human angle, unlike the psychopathic villain. The latter remains less than human. He is cowardly and attacks defenceless people, treating them like insects. After confronting and capturing the Thakur, he chains him and, in that position, hacks off his arms. The name given to the villain is nonspecific, and says nothing about his background, caste, or religion. The distinction between the two sides is stark: The dwellings of "the other" outside the village are brown, ugly, and terrifying, as are the individuals there, whereas the protagonists are human, humane, colourful, and joyous.

Kazmi (1999, p. 112) points out an interesting aspect of the film, that everyone is essentially alone, without a full-fledged, normal family life. This feeling of loneliness, of a fractured existence, becomes even more poignant when contrasted against the image of the complete and perfect family (that of the Thakur). Whereas the dacoits are loners anyway, Jai's and Veeru's (and, implicitly, Basanti's and Radha's) need for support and settling down also reflects the common person's dilemma about wanting individualism (which may well be equated with loneliness) in a sociocentric society. This paradox is evident in other aspects of the film as well. An example is the individual's (Jai's or Veeru's) need for friendship and recognition, as against his fundamental loneliness (portrayed when Veeru drinks and Jai plays the mouth organ).

In a survey of 159 males and 69 females, Dissanayake and Sahai (1992, p. 70) found that nearly 80% of the respondents found *Sholay* entertaining. Detailed interviews revealed that a majority of them enjoyed it because it related to their lives and hopes. Dissanayake and Sahai emphasized the role of social modernization and how it impinges on the values, belief systems, and lifestyles prevalent in traditional societies. It can be argued that the success of *Sholay* reflected the externalization of the inner psychological conflicts of the audience and handled their internal passions, which had been generated by the social and political process, as Nandy (1981) says.

Simply put, Gopalan (2002) argues, critics take a moralistic view of mainstream cinema, seeing little of what makes it popular; filmmakers see themselves as populist entertainers, whereas they see the critics as elitists, whose opinions rarely count in the workings of the industry. Thus, the popular culture is frowned upon and snobbery undermines any serious reading of the same. *Sholay* exemplifies the possibility of combining dominant genre principles developed in Hollywood films with conventions peculiar to Indian cinema (Gopalan, 2002). However, this is not the first film to do so but is the first in combining a western/cowboy genre with Hindi film excesses. This combination has to be seen in both a core and peripheral activity. The story of dacoits is not new but the threat to the rural idyll from gun culture and the import of similar forces to deal with the psychopaths is stunning.

Varde (n.d.) sees *Sholay* as the most popular film of the millennium. The film resembles *The Magnificent Seven* and *Mera Gaon Mera Desh*. The director made sure that each of his characters had relevant scenes and good footage. All the principal actors in the film came up with their career-best performances. Sanjeev Kumar was spectacular, Dharmendra brilliant, Bachchan walked away with all the sympathy, Jaya Bhaduri gave a silent but strong performance, while Amjad Khan was probably the most feared character even in Hindi films. In spite of censorship problems and poor draws at the box office initially, the film became a box office phenomenon. Varde saw this as a special film.

"If you had to see just one Hindi film in your life, just one, then see *Sholay*. It's deservedly considered the most perfect Hindi film ever made", says Banker (2001, p. 73). He alludes to the contention of other critics that innovation in Hindi films stopped after *Sholay*. Banker notes that not only is *Sholay* a magnificent spectacle, it also uses all the clichéd conventions and yet somehow manages to reinvent them. Packed with unforgettable characters, the film has great moments, to which Banker attributes its enduring popularity.

Themes of lawlessness, violence, vandalism, oppression, and exploitation were all articulated around the "new" villains, who became the hub of nastiness. This nastiness was markedly different from the previous villainy, in that the "new" villain was irredeemable. He worked outside the social constraints and rules. He might get his well-deserved punishment, but was generally not redeemed.

With the villain's characteristics becoming more prominent and outlandish, the audience started to empathize with the long-suffering, brooding, quiet hero, personified by Amitabh Bachchan. F. Kazmi (1998, p. 152) postulates that as these assertions became a matter of public knowledge or common sense, they also began to form the basis of a hardening of attitudes, publicly and politically, with the media recommending a legitimization of authoritarian solutions to social problems.

Several repressive laws were passed under the Emergency. These included the Terrorist and Disruptive Activities Bill, which gave unlimited powers to the police. These repressive bills resulted in an unlimited growth in gangsterism and parallel government. F. Kazmi (1998, p. 153) argues that historically, the concept of parallel government represented a challenge to the established government, with which it was necessarily in an adversarial position. The opposition parties became a parallel government supporting the existing authority: The genuine government appeared to have lost its moral authority. The government was attempting to trace the sources of all problems to clear-cut villains (terrorists, extremists, the foreign hand, smugglers, etc.), and then let the state machinery have a go at them to wipe them out. The chief aim of the 20 Point Plan let loose on the nation by Indira Gandhi and her acolytes was to protect the country from "phoren hands" and in the process justify all murders, massacres, and the suppression of rights. The president of the Congress Party, Deokant Barooah, went so far as to claim that "Indira was India and India was Indira", thus legitimizing any deed (legal or otherwise) committed to protect the honour of the state. This encouraged the citizens to tell on others, protect themselves, and take the law into their own hands. With the state encouraging vigilantism to fight its enemies, this theme became a recurrent one in Hindi cinema. The basic assumption of these films was that if the "legal State" was as strong as the "alternative" one (read: vigilante groups), there would be no problem in society (F. Kazmi, 1998, p. 153). Hence, once the heroes restored the original order, they either surrendered or were caught by the legal state.

The vigilante groups achieved what the legal state was unable to because the former worked in a more flexible manner, outside the legal framework, and had a greater degree of manoeuvrability. For them, the law, rules, rights, morality, and regulations did not count at all. The loose and immoral state had fallen in love with the vigilante, who reciprocated this love, and the political and cinematic discourses over the next 20 years or so ran a parallel course. The vigilantes needed the government and the state which, in turn, needed the former.

The irony is that this phenomenon by now has been legitimized in the Hindi-speaking states such as Uttar Predesh and Bihar. Former and active criminals have sometimes been elected to the state legislative assembly or the Lower House at the centre. They maintain their own private armies to frighten the public while the state leadership and authorities conveniently look away. This legitimization of corruption and the value of private armies are now embedded even deeper in the Indian psyche. The caste system and the backdrop of feudal landlords have only fanned its fires. Despite all this, the distinction between the hero as a villain and the villain as a villain has become more rigid. At another level, the former is still redeemable, whereas the latter is not.

Popular cinema met the challenge by recognizing the evil, finding an innocuous scapegoat (who was almost always an individual) and then having the system purged of the evil through an individual act of valour (N. Kazmi, 1996, p. 19). "The other" has never been seen as being outside the system. The existence of the "other" in cinema and elsewhere depends on how "the other" is defined. I would maintain that "the other" in the sense of Foucauldian "other" might not exist, but "the other" who is a protagonist for or against the viewer, against whom the story is measured, is extremely valid and important. However, "the other" in terms of mental illness remains an outsider, especially if one chooses the model of western classification and focuses on psychopathic disorder, which has been defined earlier. In the context of Hindi films, the psychopathy focuses on characters who show no regret at all for their wrongdoings.

F. Kazmi (1998, p. 151) says,

> Our fascination is not with crime but with the construction of a disruption, for if crime were presented in the abstract—devoid of personality, motivation and resolution—it would lose much of its popular appeal. In crime fiction, the audience is positioned in a narrative which explains the actions of its characters and constructs an outcome that we "expect" from the unfolding of the tensions in the narrative. Themes of lawlessness, anarchy, violence and exploitation are linked with villains who have to be dealt with.

In other words, the people were looking for a father figure or a super hero who could meet their needs and allow them to become dependent. N. Kazmi (1996, p. 33) suggests that the need for a messianic leader seems to be an intrinsic part of the psyche of the middle class man. The argument here is that in a patriarchal set-up, it is the father who knows best.

Insaaf ka Tarazu, directed by B. R. Chopra, antedates the avenging woman films by a decade or more. Gopalan (2002) points out that the two scenes in the beginning of the film juxtapose rape against representations of India. The heroine is called Bharati (the feminine name for India in Hindi) and although the allegory of the beleaguered nation-state is set out it is not followed through. B. R. Chopra, a journalist by training, has a well-deserved reputation for making films with social scenes. His *Naya Daur* was set in the man-versus-machine context at a time when India was rapidly moving towards industrialization. It is highly unlikely that he was not aware of the allegory. *Insaaf ka Tarazu* came a few years after the Emergency, which had set all kinds of forces loose, and the film reflected the state's failure to look after its vulnerable members. Das Gupta (1991) points out that since the purity of women is considered of paramount importance, the rapist as a polluter has to be punished in films, but in the earlier films such punishment used to be divine. From the 1980s onwards, women themselves started taking revenge, as the males around them were impotent. Also, since good girls cannot shame the family by talking about the rape and justice does not deliver, they must take things into their own hands. *Insaaf ka Tarazu* depicts the plight and trauma of a raped woman who, rather than going into a depression or a catatonic state, externalizes her anger, which makes her truly dangerous. The fact that her personal history is exposed in the open court means her self-esteem, ego, and respect are attacked, and the acquittal of her rapist demands justice on behalf of the audience (Prabhu, 2001). Once again, it is a comment on the state of women and the justice meted out (or denied?) them in a patriarchal society where rape is the right of the male. The idealization of womanhood in the film is worship of the virgin embodying Indian womanhood. Both of the sisters are strong and independent, which is obviously what makes them a threat to the male ego who, in the collective sense, sides with one of his own and abandons them. Models on the ramp are dolls decorated for the male eye and represent unethical, loose, available women. This availability is not only for visual pleasure but also for bodily pleasure. Chatterji (1998) notes that both rape scenes in *Insaaf ka Tarazu* were choreographed in detail and the lasting psychosocial impact of these representations was more derogatory to the image and ideology of women as human beings. Reflective of sexual conditions of modern India, rape films make spurious claims to document reality in order to negate accusations of exploitation, but they are exploitative. In films such as *Doosri Seeta*, *Ghar*, *Grahan*, and *Hum Paanch*, among others, the heroine goes "mad" or becomes depressed after being raped. In *Ghar*, the heroine withdraws into herself after a gang rape and, despite her husband's attempts to be sympathetic, her view of herself becomes negative and leads to attempted suicide at least twice.

Das Gupta (1991) asserts that Hinduism is the only religion in the world that declares a woman unfit to be married or to remain married if she has already been touched (or seen/thought to have been). Such a woman is considered impure. The example of Sita in the *Ramayana* is a case in point. The concept of the ritual impurity of food is extended to women, implying that a woman is an item of consumption. This subjugation of the female leads to the strengthening of bonds amongst the males. The male bonding compounds the exclusion or marginalization of the female. Das Gupta notes that in the Bachchan films of the 1970s and 1980s there is a clear psychological relationship between misogyny and male bonding.

As Bachchan obtains justice for the wronged (more often for himself), women are purely incidental and decorative. They are present for the purpose of dalliance and to highlight his heterosexuality. The success of these films may also have contributed to the rise of the female revenge films of the late 1980s, which reflected changing times.

The theme of revenge was not new. However, popular cinema was responding to the mounting disillusionment and cynicism that swept India after Nehru (Das Gupta, 1991). The anger and frustration mounted when Indira Gandhi, in her second incarnation as the prime minister, failed to live up to the public's great expectations of her and of her Garibi Hatao (remove poverty) programme. The male audience applauded the female protagonists seeking revenge in films like *Pratighaat*, *Zakhmi Aurat*, and *Be-Abroo*, some of whom were avenging their rape. Rape as shown in Hindi cinema is voyeuristic and, at times, meant for the titillation of its male audience. The attitude is clearly one of ambivalence: The male viewer "enjoys" the humiliation of the heroine, yet he also sees in her the mother goddess Kali avenging all males. In the 1970s films, the macho man did not go around hunting for women, because they fall at his feet. The distinction between avenging man and avenging woman is the distinction between society and individual honours. Men fight for social justice, although they themselves may be its symbol, but women fight to avenge personal honour.

A reviewer, Jha (n.d. b), saw *Deewar* as a slick and unforgettable adaptation of *Mother India* and *Ganga Jamuna*. *Deewar* is the ultimate product of the angry young man saga. The protagonist is full of soundless fury and his anger is so inwardly drawn that the viewer fears for his metabolism and blood pressure, noted the critic. Played by Amitabh Bachchan, the hero, Vijay, comes through as one of the most wounded heroes since Guru Dutt's Vijay in *Pyaasa*. Stylishly structured, the film conveys tremendous emotional forces that keep the drama going. Upholding old-fashioned morality, it equates wealth and material luxury with evil and negativity. Vijay's agnostic rebellion and his ultimate devoutness seem to echo the mood of anger and protest during the dreaded Emergency.

The critic notes that in both *Sholay* and *Deewar*, the hero fights personal and interpersonal demons from the wrong side of the law without seeming to twist the laws of morality beyond the conventional boundaries. Bachchan is described as being gloriously rebellious and frighteningly lonely, and as having amazingly intense eyes that seem to burn anyone who crosses his path. The direction never flounders at any level, and each component, character and shot division in the screenplay is dictated by the plot. The cinematographer is lauded for the dark, murky interiors, which have a startling authenticity. The only poor aspect is the music.

Banker (2001) suggests that the release of *Deewar* at a particularly delicate point in Indian history (which he compares to the McCarthy hearings in the US in the 1950s), when the public and producers were careful not to offend the powers that be, was aimed at giving a subliminal message. The director and writers took great care to criticize the bad guy but glamorized him. In *Deewar* for example, Vijay has a posh house, big cars, and a glamorous lifestyle, but his loneliness and that of his girlfriend is marked. Banker asserts that the device of glamour was used brilliantly to mirror the frustration of the country's working class as well. Vijay was the ideal representative of middle class aspirations, of the young, educated people who were struggling to eke out a living in a corrupt system. Meanwhile, the dishonest folk, including the police and politicians, enjoyed their ill-gotten gains. Banker emphasizes that his encounters with people in Bombay during that period attested to the fact that Vijay's frustrations were real and genuine. He also suggests that the rehabilitation of Haji Mastan, on whom the character of Vijay was said to have been based, indicated that the system had truly broken down. Banker urges the viewer to see this film, as it is a good reflection of the India of the dark and hopeless 1970s.

Zanjeer and *Deewar* consolidated the angry young man image: The hero was withdrawn and bent on revenge, not in an obviously angry manner, but in a cold, calculated rage. This reflected his isolation from the world and his loneliness, which was depicted clearly. He would not allow people to come too close to him because he was a smouldering cauldron—aggressive but unsophisticated, roguish but not cold, characteristics N. Kazmi (1996, p. 51) calls essentially all-male.

Ideologically, he is not against the law and it is only at times that he is fighting the establishment or government. Mostly, he fights evil as personified by the smuggler. At the end, he returns to his mother—dead or alive—which suggests and reflects his redemption. The polarization of the haves and have-nots is personified in several of Bachchan's films; his persona is reflective of the have-nots and calls for levelling off the inequality.

In his book *The Mass Psychology of Fascism*, Reich (1950) argues that fascism is an expression of the irrational structure of man. When the masses start looking at their aspirations and see themselves as belonging to such a mass, individuals pull together, creating a tidal wave from which a leader emerges. The reasons why people followed Hitler were many, but Reich argues that the success of Nazism lay primarily in the fact that it was supported by a mass movement and a key reason for such support was mass unemployment and poor economic conditions. Although rather simplistic, his analysis suggests that the more helpless the mass individual became (owing to his upbringing), the more pronounced was his identification with the Führer, and the greater was his childish need for protection, which was disguised by feeling of being at one with the Führer.

The texts of the films churned out by Hindi film studios in the late 1970s and throughout the 1980s were all about the characters and hardly about the plot (Sardar, 1998, p. 49). The focus increasingly shifted to the individual, their only substantive motivation being revenge. Society disappeared into a nebulous background and social justice (doled out by the establishment) was replaced with implausible, ridiculous scenarios about the avenging of personal wrongs. The angry young man personified by Amitabh Bachchan generally ignored morality (which had been instilled in him by his long suffering mother), but eventually either died or was brought to justice at the end of the film. Revenge was the most important motive and Sardar (p. 50) calls it a primeval value. The discourse of the Hindi film is limited to issues of power and survival, and violence is projected as a necessary instrument for achieving both.

The changes in the structure of the films in 1980s and 1990s have additional reasons in the way society was changing. Some of these changes are linked with the rise of Hindu fundamentalism, the persecution of Muslims, the marginalization of other Indian minorities, the fissures in and figments of the Indian psyche, and the role of western values. The obsession with revenge may be seen as a reflection of the struggle of Hindi cinema itself to fight for its rightful place in the perceptions of the people. In a study of rural people, Johnson (2000) was able to demonstrate that when television arrived in the villages, time started being defined by television programmes. He noted that the people would wake up and go to sleep according to when telecasts began and ended. The presence of television not only reduced conversation in the family, but women and men began to interact more publicly.

No cultural, social, or broader economic factors are ever shown as a cause. It is as if there is just one man against the machinery symbolized by the evil (the evil of gaining worldly goods and material possessions), whatever the guise. The capitalist versus labour struggle is a major one, often highlighted at the climax of these films. The hero remains cold but human, alone but not without family, and redeems himself in more ways than one. The Bachchan persona of the 1970s and 1980s gave way to a new persona in the 1990s—a new kind of ruthless villain.

Gopalan (2002) follows the line of avenging women and draws a clear distinction between the precipitating act and the revenge. She argues that the rape scenes, although graphic at times and symbolic at others, and the ability of these films to evoke horror, may be the major reason why others followed suit. In some of the films, the storyline is absolutely simplistic. In spite of censorship norms and strategies, the female body is still shown as an object. The rape scenes are violent and intrusive, and objectify the women even further. In *Pratighaat* and *Anjaam*, the figure of the mother goddess, Durga, provides scope for the protagonist to find a respectable way out. Leaving aside films like *Bawander*, in which a low-caste village woman is raped and has to go all the way to Delhi to seek justice, the shortcut taken by most of these films is to allow the protagonist to explode in anger. The role of women in the social order has to be taken on board if this avenging creature is to be understood.

In a sense, the popular Hindi cinema of the 1970s and 1980s explored the primordial Nietzschian belief in the existence of men and super men, the herd and the heroes, by creating the persona of a superhero. However, interestingly, and perhaps paradoxically, this persona also incorporated the human (fallible, loveable) component on one side and the irredeemable inhuman individual as the psychopath on the other side.

Like *Damini*, *Grahan* was also a film with the theme of justice. The story involves the rape of a woman by the son of the Chief Minister of a state. On hearing this, the Chief Minister dies and his daughter becomes the Chief Minister (art imitating real life). Her lover, an astute dynastic and able lawyer, defends the rapist by proving the rape victim to be a girl of loose character but is unaware of her innocence. This leads to her becoming insane and, when she recovers after being treated, her potential in-laws refuse to accept her. The rape victim shoots the rapist after the elections and the lawyer then defends her. The film was seen to have an ennobling theme but was viewed as dull with a slow pace. The drama was noted to be a switch on/switch off type. The acting honours were mixed and the technical aspects were seen as fair.

On a similar theme is *Ghar*, where the heroine becomes mute after a rape. A newly married wife is raped and she has to face the world with this blemish. The method she and her husband use to overcome this tragedy is shown as delicate and moving. The reviewer for *Picture Post* (1976) praised this as an offbeat movie that was well made and well acted, but noted that the story might not appeal to the ladies and family audiences.

The aftermath of rape explored in *Ghar* indicates the psychological implications of gang rape on a newly married woman who withdraws into herself and stops "feeling". Tellingly, the film was a flop at the box office, underscoring the fact that rape in cinema is indeed a titillating instrument of entertainment; the sex-starved and sex-hungry Indian audience is just not interested in psychology but only in graphic visuals (Chatterji, 1998, p. 159). Chatterji (p. 160) notes that a filmic text often gets transformed from a serious film to a titillating one by a set of institutional procedures where text and context start to diverge. The expectations of the viewer and the distributor may well differ from those of the author and the director, and the manipulation of the visual images may change the meaning of the film as well.

Bikram Singh in *Filmfare* saw *Ghar* as a half-hearted attempt to deal with the shattering trauma under which the victim continues to reel for a long time after the event. The story was plausible and the heroine's catatonic state after the outrage also leads her to believe that she is too unclean to resume normal relations with her husband. The director was criticized for not marshalling the resources of the camera, though he was praised for dealing with the heroine's hallucinations and snatches of memory. The acting of the heroine was praised, although overall the film scored two stars out of five by *Filmfare*.

Sadma, a remake of the Tamil film *Moondram Pirai*, is the story of a teenage girl who regresses to childhood following a road-traffic accident. A schoolteacher is visiting a brothel with a friend of his where the girl has been forcibly taken. Left alone in the dingy room, she reacts violently; the teacher notices the fright in her eyes and eventually takes her away from the brothel and looks after her. When she recovers her memory, she refuses to recognize him. The reviewer in *Movietitle* praised the direction and the acting, whereas Pradhan in *Filmfare* felt the acting made the film soar. The relationship between the two was noted to be similar to that of the prostitute and the madman in *Khilona*. The latter ended happily, but *Sadma* does not; and whereas the relationship of the protagonists was sexual in *Khilona*, it was emotional in *Sadma*.

CONCLUSIONS

The lawless 1970s and early 1980s gave direction to revenge films and the revenge was both male and female. Males were lonely rootless characters, whereas females even in their family settings demonstrated that males supposedly looking after them were impotent, inadequate, and weak. The trauma of rape was a reflection of the rape of the nation and the fact that the general populace had no one to rely on except themselves to obtain any comfort. The role of trauma in developing emotional and psychological disorders became more populist and evident.

CHAPTER ELEVEN

Rootless 1980s and fundamentalist 1990s

Masood (1982) states that the films of 1981–82 had a new rootless hero, self-parody, and success as a reward for being smart (but perhaps not too smart): "Exactly the mixture that the doctor prescribed for the huge uprooted urban 'proles' which will also keep them in the lumpen state they are in" (p. 11). In the 1980s the old family dramas, which had an easygoing spontaneous charm, gave way to aggressively conservative and frantic worship of divinities. Hindi films showed individual violence which however never endangered the social status quo.

Basu et al. (1981) analyse the films by using binary oppositions from a myth. The coding of particular genre of films was rich/poor, inside/outside society and strong/weak. They argue that in the late 1970s, with the advent of multi-starrer films, each film had a group of heroes, who shared strong emotional ties but did not always have family links, and who were exceptionally able and yet outsiders, whereas heroines were unorthodox and paired up with heroes. When alone, both hero and heroine were vulnerable, whereas the villains headed powerful organizations and preyed on society but harmed someone close to the hero. As the society was weak and could not ensure justice, the heroes sought revenge, with the heroes and heroines fighting together, and after the villain is defeated the heroes are vindicated. Basu et al. point out that the strong social group inhabited by the heroes is the ideal (perhaps democratic, equated with Ram Rajya) but the villain's groups are rigid, hierarchical, despotic, cruel, and ultimately unsuccessful. Yet in the 1990s and beyond this was taken even further.

After her re-election in 1980, Indira Gandhi had started to rely increasingly on her younger son. This led to a change in her approach to decision making. She became more hesitant and cautious. She was surrounded by either yes-men or inexperienced politicians, and her hesitancy in making decisions was further compounded by the sudden death of her younger son, adviser, and confidant Sanjay Gandhi. She then managed to convince Rajiv, the older son, to come into politics.

Chandra et al. (2000) highlight the fact that one major weakness in her functioning was compounded by the weak organizational nature of the party and her failure to rebuild it and strengthen its purpose and structures. They attributed poor performance of the government and its popularity to blocking of channels of communication within the party cadres, through which party members could feed back to the leadership the concerns of the populace and in turn the nature and rationale of government policies to the populace. Despite domination of the party and the government, factionalism and infighting within the party continued, especially at the state level. In addition, the continuing problems in the country related to linguistic and caste conflicts, producing communal riots from 1980 to 1984. Although the rate of inflation was reduced to 7%, the growth rate was up by 4%, and the perceived problems related to multinational companies entering the country led to an increase in red tape. This role of government against democracy became evident at individual and state levels (Kothari, 1995).

Indira Gandhi's assassination in 1984 at the hands of her own security guards followed her decision to send the Army into the Golden Temple to flush out Bhindrawale and this led his associates to mass scale anti-Sikh riots. Only in 2005 did the government apologize for the massacre—some 21 years later!

In their evaluation of Indira Gandhi, Chandra et al. (2000) emphasize that one of her key achievements was politicization of the people, especially women and the poor, by making them more aware of their social conditions and the underlying unjust nature of society, and in arousing the consciousness of their interests and their political power. The strategic failure in long-term planning and policy making not only let the electorate down but also affected her status and reputation.

Raychaudhuri (1999, p. 221) observes that the erosions of consensus (in Indian politics) happened in the last phase of Indira Gandhi's government. He blames this on an anxiety to retain personal power and a desire to establish a dynasty. Gandhi played shortsighted political games, dangerously undermining the national consensus. The power inherent in the hands of one individual meant the erosion of confidence in the government at the centre. Cinema responded by showing ideal family structures where joint families lived happily together. This contrast with the reality on the street may have led to massive Oedipal disillusionment. Raychaudhuri's (p. 233) argument about the role of nationalism and the construction of nationhood wrapped around the notions of ethnicity and religion raises interesting points. Deep-seated feudalism and belated empowerment of those pre-viously excluded from even the political process have led to a complex shift in the governing structure (Malhotra, 2003). Kinship and dynastic control permeate the entire national life including cinema and how stories are portrayed.

Tarlo (2001) concludes that memories of the Emergency have given way to alternative memories. There is no doubt that, despite being recognized as a moment of crisis, the act of Emergency has been almost forgotten. She explains that first the re-election of Indira Gandhi was an act of forgiveness; second, Sanjay Gandhi's death, as he was one of the key figures of that period and, lastly, Indira Gandhi's own assassination, were all factors indicating that Indira Gandhi's actions were subsumed by the fact that she and other members of her family died for the nation. The Emergency thereby becomes a forgivable aberration.

Political upheaval caused by Indira's death and Rajiv becoming the Prime Minister did not provide any respite to the common people. The Bhopal gas tragedy was followed by the Bofors scandal and in 1989 Congress was voted out of power. The leaders who inherited political power lacked vision and charisma. Rajiv Gandhi was assassinated in 1991. The economic changes were slow. Inflation was high, the national debt even higher.

The results of Indira Gandhi's failure to develop strategic thinking in other areas such as institutional changes and political governmental aper-tures, the emphasis on personal power and negotiations with individuals like Bhindrawale and her ability to centralize authority and decision making in the party to herself, especially after Sanjay's death, meant that her time was employed on firefighting and dealing with factions in her party and in the country at large. The party gradually lost contact with its grassroots, which was the biggest tragedy in its history. As a result there was every likelihood that the party would become a shell of its former self, and this is exactly what happened over the following decade or so. There is little doubt that she was a tactician *par excellence*, but her inability to reach out to people directly and establish direct contact meant that she was hampered by being able to listen to only a few rather than many.

Much against his own wishes, and with an almost unseemly rush, Rajiv Gandhi became the Prime Minister on 31 October 1984. The anti-Sikh riots immediately after Indira's death did not provide any succour to any of the minorities and instead gave a clear signal of fear and oppression. Rajiv led the Congress to a massive majority focusing on the threat to India's stability and integrity. The government's delay in providing refuge and succour to the Sikhs has been attributed to confusion following Indira's death. This was followed by the Bhopal gas tragedy, when thousands of people lost their lives and many more thousands were injured and taken ill. Union Carbide, the owners of the plant, got away virtually scot-free and the compensation to the poor and the deserving was inadequate and late. Rajiv led on modernization, using computers and telecom as a significant step forward. Introducing employment plans, literacy plans, clean water for villages, and immunization of pregnant women and for children meant that a technological push of all kinds was on the way. His government also pushed very heavily to deepen and strengthen *panchayati raj* (local self-government at the village level). The Rajiv Gandhi government also managed to set up seven zonal cultural centres with cultural festivals abroad. In spite of serious attempts to clean up the political and bureaucratic system, the party organization remained weak and eventually defeated him.

However, the Bofors scandal, linked with allegations that various friends of Rajiv had received commissions, ruined his "Mr Clean" image and reputation. When the former finance minister and subsequent defence Minister V. P. Singh resigned, the scandal became public and the attacks on Rajiv Gandhi snowballed. In the election year it resurfaced. Chandra et al. (2000) point out that Rajiv shuffled his cabinet once every 2 months on average. His flashes of anger, lack of political experience, and unfamiliarity with nuances of grassroots mobilization made him vulnerable to attacks, personal and political. Losing the 1989 elections, even though Congress was the single largest party, Rajiv chose to remain in opposition. V. P. Singh became the Prime Minister on 2 December 1989. Devi Lal was said to be the choice of the coalition but in the meeting Devi Lal chose to nominate and support V. P. Singh. This was a coalition government; once again there was no unity and most of the energy was spent on resolving differences rather than governing. The day before Deputy Prime Minister Devi Lal was to speak at a farmers' rally, V. P. Singh announced that the Mandal commission report, appointed by the first Janata government (1977–1979) and quietly buried by Indira Gandhi, would be fully implemented. This meant that a total of 49.5% of all government jobs would be reserved for backward castes and other scheduled castes and tribes. This would be followed by reservations in educational institutions. The sudden and arbitrary decision, without consultation with constituent parties, led to a level of social division not seen before. The inability to identify backward castes was only one factor. The strong and violent reaction among students specifically led to several immolating themselves publicly in protest of the decision. Attacks on public property and riots continued till a stay was granted by the Supreme Court. The right-wing Hindu fundamentalist party, Bharatiya Janata Party, saw an opportunity. One of its leaders, L. K. Advani, set out on a 6000 mile "rath yatra" (journey on a vehicle made up as a chariot) from Somnath on the west coast to Ayodhya to push for establishing a temple at the birthplace of Ram, where a mosque stood. The government of V. P. Singh fell and the short-lived Chandra Shekhar government took its place, lasting barely 6 months.

Rajiv Gandhi was assassinated by a suicide bomber in the middle of campaigning. Congress emerged as the largest party, gaining an additional 35 seats. P. V. Narasimha Rao, who had previously been in the Rajiv Gandhi Cabinet but did not stand in elections, formed a minority government but managed to last for 5 years. With full-scale economic reforms and liberalization it meant that initial economic growth was significant, but corruption hit the government. The elections in 1996 led to a further reduction in Congress seats; it was no longer the single largest party. BJP led an alliance that lasted only a short while, to April. Subsequent elections produced BJP as leading the National Democratic Alliance and it survived the full 5-year term. India's conduct of nuclear tests in May 1998 led to Pakistan detonating the Islamic bomb and the vibrations, both political and economic, are still being felt. The Pakistani invasion of Kargil in 1999 further complicated the domestic and foreign policy. It has been alleged that under the BJP, saffronization (making changes due to politicization bringing in the Hindu agenda) of both educational system and civil service (including the Armed Forces) started. This has meant that the views of people in the country are beginning to become more rigid. This relationship of religion and religious orthodoxy, scientific advances in nuclear proliferation and space missions, and economic liberalization has created a potent cocktail of very high expectations with little achievement at personal level, especially in the lower middle classes and rural populations.

The economic changes, on the other hand, were slow in coming; when they did, they transformed the face of the nation. Following on from the ravaged economy at the time of the independence as a result of colonialism the Nehruvian experiment in socialist economy led to some changes, but these were not seen as fast enough or significant enough. The industrial growth between 1951 and 1961 was 7.1% and the agricultural growth was around 3%. Although expectations were high, the delivery flopped because of the over-reliance of agriculture on monsoons, which failed, and the two wars with China and Pakistan in 1962 and 1965 respectively. The Green Revolution in the 1970s led to India being self-sufficient in food output, which continued in spite of the further wars with Pakistan. India's poor growth in exports had implications regarding the productivity levels achieved in the country. The fiscal prudence was gradually abandoned as a result of persisting and competing demands from interested groups. The increase in government expenditure had to be met somehow.

Combined with political instability, the general public started to feel that they had to rely on hidden resources leading to black money and a black economy. The relaxation of fiscal prudence meant that inflation reached absurd levels towards the late 1970s. The budget deficit expanded as well and the growth in late 1980s, although impressive on the surface, was debt led. Chandra et al. (2000) observed that, although the need for reform was justified and identified since the 1980s, for various reasons this could not be carried out. In 1991 the government decided to break through the traditional mindset and attempt an unprecedented, comprehensive change at a time when both the ideological opposition and the resistance of the vested interests was at a weak point (Chandra et al., 2000).

Increase of capitalist policies, together with decreased restriction on foreign investment, led to an outwardly improved social and financial picture. Communalism raised its ugly head. The destruction of Babri Masjid in Ayodhya and the Hindu cry for a temple shook the Indian secular foundations deeply.

Immediate fiscal correction, liberalization of trade, and industrial controls such as free access to imports, a significant dismantling of the permit raj, and reforms of the public sector and capital markets with removal of restrictions on foreign investment led to freeing of the economy from the controls. This led to a significant growth in GDP and industrial output increased by 12%. There is little doubt that critics of the reform saw the changes as anti-poor. The social perspective of such a rapid change means that those who are left behind may well resent the holding of the money power in some hands and feel alienated. The revival of communalism may be linked with the rise of BJP and by concentration of economic power in the dominant community (be it because of caste or religion). The legacy of the national movement led to the formulation of the democratic state, which had multiple religions and classes. The danger to national sovereignty is communalism hiding behind other agendas of political opportunism.

Raychaudhuri (1999, p. 208) points out that the Sangha parivar (i.e., the family, which also has Sicilian resonance) of organizations built around the Hindu fundamentalist Rashtriya Swyamsevak Sangh (National Volunteer Organization) involved in the destruction of the mosque in Ayodhya had led to the imposition of a type of secularism that does not necessarily fall smoothly in a society as illiterate and as committed to *vita religiosa* as the Indian. This sustained campaign to build a temple has converted an issue of little or no relevance to millions of people who face multiple problems of contemporary Indian daily life into the central concern of Indian politics. Raychaudhuri raises the question that if the temple site was so important, why did the agitations stay so low-key for nearly 50 years after Independence? He observes that the urban petty bourgeois shopkeepers, small businesspeople, clerks, lower level professionals, and the like are highly politicized by now and share the multiple aspirations of their more fortunate fellow citizens. Excluded from the higher echelons of political and administrative power and social privilege by virtue of their relative disadvantage in education and resources, they obviously latched onto BJP and its parivar, thereby giving it electoral validity. In the 1990s the nature of films changed in order to attract this audience.

The prevalence of poverty, inequality, and social injustice, in addition to the insidious impact of the caste system and communalism, especially in the cow belt states of the country has led to illiteracy and poor achievement in these states. As most Hindi films target the same northern states, it is also likely that the influence is a two-way process. Poverty, quality of life, social inequality, and acknowledged poor health care and sanitation, high infant mortality, and illiteracy (especially for women) have marked out the difference between the ever-burgeoning middle class and the poor. This is also reflected in the consumption of cinema, in that the expanding middle class has taken recent multiplexes to heart with producers and directors attempting to fill this gap with other films, either in Indian English or focused on the middle class patrons. Directors such as Subhash Ghai with films like *Krishna Cottage* and Ram Gopal Varma with films such as *Ek Hasina Thi*, *Jungle*, etc., are clearly targeting the multiplex market.

In the 1990s, with gradual economic liberalization emerging both in the media, through access to satellite and cable with reduced control, and through importing consumer goods, the society's attitudes started to shift very rapidly and the films started to reflect these changes.

Following the second assassination in the Nehru-Gandhi dynasty, that of Rajiv, the Gandhi Congress Party formed a government led by P. V. Narsimha Rao, who had not planned to stand in the elections. His subsequent election, both as Prime Minister and then to the Parliament, and his gradually tightening grip on power by allegedly bribing members of other parties to join his government, obviously sent a very clear message to the populace that corruption is acceptable. To date he is the only ex-Prime Minister to have been convicted of corruption. The liberalization let loose made consumerism respectable. It also allowed women to be treated as commodities and the notions of self-aggrandisement and revenge spearheaded by the angry young man in the 1970s went one step ahead two decades later.

Mishra (1985) points out that films in the 1960s were largely romantic and comic. After 1970, the influence of Hollywood became more marked. In the 1970s and 1980s, Hindi films were influenced by the sociopolitical climate as well as Hollywood films of the contemporary period. Films became more permissive. In the late 1980s and 1990s villains in Hindi film started to be more psychotic and more psychopathic. In the 1990s the influence of Hollywood took another turn. Mishra identifies three films in this context: *Baazigar*, *Khalnayak*, and *Anjaam*. Mishra (2002) acknowledges that violence, which was suggested in *The Silence of the Lambs*, became more prominent in *Anjaam*, which presented a number of passionate violent deaths. *Anjaam* is seen as a remarkable film for its Hollywood-type physical violence, which also constitutes the core of *Khalnayak*.

Khalnayak ("The Villain"), a huge hit in 1993, gave the hero a chance to become not only the anti-hero but also an opportunity to play a multi-faceted role. *Khalnayak* is the director's paean to the wayward youth of the 1990s. Portrayed by Sanjay Dutt, the character Ballu Balram is the son of an idealist lawyer and an indulgent mother. On a Diwali day, when the villain visits Ballu's parents and offers gifts, Ballu's father declines. Ballu accepts firecrackers; his father chides him, whereas his mother continues to protect him. After a materially deprived childhood, Ballu (the grandson of a freedom fighter) joins the local mafia gang of Roshi Mahanta. The film opens with Aarti (Ballu's mother) hiding Ballu's photograph in the pages of *Ramayana*. Ballu shoots a politician at the behest of Roshi and is arrested while trying to escape. He is tortured by the police. The Central Bureau of Investigation (CBI) sends Ram Sinha, an officer, to investigate Ballu's crimes. Ballu manages to strangle a gang mate in the presence of a dozen policemen. Ballu challenges Ram by saying that government officers and leaders shout slogans about motherland and yet continue to line their pockets at the cost of the poor people. He insists that right and wrong are subjective. Ballu escapes from prison after killing a police officer and stealing his uniform. Ram's fiancée, Ganga, also a police officer, vows to retrieve Ram's reputation by catching Ballu. She pretends to be a dancing girl in order to find out Ballu's whereabouts and is forced to accompany him when he is on the run.

During the course of the journey Ballu falls in love with Ganga but uses her as a shield to escape again. In order to catch Ballu, the police trace his mother and arrest her. While she is being tortured, Ram realizes that she is his old teacher and that Ballu happens to be his old schoolfriend. She explains to Ram how she feels responsible for spoiling Ballu.

Her husband, a prosecution attorney, had been insulted by Roshi when the latter attempted to bribe him, thus representing some idealism. Roshi kills Ballu's sister when she leads a march against Roshi's drug peddling business. Ballu justifies his decision to join Roshi's gang, by saying, "I prefer being a slave to Roshi than being a slave to poverty." While on the run, he becomes close to Ganga. Ballu hides in a church, where he is trapped by the police. This relationship may reflect a parallel with the Khalistani separatist and terrorist Bhindrawale and his group being trapped in the Golden Temple in Amritsar. In both cases villains use religious places to hide and are challenged by the police. The use of the church here indicates forgiveness by the religion but more importantly also allows Ballu to be the son of God and his relationship with his mother to be seen as similar to that of Christ and the Madonna. His mother has also been brought in by the police. She attempts to persuade him to give himself up, but to no avail. After another fight with Ram, Ballu escapes to Roshi's den. Roshi then kidnaps Ballu's mother and brings her over. While trying to escape to Singapore, Ballu realizes that Roshi has doublecrossed him and abandoned his mother in the sea, where Ram saves her. Meanwhile Ganga is prosecuted for allegedly helping Ballu and is sentenced to 7 years of hard labour in gaol.

Ballu discovers that Ganga is engaged to Ram. He shows up in the court to admit his villainy and hand over his weapons to the police. Although there is a sense of reconciliation, the stark images of the police torturing the hero/villain and his mother are revealing. The film has parallels with a classic film, *Mother India*, in which the mother shoots her much loved errant son, incidentally played by Sunil Dutt—Sanjay's father. The running away with Ganga also has elements of *Ramayana*, where Sita is brought back in and she has to prove her innocence. Here Ballu provides that evidence.

Through the 1980s and 1990s the key factor in social polity was the frightening climate in various states, including Punjab, Kashmir, Assam, and Nagaland, in terms of terrorist and separatist activities that were encouraged and abetted by Pakistan and China. The second observation is that of the economic state of the country as a whole. The separatist movements, possibly encouraged by Pakistan and China, have their roots in the alienation of the people; they did not feel part of the country and felt that they were lagging behind. The economic growth in Punjab was the highest in the country; communal underpinnings of decision in dividing Punjab into two states; Punjab and Haryana on the basis of language and ongoing demand from both states to retain its newly constructed capital, Chandigarh, meant that the central government was constantly under pressure from politicians of both states to let one have the capital. The pressures related to Gurudwaras and the potent mixture of religion and politics meant that the Sikh demand for a separate home state never really went away. Reclaiming Gurudwaras and using these holy places to hide terrorists meant that from 1981 onwards Punjab became a bubbling cauldron with a clear but unstated threat to move Hindus out by intimidation. This ambition for general insurgency was handled indecisively by Indira Gandhi and sent the wrong messages to terrorists. Similar messages were being given to terrorists in other states. In Punjab, the military action against the Sikhs when it happened angered the Sikhs in the rest of the country. The mother who was supposed to be protective turned out to be destructive, like the goddess Kali, as Indira Gandhi had been portrayed by the famous painter M. F. Husain.

Terrorists took to extortion, robbery, smuggling, drugs, abduction, rape, landgrabbing, and kidnapping, and had a lavish lifestyle (Chandra et al., 2000). People felt oppressed and the common man lost all faith in law and justice. It was not surprising that communal and religious ideologies became dominant.

In his anger and irreverence, Khalnayak (the villain) takes over from the angry young man. This villain is more extreme, overturning the existing concepts of good and evil. The hero and the anti-hero respond to personal and social injustice through glamorized violence; the aim is destruction, not redemption. N. Kazmi (1996, p. 65) compares *Khalnayak* with Ravana, the demon king in *Ramayana* who kidnapped Sita, but here Ram's Ganga voluntarily goes with evil to protect her fiancé's reputation. Ballu believes in the righteousness of his actions and his drift is not circumstantial but voluntary and well-chosen. He likes materialistic things and hates the pseudo pride of suffering poverty, unemployment, and hopelessness. He discards abstractions like family lineage, past heritage, and honour for the sake of basic necessities, upward mobility, and economic betterment (N. Kazmi, 1996, p. 68). He is not ashamed of being a villain; it is his choice. He represents an alienated generation which has to take action on its own behalf.

The anti-hero is acceptable because society deserves such an "anti-hero" hero. He deserves to be applauded because he takes a positive decision rather than simply be pushed around by the poverty and his circumstances. This almost western view of the egocentric self and hero as rebel indicates the influence the west was able to spread. An additional observation concerns the role of the mother, who is used as a pawn by the police and later by the villain Roshi. There is no difference between the two sides, both of which are using a teacher as disposable. Perhaps she is being punished for protecting her son! It may also be that her punishment reflects a general sense of punishment to women, who by their style of nurturing are seen as responsible for deterioration of society's standards.

Mishra (2002, p. 203) argues that the Hindu fundamentalism of the 1990s is symptomatic of an authorized silence or repression located at the very heart of national culture. The object of such fundamentalism is to express a whole set of political, social, economic and religious conditions.

He attributed its rise to several factors, including the Iranian revolution and Iranian fatwa on Salman Rushdie, which on the surface appear to "give" more power to the Muslims. Mishra (2002, p. 205) suggests that the rise of Rama as an avatar and his being turned into a temple cult was a significant factor in the rise of Hindu fundamentalism. Gandhi had to pay with his life for giving away land to Pakistan. Mishra (p. 210) suggests that Partition is the modern demonic with which the North Indians generally overcode the Muslim "other". He is right to note that people in the middle of that tension "forget" what went on. The search for identity meant that the difficult and the unpalatable had to be hidden away deep in one's unconscious. In the late 1980s and 1990s this agony of the partition and its "encrypting" took a slightly different and politically dangerous form through the redefinition of the concept of Hindutva (p. 211).

In *Khalnayak*, Mishra (2002, p. 224) also sees the symbolism of *Ramayana* as religion. The return of Ganga to Ram after spending time with the anti-hero suggests questions about the purity of Sita. But as we know, Ganga never gets polluted, because the name has a symbolic significance. Mishra (p. 226) notes that this film has two levels of spectatorial complicity: On the surface the dharmik (religious) code is affirmed, and on the level of spectatorial involvement responses become varied.

Mishra (2002, p. 227) goes on to argue that the final scene of *Khalnayak* illustrates the filmmaker and the hero's response to the sociopolitical events. Mishra sees the film not as being about the spectator's attraction to the figure of the anti-hero but a statement about the demon within of both the spectator and the nation.

The differences between *Khalnayak* and *Sholay* are relevant, as are the similarities between Ballu Balram and Gabbar Singh. Both are on the wrong side of the law and boastful about it; both run their gangs in a ruthless manner and do not hesitate to kill their gang members. Ballu is a well-crafted character in that he is able to stand and look at the reasons for his psychopathy and in the end is reformed—at least he has some maternal connections and support. However, the contrast between Ballu and Ram Sinha in *Khalnayak* is not as marked as that between Gabbar and Thakur in *Sholay*. The Thakur, as a police officer in *Sholay*, appears to uphold the law, whereas for Ram Sinha it appears very muddled. He does not even hesitate in torturing an old woman, perhaps a reflection of the times where police itself has taken on the mantle of the villain.

Both films represent modern India in an anarchic way where modern values are infringing upon the rural idyll, the traditional values and idealism. When Ballu walks off to join Roshi he very clearly declares to his father that he is rejecting the Gandhian philosophy and he can't see why he should not have what he wants because everyone around him is doing exactly the same. The sense of alienation is reflected in the voiceover later on in the first half of *Khalnayak* where Ram Sinha is seen addressing a press conference: "This is our nation's youth . . . one who has blood in his eyes, who has murdered four leaders, committed nine dacoities, looted 20 polling booths. So many crimes at such a young age . . .", thereby highlighting the criminality of the central character and embedding it very strongly and essentially into the social/political/criminal nexus. Ballu is not a typical Hindi film villain. He believes in his unlawful actions and hits his mother when he thinks that she is responsible for bringing the police with her. He feels let down by the fact (not clearly stated, but only implied) that his grandfather's sacrifice in the Indian independence struggle has not enabled them to pay their rent or facilitated him in getting a college education or his sister in getting a job. There is an underlying lust for reward. This also indicates the alienation younger generations feel towards the struggle for freedom.

The younger generations' search for personal goods is not related to that of national or kinship achievement. Ballu's reaction to the past heritage, lineage, and entry into the crime world of Roshi Mahanta allows him to justify his actions at every step. He illustrates his badness by using chosen negative adjectives with a sense of achievement. His villainy, his lust for material things, is not dissimilar to the villainy and the psychopathy of three characters which established Shah Rukh Khan at the apex of psychopathic behaviour before he graduated to romantic roles as a hero. Masud (1997) sees Sanjay Dutt's performance in *Khalnayak* as extraordinary, classic, brooding, mournful, crackling with wit.

Krutnik (1991) posits male masochism as manifesting a desire to escape from the regimentation of masculine (cultural) identity effected through the Oedipal complex. Hence the relations between the hero and the women in his life are either overinvolved or alienated; there is no midpoint. The relationships with girlfriend, sister, mother, or maternal figures are coloured by self-doubts regarding his own masculinity. The dread implicit in throwing away the paternal rule or law and masochism in it and yet the dread of emasculation make these masquerades intriguing, yet problematic. The lesson is (1991, p. 85):

> [This] dramatic is articulated, and elaborated and results in various ways but these are all unified by what can be seen as an obsession with the non correspondence between the desires of the individual male subject and the cultural regime of masculine identification.

Krutnik then goes on to postulate that masochism, paranoia, psychosis, homosexuality, various forms of "corruptive" sexuality are some of the principal ways in which this crisis of confidence in the possibilities of masculine identity is articulated within the tough thrillers as culturally conventional parameters of masculine identity.

Anjaam, *Darr*, and *Baazigar* can be seen as three key films of Shah Rukh Khan's dealing with the hero's obsession. Along with these films Shah Rukh Khan also appeared in *Deewana*, which had a similar theme. With the 1990s emerged the hero who cannot accept refusal from the woman he loves. This preoccupation with lust and possession reaches its climax through these three early films of Shah Rukh Khan, who epitomized the crazed, obsessive, possessive lover. The characters portrayed are ruthless and remorseless. This behaviour on the part of the anti-hero stands out in stark contrast to the traditional hero's messianic bids (N. Kazmi, 1996, p. 79).

The traditional Hindi film stories have been boy meets girl, boy falls in love with girl, some personal social or familial misunderstanding occurs; a rift is created, but the misunderstanding is eventually resolved, and the boy gets girl. Villains did everything they could, often using the vamps, but eventually gave in gracefully and redeemed themselves, often by apologizing publicly. In the 1990s this change became more apparent. Although villainy changed its shape and form in the 1970s, it reached its apotheosis in the 1990s when the crazed lover—who was almost psychotic, with no regrets and no redemption in sight—emerged, and continues to hold sway. This in the context of kinship-led society raises important questions.

The development of an egocentric individual who paints himself as above everyone, unable to understand why the heroine rejects him, is far removed from the conventional sociocentric or kinship/family-oriented individual. These demarcations between good and bad were blurred in the cinema of the anti-hero. In *Baazigar*, *Darr*, and *Anjaam* the hero makes a virtue of his obsessional love. The murder of various friends and acquaintances who are perceived as obstacles is customarily wrong and reprehensible, but the hero validates it repeatedly (N. Kazmi, 1996, p. 79). The psychopathic hero and his personal gratification become important purely for the personal gain of the anti-hero; societal opprobrium means nothing.

Kasbekar (2001) notes that Hindi films have used various strategies and subterfuges in order to uphold the vision of the Indian woman as a muse rather than an erotic spectacle, yet still provide erotic pleasure to the viewership. Female chastity is prized. Cabaret performance and disavowal of voyeurism are two other factors identified by Kasbekar on the perception of the female. The cabaret dances and the vamps in Hindi cinema are often Anglo-Indian, indicating a racial stereotype. The new heroines of the 1970s and 1980s, influenced by Indira Gandhi's position of power, portrayed modern independent women who uphold family values and the virtue of chastity. Ford and Chanda (2002) illustrate similar themes in relationship to Hong Kong and other Asian cinema. They claim that films have certain gendered geographies, histories, and ideologies across several generations of films.

In the early 1980s, Hrishikesh Mukherjee directed *Bemisaal*, a story of two very close friends who fall for the same girl. The hero, Sudhir (Amitabh Bachchan), encourages the girl to marry his best friend because he owes a debt to his friend's family, as they were responsible for him becoming a doctor. A *ménage à trois* develops, and then suddenly a lunatic brother of Sudhir (played by the same actor in a double role) appears. He wants revenge on a girl who rejected him after having seduced him. Sudhir tries to avenge his brother by seducing the girl in return and informing her fiancé about her evil deeds. In order to protect his friend after a case goes wrong in the clinic, Sudhir manufactures evidence and hands himself over to the police.

The reviewer in *Filmfare* castigates the director, even though the film occasionally comments on foreign qualified doctors and distorted professional ethics, the need for doctors to go to the villages, and the weird goings-on in the nursing home. She comments that the portrayal of madness is hackneyed. The mad brother gets better, as usual the blame is on the girl and the avenging rejected love causes the individual to become well.

Dilwale opens at night with a group of psychiatrists discussing Arun (Ajay Devgan). While they are discussing whether the full moon influences the mental state of insane individuals, in a dramatic scene under the influence of the full moon Arun becomes agitated. He breaks through the prison-style bars and runs away from the hospital, thus proving the psychiatrists and the modern psychiatric theory wrong. It transpires that he was in love with Sapna (Raveena Tandon); but her uncle and cousins (Paresh Rawal and Gulshan Grover) are against the match for several reasons and do their best to keep the two lovers apart. Arun has flashbacks of fires in which he had suffered severe losses, reminiscent of Post Traumatic Stress Disorder. True love wins in the end. An incredibly tedious film, there appears to be no discussion of diagnosis, aetiology, or management strategies. Madness allows the hero to "misbehave"!

Anjaam is the story of Vijay Agnihotri (the name Vijay had earlier been synonymous with characters played by Amitabh Bachchan) played by Shah Rukh Khan who took over from him as the new incarnation of the angry young man in the 1990s. Vijay meets Shivani, an air hostess, and falls in love with her. He tries to woo her but without success. She is not in love with him and that is what tips him over the edge. The first 20 minutes or so of the film are like any conventional film: hero sees heroine, hero falls for her and serenades her, but she does not respond. After seeing her model for Air India in a TV commercial he wants her to do the modelling for his business, though exactly what business he runs is unclear.

Vijay is arrogant, boastful, and very aware of the power of money, making remarks like, "I have the power because I have the money." When he tries to "buy" Shivani and she turns him down, he becomes aggressive. At times of stress he regresses into a child, his voice changes, and he sings a nursery rhyme. We know little of his father, and even though his mother appears to run the business she seems to spend most of her time at home. When Vijay tells his mother that he is in love and they go to Shivani's house with the marriage proposal, they discover that her marriage is already in progress. Shivani is marrying Ashok, an airline pilot. An obviously upset Vijay goes deer hunting. His mother tells an employee that he has gone hunting and that he has become angry at life in the past 4 years. Later, Vijay meets Shivani and Ashok at a party and returns home drunk, having observed their happiness. A lack of control and tendency to injure animals is often a key feature of psychopaths.

Shivani and Ashok go to Mauritius and Vijay follows them with the excuse that he has to have Ashok's signature on the agreement to become Managing Director of the airline that he is setting up. Much against Shivani's advice, Ashok signs the agreement. To publicize the airline, Vijay wants to use Shivani's photograph, which makes her angry. It is clear that she is much more aware of his character than her husband is. Vijay mercilessly beats a thief who appears to have stolen Shivani's mangalsutra (a necklace that symbolizes marriage), which also upsets Shivani. It is paradoxical that the dread of the loss of the symbol of her marriage should upset him, whereas that is exactly what he is trying to do. He seems to ignore the implications of his act and in the selfish narcissistic state is unable or unwilling to see what his actions could mean.

During a disagreement, Ashok hits Shivani. As a result of this Vijay beats Ashok unconscious. Vijay then visits Ashok in the hospital and asks Shivani to sign the divorce papers so that they can get married. When she refuses, he removes the oxygen tubing and thereby kills Ashok. Shivani lodges a complaint but Vijay produces an alibi. Vijay pretends to police that he was having an affair with Shivani and she was blackmailing him. When the police inspector challenges Vijay, he is enraged and talks of an incident in his childhood. He had seen a beautiful glass doll belonging to a girl who refused to let Vijay play with it and he then broke it. While narrating this story he breaks another glass ornament, causing bleeding (again a symbol of borderline behaviour). Between the police inspector and Vijay, they get Shivani arrested by falsely alleging that when Vijay refused to comply with her blackmail she decided to attack him. She is sentenced to 3 years' hard labour in prison. While in prison she is beaten by the sadistic female warden who is having an affair with the same corrupt police officer. Political leaders pick up women for sex from the prison. Shivani is recommended by the warden but because she is pregnant she vomits on the politician. Instead, her cellmate is taken for the politician's pleasure and is raped. Shivani complains to the Home Ministry about the warden, but the warden beats her and causes her to have a miscarriage. Meanwhile, in a drunken state, Vijay kills Shivani's immediate family in a car accident. At this point Shivani decides to avenge herself, by killing the gaoler first and then the arresting police officer.

When Shivani discovers that Vijay and his mother have moved, she finds a job as a "nurse" in a nursing home in another town; this happens to be where Vijay is admitted, having sustained injuries in the car accident. Her development from an air hostess to a nurse is never explained, but must represent the nurturing/caring role of the woman. With her devotion and love she gets him back to his normal self, but then she kills both him and herself. She nurtures him to health first because she does not want to kill a disabled person, which she would see as a sinful act. Shah Rukh Khan went on to play psychopaths in *Darr* and *Baazigar* with different levels of psychopathy, obsessive love, and stalking.

The avenging women genre relies on the generating of sadomasochistic pleasure, which unwittingly challenges the sadistic impulses of rape.

Gopalan (2002) argues that rape scenes are inextricably enmeshed; the masochistic dimensions outweigh the sadistic associations. The male viewer watching sadistic exploitation then can switch fantasy to masochistic exploitation. The question arises whether this is a son/mother relationship fantasy where the male may want to punish the mother for his having sexual thoughts about her and then feeling guilty about it. The female's revenge in the guise of goddess Kali allows the male to "receive" the punishment in order to expunge the sinful feeling that he may have had towards her. The interpretation may not be conscious but the confusion in the male mind about mother/Madonna/whore, someone who deserves what she gets, especially if she chooses to transgress the expected role and power attributed to her, is what is still portrayed in Hindi films. The number of times women, whether in the role of heroine or otherwise, are hit/slapped/ physically assaulted in modern Hindi films is too numerous to be mentioned.

Chatterji (1998) highlights that, in addition to the portrayal of women as the goddess Durga, the relationship between Radha, Meera, and Krishna have also led to multiple portrayals in popular Indian cinema. While Meera's love is devotional, spiritual, and somewhat distant, the love of Radha is here-and-now, passionate, intense, and physical. Many songs use these symbols to express love. The courtesan's unrequited love for the hero is often identified with Radha's love for Krishna, thereby legitimizing the role. This ambivalence in the male mind in relation to the mother/lover relationship is striking in these films.

Gopalan (2002) makes a significant point that rape revenge narratives stage aggressive and contradictory contours of sexual identity and pleasure. She suggests that both public and private unacknowledged aggressiveness underscores understanding and articulation of sexual identities.

The possibility is that avenging woman is a "male", ergo atypical female, who without a phallus can (almost) beat the male; when violent she is uncontrollable and the so-called masculinity hides behind a kind, generous, and otherwise simple female persona. These interpretations reflect the avenging woman as seen through the eyes of the male auteur and male viewer. However, that is not to say that female auteurs and viewers do not see it the same way. Gopalan (2002) observes that masquerade (the difference between genuine womanliness and the "masquerade" is defined by Rivière, 1986) can be extended to both masculine and feminine subjects. If this masquerade is then turned to the mad, the other, the deviant, it becomes apparent that the portrayal in that genuineness of the individual and their madness provokes the viewer into a false sense of security.

Darr was produced and directed by Yash Chopra, who can be called a romanticist in his portrayal of love and women and perceptions and meaning of love. *Darr* was released in 1993 and was perceived as an important step for Yash Chopra, Juhi Chawla, and others. Inspired by *Cape Fear*, the director was seen to treat the psychopath with kid gloves. *Darr* is the story of a naval officer, Sunil (Sunny Deol), who loves Kiran (Juhi Chawla), who is being stalked by Rahul (Shah Rukh Khan). Rahul and Kiran had been classmates but she had never acknowledged his existence. Rahul has loved her ever since, and followed her and left messages for her. As the film progresses his stalking increases dramatically.

Rahul says "I love you Kiran" in the same tone used by Hannibal Lecter in *The Silence of the Lambs*. Khan explained it by saying that he copied the director's (Yash Chopra's) stammer (Dwyer, 2002). Kiran then starts to get phone calls and receives a batch of photographs that had been taken by Rahul without her being aware. Meanwhile, Rahul is seen talking to his mother on the phone, telling her how beautiful Kiran is and how he is going to marry her. He is also surrounded by Kiran's pictures. Rahul's father, who also happens to be Sunil's boss, walks in and asks Rahul who he was talking to. Capt Mehra (Rahul's father) then goes to the doctor and we learn that Rahul's mother has been dead for 18 years. Capt Mehra was driving the car in which Rahul's mother died. The doctor asks whether Rahul holds him responsible for his mother's death. Capt Mehra explains that Rahul was always lonely and shy and spent most of the time lost in his own world. The frequency of phone calls by Rahul to Kiran increases. He is seen walking on the edge of a wall on top of a multistorey building picking petals off a flower while chanting ". . . she loves me, she loves me not . . ." and ends with "she loves me". Rahul "rings" his (dead) mother after hearing that Sunil and Kiran have decided to get married and declares, "I have no objections to Sunil's marriage, I am not his enemy, he is a very good person, but how can he marry Kiran? [She] is mine, only mine. How can he steal Kiran from me. He is mad . . . totally mad." This projection of madness on to the other becomes interesting in creating the "other".

Rahul severs the brake lining of Sunil's car; his phone calls to Kiran become longer and more threatening. Rahul tells her that he will come to her house the next day for the festival of Holi, which he does, dressed as a drummer. Sunil chases him and manages to hit him with a stone, at which point Rahul says, "You did not do the right thing Sunil. You should not have hit me but now you'll have to pay for every single drop of blood." He then sends a handkerchief stained with his blood and with a message written in blood.

On being invited to their wedding, Rahul's angry and destructive response is: "I am living on the strength of your love and your pictures. If you snatch these what will I do? I have nothing except your love . . . ." Of course, Kiran does not love him and never has, but the sense of unreality in Rahul's life is deep-rooted. Sunil and Kiran get married and have police protection. Rahul manages to kill two police constables by cutting lift cables. The couple's new flat is full of graffiti in Rahul's writing, "I love you, Kiran", "Kiran, congratulations on your marriage." She starts to hallucinate that the telephone is ringing, though it is disconnected. "Sunil, save me. I don't want to go mad", she repeats. Sunil and Kiran leave for Switzerland but pretend that they are going to Goa. Rahul goes to Goa but can't find them.

Vicky is an old college friend of Rahul's, and is dying of cirrhosis of the liver. Rahul kills Vicky, then scatters his unsent letters to Kiran and some of Vicky's belongings in order to convince the police and family that Vicky was responsible for harassing Kiran. He manages to find out that Kiran and Sunil are in Switzerland and arrives there. Kiran recognizes him from their college days and tells him, "You have remained a jhempu [nerd]." Sunil talks to Rahul and notes his violent behaviour. He is convinced that Rahul is the stalker. He lures Rahul into the forest where Rahul stabs him and leaves him for dead. Rahul kidnaps Kiran and wants her to marry him, all the while telling his dead mother that he is marrying Kiran. He tells Kiran: "I am mad for you. You are my madness. You are my obsession. I love you Kiran." He then boasts about all the killings and hands her his mother's wedding sari to get dressed in. Meanwhile, Sunil manages to reach them and after a fight he kills Rahul. Rahul's dying words are, "Kiran, my life began with your love and ended with your love. I know I have sinned but don't hate me, I love you." This is a love triangle with marked psychopathology of obsession, possession, and morbid jealousy.

Yash Chopra, in an interview with Dwyer (2002), acknowledged that originally *Darr* was to be made by his assistant Naresh Malhotra. The role eventually played by Shah Rukh Khan was offered first to Rishi Kapoor, who turned it down saying that it would damage his romantic image. The role was then accepted by Aamir Khan, but he later withdrew. Yash Chopra emphasizes that his film was about obsessive love. Shah Rukh Khan told the director that he was already playing two negative roles in *Baazigar* and *Anjaam*, but if this role was different from those two he would do it (Somaaya, 2002). Chopra states (Somaaya, 2002, p. 576):

Selective stammering was part of Rahul's [Shah Rukh Khan] characterization. Rahul is a normal boy but gets hysterical only when he mentioned Kiran's name . . . The audience applauds Sunny Deol for killing Shah Rukh Khan . . . in a strange inexplicable way they are also attracted to the villain and mourn his death.

Similar problems occurred in casting the heroine. In the end Juhi Chawla, who had acted in another film, *Aaina*, with Yash Chopra's wife as producer, accepted the role. *Aaina* also had an interesting romantic triangle with Amrita Singh as the older sister to Chawla and the male lead being played by Jackie Shroff. Amrita Singh played a borderline personality, threatening to kill herself and taking overdoses, but exaggerating claims by acting histrionically and in an attention-seeking manner.

Shah Rukh Khan played the obsessive, verging on psychotic, stalker with great success. His obsessive nature and strange state of mind are made clear in a sequence of looks in the film (Dwyer, 2002). In the first song of the film, *Jadoo teri nazar*, the heroine runs around the campus looking for her lover. It is only later that the audience discovers that the singer is the stalker. Shah Rukh Khan is able to enter into the private estate of the family unobserved, whether in disguise or as himself. It is also unusual in that the distinction between private and public space is clearer in this film than it is in reality. Very often, even in modern urban India, the distinction between private and public space is blurred.

Yash Chopra highlighted the fact that he appeared to be making a film which fed on people's fears, especially in the context of excessive and obsessive love (Dwyer, 2002, p. 150):

> There is no vamp or villain. The villain is your weakness. Love may be the weakness but the villain . . . [Shah Rukh Khan's character] is a positive character; he's a man who is obsessed with a girl. He does not rape; his crime is that he loves someone who doesn't reciprocate. The villain (generally) harms people morally or emotionally.

There is little doubt that the audience sympathized with the deranged obsession of Shah Rukh Khan rather than the alternative masculinity offered by Sunny Deol, the brave naval officer who single-handedly managed to save a minister's daughter from her captors.

Dwyer (2002) notes that it is also hard to draw the line between the pursuit of women as depicted in many other Hindi films from that in *Darr*, although the anonymous phone calls to the dead mother are much more disturbing than anything else in earlier films. Dwyer observes that *Darr* uses little outdoor space in India, except as a place of fear. The idyllic Switzerland is also "invaded" by the villain, even in outdoor space. The control of these spaces by the obsessive lover is possessive and frightening by itself.

Baazigar, inspired by the Hollywood film *A Kiss Before Dying*, with Shah Rukh Khan playing the Matt Dillon role (earlier played by Robert Wagner), was also a huge hit. The portrayals of psychopaths in *Baazigar* and *Darr* made Shah Rukh Khan a popular star and he won the *Filmfare* award for Best Actor over Sanjay Dutt, who was a popular choice for his role in *Khalnayak*. Reviews on the internet (see www.rediff.com) hailed *Baazigar* and Shah Rukh Khan but sounded a note of caution: "if you dig deep it can be found that it is only a reinvention of the past, a beautiful decorated exterior for essentially the same interior, just like a bride choosing to wear an ensemble outfit in a wedding when the wedding is all the same".

There were other reasons for the success of the film. The producers took advantage of satellite television and promotional trailers (promos) were aired every 5 minutes. When the film opened in November 1993, the audience flocked to see it.

There were, however, structural problems with the film. For example, the heroine, despite knowing how bad the hero was, cries buckets on his death. It may have been cathartic or it may have been genuine grief, but the fact that the hero had killed several people close to her did not appear to cause her even remorse! She is in love with the hero, who has killed her sister and her friend, and her response to this discovery is surprising.

Shah Rukh Khan was noted by a reviewer on the internet (www.imdb. com) to have delivered a raw and fresh performance but "it still has series of rough edges to take care of especially in the blatant candour that makes some of the romantic and emotional scenes. He portrays the evil well and does scare you." Another reviewer (www.imdb.com) saw it as a disappointing thriller with an unrealistic ending. The story reflected the sense of revenge by the son on behalf of his parents, a series set in motion by Amitabh Bachchan.

Baazigar is the story of Ajay Sharma (Shah Rukh Khan), whose father lost his business to Mr Chopra (Dalip Tahil). Mr Chopra has two daughters, Seema (Shilpa Shetty) and Priya (Kajol). The film opens with Ajay as a child; he takes on menial jobs and looks after his ill mother who keeps talking about her dead daughter and husband. He then leaves home to go to Bombay where he pursues Seema but refuses to be seen with her in public. At the same time he is also pretending to be Vicky, in order to woo the younger daughter, Priya. After much manipulation he persuades Seema to write a suicide note. He then takes her to the Registrar's office to marry her. The office is closed for lunch; he takes her to the rooftop and throws her off.

He then ensures that Priya falls in love with him. Priya is aware of her sister's fear of heights and refuses to believe that she would have jumped. She starts asking questions and finds out that Ravi, a classmate of Seema's, had seen her with a boy. When Ravi goes to his hostel room to collect the photograph of a function at which the said boy was present, Ajay/Vicky is waiting for him; he gets Ravi to sign a confession that he was Seema's lover and killer. Ajay/Vicky then kills Ravi and leaves his body hanging for Priya to discover.

By emotionally supporting Priya he is able to gain the trust of her father, who in turn makes him an equal partner in the same business that at one time was owned by Ajay's father. Madan Chopra gives power of attorney to Vicky before going abroad on business and Vicky gradually takes over all the property, using exactly the same technique Chopra had used on his father. Meanwhile, Vicky and Priya meet Anjali, an old friend of Seema who seems to recognize Vicky as the person whose identity Ajay had taken. Priya becomes suspicious; she traces Vicky's mother and finds evidence of Vicky's true identity. While Priya is going through the evidence Ajay returns, pursued by Madan Chopra and his gang. In the end Chopra and Ajay are both killed. Before dying, Ajay tells his mother that he is dying content in her lap.

Baazigar is an interesting film not only because Shah Rukh Khan carries on the Bachchan tradition but also because he does so in an incredibly hard, violent, and ugly manner. The last scene, where Madan Chopra impales Ajay on an iron rod and in turn is impaled on the same rod as both of them plunge to their deaths, signifies the union of the hero and the villain. Although there is indiscriminate murder and revenge, the redemption appears finally to lie in the mother's lap.

Madan Chopra is a psychopath, too; he has no scruples in embezzling money from Ajay's father but scorns that he had taken only 500,000 rupees, as if the amount of money and not the act itself is relevant. There are several scenes in the film where the police appear to be standing by idly while the protagonists are fighting or bleeding to death.

Such dramatic narrative convinces the viewer that it is acceptable to be an avenging death angel and take the law into one's own hands. There is no attempt in either case to seek redress from the courts. The personality trait here suggests to the viewer that it is acceptable and even laudable that such things happen. Rather amusingly, there is a television news report where it is announced that as crime rates are going up in Mumbai, police constables are being given rifles. This indicates that the police are being armed to deal with increasing violence but are impotent. The sense of helplessness generated by the criminal-politician-businessman nexus in the minds and actions of the police is remarkably obvious.

A clear-cut demarcation between good and bad appears less distinct. In all three films the protagonist shows no remorse in killing people. N. Kazmi (1996, p. 79) opines,

> Nobody ought to kill four people, including his best friend and his beloved's husband (as in *Darr* and *Anjaam*), however strong the passion for the object of his desire. And nobody ought to throw his beloved off a high-rise building on the eve of his wedding or with the innocent witnesses (as in *Baazigar*) even though it may all be part of a grandiose scheme of vendetta. But that which is customarily wrong is held as right and proper by these protagonists.

This obsessionality, with elements of a borderline personality disorder and narcissistic all-encompassing personality traits, suggests that external and internal factors are at interplay. The absence of guilt and remorse is striking.

Baazigar has spawned the genre of anti-hero films where the hero is permitted to do anything. Heroes who killed dominated the films of the 1980s, but there were always some legal constraints. *Anjaam*, *Baazigar*, and *Darr* defined the roles for Shah Rukh Khan the same way that Amitabh Bachchan has been defined by his films. Shah Rukh Khan turned a revenge-obsessed, murdering psychopath into a sympathetic, even desirable hero. Shah Rukh Khan's image underwent a transformation in *Baazigar* and *Darr* and established him as an anti-hero hero!

The Shah Rukh Khan persona can be the extension of the Amitabh Bachchan (angry young man) phenomenon with changing social realities (Majumdar, 2000). One can argue that the psychotic hero is the "other" of the Bachchan phenomena and, even though he has no sense or context of social realities, he plunges the depths of hitherto unknown territories of desire—a deeper exploration on interiority (defined as inner/outer distinction by drawing attention to how regulatory practices working on the inner hidden space of the body are manifested on the surface of the body). Majumdar uses the term "interiority" to depict the struggle of representation of an imagined interiority, however unstable that might be. The representation of Foucauldian interiority in its most concrete form is illustrated by the psychotic or the psychopath who cuts parts of the body and demonstrates the bleeding wounds as reflected in the darkness of their desire and interiority. This darkness is evident in that the evil nature is both externalized and internalized with little scope for any redemption.

The personae of the heroes played by Amitabh Bachchan in the 1970s and Shah Rukh Khan in the 1990s and onwards deal not only with the question of identity/subjectivity, but also with the discourse of pain experienced by the body on screen and the reinvention of the city of Bombay (now called Mumbai) in the 1990s (Majumdar, 2000). The embedding of these persona dates to the imposition of the Emergency rule and the changing of the city into becoming a more focused reference point. These characters are urban, therefore more modern and perhaps more sophisticated. The shift from destruction of rural idyll to lonely alien urban landscape is striking.

The stalking theme continues in a new guise in three films released in the 1990s: *Agnisakshi*, *Dastak*, and *Daraar*, all of which are said to be loosely based on the plot of *Sleeping with the Enemy*. In both *Agnisakshi* and *Daraar*, the ex-husband is the psychotic stalker who is unable to let go of his wife. In *Agnisakshi*, Suraj (Jackie Shroff), a multibillionaire falls in love with Shubhangi (Manisha Koirala) and eventually, when he saves her from a fire in an auditorium, she reciprocates his love and they get married. On their honeymoon she meets Vishwanath (Nana Patekar), who follows her around and starts telling her that she is his wife, showing her a video and photographs of the wedding ceremony. The stalking continues unabated. We learn that Vishwanath had been in the Army, had been court-martialled for disobeying orders, and was considered too violent even for the Army.

Eventually, Shubhangi admits that Vishwanath had blackmailed her father and during their marriage had kept her under severe control, showing evidence of clinical morbid jealousy. Once, when she goes shopping for 2 hours, he is waiting for her at home, convinced she is seeing someone else. He then takes the same trip with her to measure the exact time taken to finish her shopping, thereby emphasizing his possessiveness and control over her. The psychopathic behaviour verging on the psychotic with morbid jealousy portrayed by Vishwanath is extreme. He is ruthless, irritable, unpredictable, and lacks any sense of social guilt. He wants to own her as a piece of property. Similar pictures emerge in *Daraar* and *Dastak*.

In *Agnisakshi*, Nana Patekar's performance was praised. The film was seen as being reasonably successful, especially in the first half, with good songs, but the second half of the film was seen as boring and repetitious. Patekar was seen as extraordinary, without compare. Others were noted to act well and the direction was praised as good with technical values above average. It was noted as an entertaining film intended mainly for an urban market.

Nana Patekar's outing in *Yugpurush* relates the unusual story of a young man being released from the asylum 25 years after admission, in spite of his ability to see through people. He is pure at heart, extremely simple in looks, and not worldly wise, which leads him into all kinds of difficulty. Intriguingly, there is a strong political subtext. Not only are there snide remarks made about dynastic roles but also a politician is heard to acknowledge that he is interested in politics because of his desire to do good for the country and for himself. This is a fairly accurate representation of politicians. Patekar finds it difficult to settle in the community. Notwithstanding that he is not prepared for the transition, the psychiatrist types up his sanity certificate, takes him to the railway station, and puts him in a first class compartment. The pace of the film was seen as slow, with the second half being grim and too tense. A major criticism of the film was that the central character is someone that the layperson could not identify with. Patekar's performance was seen as award winning, although, interestingly, it was noted that his fans would be disappointed. Technical aspects were noted to be of an average standard.

Dastak was the first film for Miss Universe, Sushmita Sen, where she plays herself. While being crowned Miss Universe, a psychotic patient, Sharad, is watching her on TV in his room. He stalks her, writes to her and wants her to sign her name on his body with a blade. Like Shah Rukh Khan in *Anjaam* and *Darr*, he cuts himself with a razor blade, which seems to give him pleasure. The female protagonist falls in love with Rohit, the police officer who has been sent to guard her. The stalker manages to kill her best friend and others in a psychotic manner. When the police find out that he had been an inpatient in a psychiatric hospital, the nature of the obsession becomes clearer. The doctor tells the police that "he was the most intelligent patient I have ever seen". The stalker manages to kidnap Sushmita Sen while she is visiting the Seychelles. In the end, the stalker is shot dead and the police officer and Sushmita Sen unite. The bodyguard falling in love with the subject he has been sent to protect is a not uncommon theme in both Hindi and Hollywood films. The two poles of madness and stalking with obsession on one end and security offered by the police bodyguard on the other indicate that the creation of the "other" and balancing the hero with the villain is of interest to the viewer.

Dastak was recognized in a review as being well made but reminiscent of *Darr*, *Agnisakshi*, *Daraar*, and *Fareb*. The reviewer noted that the incidents in the drama may be different but the story is the same, and the film that is released last suffers, which was the case in point as far as the box office success of *Dastak* was concerned. The reviewer noted that there were several points where the film shocked viewers and its shock value led to excitement and interest on part of the audience. The screenplay was noted to be tight and dialogue as appropriate with an effective climax. All the actors were noted to have made a good impact. Although the direction was also noted to be good, the choice of subject was disappointing. Technically, it was seen to have good cinematography, good background music, and appropriate foreign locations. The songs were seen as disappointing but the target audience of the film was city-based and not rural. It did not set the box office alight.

In *Daraar*, a rich painter Raj (Rishi Kapoor) falls in love with Priya (Juhi Chawla), who has brought her blind mother to Shimla for treatment. When she discovers that Raj loves her, she writes to him with details of her earlier life but the letter does not reach him. His servant gets another letter written by a poet and delivers it instead, and Raj thinks that Priya has agreed to marry him. Priya's mother tells him that it is very brave of him to marry a married woman, at which point he returns to Bombay. When his servant delivers the correct letter to him, he discovers that Priya had been married to Vikram (Arbaaz Khan), who had settled down in Goa in an isolated house. If Vikram saw her talking to a man he would beat her; on several occasions he fantasizes that other men are sexually interested in Priya and he also feels that she likes to flaunt herself in front of strange men. He threatens her by saying, "If a stranger talks to me of your beauty I will throw acid on your face."

When a neighbouring doctor helps Priya with her mother's condition, Vikram fantasizes that the doctor and Priya are having sex and seeing each other while he is at work. He murders the doctor but makes it look like suicide. On her birthday, the two of them are on a boat when a storm breaks. Priya then escapes to Shimla with her mother. When Vikram sees a painting of her done by Raj, which appears in the newspapers and for which Raj has won an award, he follows Raj to Shimla. He kills Raj's assistant and tries to kill Raj; but Raj is arrested instead.

It could be argued that the angry young man has become psychopathic over these two decades because his controlled anger and fury have not resolved anything and the failure to achieve has changed to a behaviour linked with deliberate self-harm. The psychopath wants to rule the world not because he deserves it but simply because he wants to. Chatterji (1998) acknowledges that in the mid-1990s the obsessive lover within and without marriage made his entry in to mainstream Hindi cinema (to be quickly picked up by regional cinema). She raised the question: Where did these lovers come from? Of course Hollywood was a source of inspiration, especially, as noted earlier, with *Sleeping with the Enemy*. The three films discussed are *Agnisakshi*, *Daraar*, and *Dastak*, in addition to *Yaarana*, *Anjaam*, and others. The first three portray the husband as a jealous and obsessive lover who will go to extremes to hang on to his property, even if it means trying to kill his wife if she decides to leave him. Within marriage, too, the control and terror, reflecting his suspicious paranoid fantasy, is extreme, leading to physical abuse and emotional blackmail. The husband has the social approval to control his wayward wife even though that means she has to be controlled physically. In *Agnisakshi*, Nana Patekar's violence is explained by his mother's behaviour when he was a child, when his behaviour could not be controlled even by the extremes of military discipline. When he beats his wife because she is dancing alone in the house, it would appear that her dance is, or should be, only for his pleasure. The audience acknowledges that he loved his wife to distraction.

Chatterji (1998) notes that it is the husband who has the viewer's sympathy. His death, rather than a legal reprisal, indicates where the director's sympathies lie. Chatterji wrote that *Agnisakshi*'s box office success, in contrast with the failure of *Yaarana*, might lie in the fact that the male protagonists in the latter are older and not box office draws. The voyeuristic vulgar violence in both films indicates a male perspective, which is alluring but also becomes obsessive and possessive. In contrast to the selfish, demanding, irrational, violent, and overpowering male, the females are subdued and sensitive creatures but beautiful alluring Eves who bring the violence upon themselves. The dependent woman whose life and identity are incomplete without a husband, no matter how abusive and obsessive he is, is the reflection of the Bharatiya naari (traditional Indian woman), who is all-suffering. Citing a psychiatric opinion, Chatterji notes that this scary irrational phenomenon marks a thin line between love and obsession; men, being extroverts, are more expressive compared with introverted women who do not show what they feel. No doubt this is a gross generalization and caricature, but as ever there is a kernel of truth in it. Although this obsessive love had existed and been portrayed in Hindi films, it is only recently that it has become violent, controlling, and vicious. The invasion of personal space and altered materialistic possessive values have made it acceptable.

Chatterji (1998, p. 103) cites a psychoanalyst who observes that obsession is a serious personality disorder—an extreme form of narcissism in which the person experiences emotions which are not within the realm of reason and over which they have no control. Chatterji notes that these films do not probe psychological motives but perpetuate the myths that obsessive husbands have some reasonable explanation for behaving the way they do, and also that such obsession is linked to the physical beauty, desirability, and sexuality of the woman. The husbands are psychopathic jealous possessive lovers, which, in spite of their villainy, is shown as rare; the patriarchal message of control is clear.

The portrayal of rape is often related to visual titillation and also to visual gratification. The act itself lends credence to the abuse of power rather than to sexual pleasure, but that is not how the viewer sees it.

The role of depression and its relationship with suicide is not part of this book but will be explored further later. Suicide itself is a dramatic act and often employed as a point of reference in the storytelling.

Another possible explanation that can be put forward is that the definition of self in deliberate self-harm varies across cultures (see Bhugra, 2004). The sociocentric self involves others, in which case the act of deliberate self-harm is also meant to hurt others around the individual rather than the individual himself/herself. Under these circumstances the act takes on a much broader significance. The introjection of the anger can lead to depression and one way of dealing with it is to externalize the anger by self-hurting.

The portrayal of the anger has changed dramatically and allows the viewer to have a set of emotions that are disjointed, fractured, and difficult to comprehend. The sense of anger, lack of guilt, and fervent desire to possess either material things or women is obvious. The two personas of the angry young man and the psychopath are differentiated by an area controlled by society.

In *Anjaam*, *Darr*, and *Baazigar* the villain is the hero and in an egoistic manner he is not at all interested in social norms and morals. He is interested in lust and he wants the heroine for himself, not because it is love but because it is love combined with lust and obsession. Such an obsession for the first time is public and open. In *Dastak* too, the villain is known to be mentally ill as well as being highly intelligent, but he kills people considered close to his obsession and then eventually kidnaps a woman. There is no evidence of medical involvement or treatment. The characters played in these films are remorseless and ruthless, with no respect for human life. They are not interested in money, glory, or political advancement; all they want is a sexualized object they lust after. The villains in the romantic films of the 1950s and 1960s also lusted after the heroine, but were restrained. They were not portrayed as conventional villains; their evil was enticing for the audience. The current lust to kill is for their own ego, self-esteem, and possession.

The evil portrayed by heroes in Hindi cinema in the 1990s had very strong parallels with Hollywood's *Natural Born Killers*, *The Silence of the Lambs*, *Cape Fear*, *Sleeping with the Enemy*, etc. In 1991 and 1992, Anthony Hopkins and Jodie Foster won Academy awards for *The Silence of the Lambs*; Kathy Bates won the best supporting actress award for *Misery* as a female psychopath holding her favourite author hostage; Jeremy Irons got the best actor award for *Reversal of Fortune* as an alleged wife killer; and Joe Pesci won the best supporting actor award as a sadistic psychopath in *Goodfellas*. The characters being put up and revered in awards are perfectly horrible people who have no saving grace. This too is a reflection of the society where the then President (Clinton) faced impeachment and the general attitude was that "anything goes".

In India in the 1990s, the economic liberalization and expansion of television outlets from cable to satellite TV suggest that traditional values were under a lot of pressure from modernity, which is not defined by India but is being defined by others outside. The "other" has become respectable and more acceptable; the psychopathy itself has become respectable. This generation is being represented by heroes who have nothing to give except hate, venom, and bile, which is destructive. It is not surprising then that, in Hindi cinema at least, women are following the trends set by their male counterparts.

The mother in *Mother India* did not hesitate to shoot down her younger son when she felt he had crossed the line. In current films, the mother rarely takes control or stops the wayward son. In *Khalnayak* the mother does tell the hero Ballu that she wished she had slapped him when he stole someone's pencil, but in *Anjaam* and *Baazigar* the mother "pretends" that she does not know what her son is up to and turns a blind eye to his transgressions and criminal activities. In *Anjaam*, the mother is rich and runs her own business but is not able to tell her son that he can't set up an airline, or that he would require a manager rather than a pilot to run the company.

The mother is missing in *Darr*, *Daraar*, and *Agnisakshi*, suggesting that the absence of the mother is giving in to the "villain hero" protagonist. The mother had always been an important symbol of conscience; she guided her misguided son back to sanity but, in the 1990s, having asked the question, "Is the voice of conscience then singing a different tune in the turbulent 1990s?", N. Kazmi (1996, p. 83) suggests that the answer is in the affirmative.

CONCLUSIONS

Upheaval in the country, with the collapse of consensual politics, short-lived unstable central governments, increased value on regionalism and regional parties, and the destruction of Babri Masjid all contributed to a sense of chaos, rebellion, and selfish mentality, which is reflected in the films of this era. The struggle between the adoption of western values and the fear of losing one's own culture and identity continues to this day.

The heroes of these films portray and reflect what they see in their leaders and in their establishment. The representation here is that possession by might is right.

CHAPTER TWELVE

Why should women remain behind?

While Amitabh Bachchan and Sunjay Dutt were at their peak, the roles given to women in their films were feeble to say the least. They played docile, doting, and overinvolved mothers. The heroines were decorative pieces with small perfunctory lines and roles. In *Deewar* as well as *Zanjeer* the romantic female lead is secondary. In *Deewar*, Parveen Babi plays a prostitute with a golden heart who is lusting to become respectable by marrying the hero and, in *Zanjeer*, Jaya Bhaduri virtually disappears from the screen after the first half of the film. *Deewar* was inspired by *Mother India*, acknowledges its director, Yash Chopra (Dwyer, 2002). The success of *Deewar* also relied on breaking many rules: There were few songs, little romance, the heroine is a nonvirgin and dies, and the father dies before the family reunion takes place. The seamy side of Bombay was shown unflinchingly and the real threat of smuggling was highlighted.

Somaaya (2004) argues that in the 1950s and 1960s the hero of Hindi films was up to some mischief but it was gentle and not at the cost of others. The 1970s hero reflected the turbulence of the volatile decade. The heroes were repressed and transmitted their restlessness to the audience. The mood was introspective. In the 1980s, young heroes followed the restlessness of their seniors. The following decade emphasized form rather than substance. The hero of the 1990s was fixated on himself, like a selfish adolescent, and a rocking youngster emerged. Somaaya observes that the hero's costume designer and personal trainer have jumped centre stage. The cosmetically perfect hero urgently needs a soul. The hero's image was cocooned and protected from any external factors.

To target the NRI market, the hero became a world traveller with bits of India to tie him to the mother country, but the emptiness of the soul is clearly discernible. Somaaya (2004) argues that post-Independence ideals of social consciousness started to fade and while the films became frivolous the hero became self-absorbed. In recent times, she notes, the hero has two goals: to be rich and to conquer love. She sees wealth as the primary goal. Her argument that the oppressed has become the oppressor is worth noting.

However, the emergence of *Khalnayak* as the nayak (hero) also brought about another challenge in the Hindi cinema where the heroine (as in *Khalnayak*) decides to stand by her man to fight alongside him. However, the female psychopath is a relatively recent incarnation. The contemporary female represents a perfect combination of traditionalism and modernity. She is aggressive, demanding, assertive, and able to flaunt her sexuality. The extension of the heroine to this level has led to the vamp as obvious next step. The vamp used to be the outsider, a glamorous presence who represented either the western perspective in juxtaposition to the traditional heroine or the extreme Indian perspective of sister-in-law or mother-in-law torturing the heroine. The role of the vamp in the glamour tradition was in competition to the heroine, providing an attractive counterpoint for the audience, who tended to hate her anyway and to characterize her as a loose woman. Such a loose woman offered a potential for sexual titillation to the male audience and a cautionary reminder to the female as to what they could end up being if they gave up their traditional and Indian cultures.

The role of the vamp and the consideration of this role cannot be viewed in isolation from the roles women have portrayed in Hindi cinema and their development up to the level of psychopathy. Vasudev (1988) argues that the role of women in society as well as in films is dictated by mythological depictions of the goddesses. Although they are *ardhangini* (half body of the male), they are submissive and subjugated. This was borne out literally in *Ardhangini*, where Chhaya (Meena Kumain) as the heroine goes through agony because she is seen to be submissive and inauspicious. Her husband, an airline pilot (Raaj Kumar), goes mad and is nursed back to normality. Vasudev suggests that when Manu, the lawgiver for Hindus, wrote that a female must be subject to her father in childhood, to her husband in youth and after that to her sons and that she should never be independent, he condemned women to millennia of being treated like chattel. She adds that the perceived Victorian values and hypocrisy as a legacy of the Raj allow men to keep double standards. Hindi films have reiterated and reinforced these values.

The heroine in Hindi films was seen as a very important person by P. Chatterjee (1995a). He argues that the woman was never a foil to the hero but it was the other way around, even if the heroine was paid less and had less important dialogue in the film and a lower place in the credit list.

In the 1980s, the heroine in her new incarnation was an oversexed Jackie Collins-type of woman, crossed with pseudo Kung-fu training, possessing a murderous, vengeful temperament too and the hypothetical eloquence of the religiosocial feminist crusader found only in India (P. Chatterjee, 1995b). Discussing the saffronization of the silver screen in the 1990s, Viswanath (2002) observes that a growing disillusionment with the inadequacies of the Nehruvian interventionist and tutelary state, coupled with technological advances and economic imperatives, forced India to open its doors to western market forces (again! after the imperialist rule); and the resurgence of religious factors helped foster the growth of Hindu nationalism. Hindu nationalism equated Hindu with India, and the films of the 1990s reflect this. Hindutva represented an ethnic, monoculturalistic, homogenized racist premise and was a clear response to a number of factors. Viswanath points out that in the 1990s there were two types of film—action films and family drama. Both genres tackled an imagined enemy and right wing ideologues created paranoia about the enemy, whether a terrorist foreigner or an enemy of family values.

The paradox in Hindi film, as in society, is that women may be victimized as wife on the one hand and venerated as the mother goddess on the other. Mother figures are important even in angry young man films. Vasudev (1988) highlights the fact that even with sons the relationship is not explored, but the mother fights fiercely and protectively and somehow her identity and existence are subsumed within this all-engulfing relationship.

Sisters too have a role in the Hindu context and they pray for their brothers' welfare and protection. However, they are weak and sidelined in the story and do not have a tremendous degree of freedom or an independent existence. The dancing girl is another stereotype vamp, or golden hearted call girl dealt a rough hand by fate. Men go to the dancing girls either for relaxation (if they are rich feudal landlords) or to drown their sorrows. Once again few films have a dancing girl as heroine and, if she succeeds in settling down by getting married, it is because she is pure or because she is not a *real* prostitute (a case of mistaken identity).

Prabhu (2001, p. 77) points out that in *Mausam*, Chanda (played by Sharmila Tagore) goes mad after being abandoned by Amarnath (Sanjeev Kumar); the daughter born by her becomes a prostitute after she is raped. The feelings of rejection and hatred the young daughter holds towards her father are greater than those she holds against her rapist. However, a love gradually develops for her father, whom she initially sees as her customer. The Electra complex is resolved to a degree but the abandonment of the innocent, uneducated rural woman by the educated, wandering, foreign man is a not uncommon theme in Hindi cinema. *Mausam* brings out the consequences of a broken, incomplete relationship, and promises the irreparability of certain decisions: Memories and nostalgia connect the irreparable past to the present (Prabhu, 2001, p. 80). There is no doubt that, like many other Hindi films in a similar vein, this film depicts the patriarchal nature of Hindu society. Men dictate to women and "modify" their behaviour by "breaking" them. The older woman certainly has no individual existence. She is the daughter of the widowed father and exists for the father, and then pines away for her lover. Gulzar, the writer/director, in his interview with Prabhu (2001), sees *Mausam* as a film related to nostalgia in human beings and intricacies of relationships.

Gopalan (2002) asserts that a standard narrative has a happy and normal family setting with an absence of marked paternal figures. The female protagonist is a working woman with a strong presence; she is raped and a miscarriage of justice at one level or another allows her to become an avenging woman, because men who run establishments, be it government or judiciary, are impotent and inadequate. The women also evoke figures of Hindu shakti goddesses to give legitimacy to their revenge. *Anjaam* is different, as the rape here is not physical but a psychological intrusion and destruction of her life.

Gopalan (2002) suggests that the state of Emergency is the origin for the crisis of legitimacy of the Indian state. At the very least it did set into motion contestations between power and authority that have pressed upon a more thorough exploration of hegemony, citizenship, community, nationalism, and democracy in India, but Gopalan emphasizes that discussions of violence have to consider how films, replete with violent women, gangsters, and vigilante closures, stage some of the most volatile struggles over representations that shape our public and private fantasies of national communal, regional, or sexual identities.

The image of the working girl in Hindi cinema shifted in the 1980s. They could be working girls but they still paid homage to the male values or their families. They handed their salaries to their fathers and mothers, and looked after sisters and brothers; if they were working, marriage was somehow contraindicated. The roles of nurses or doctors for women existed largely on the margins.

Whereas in the early 1970s stars like Sharmila Tagore and Asha Parekh were seen to play a doctor or surgeon in films like *Safar* and *Upkar* respectively, the modern emphasis is on filmstars playing models, dancers, actors, etc. These changes reflect the materialistic and capitalist changes prevalent in the country at the present time. Although women are still being presented as traditional, there have been changes in the ways in which they are portrayed.

Bandini is the story of Kalyani, a woman convict serving life imprisonment for committing the murder of her lover's wife. The repression conveyed by the blacksmith's hammer and the hysterical illness of the wife drives Kalyani (played by Nutan) over the edge. The film beautifully portrays how oppression leads to the metamorphosis of a gentle creature who sings love songs into a murderer. The message is that anyone is capable of murder. In addition, the destruction of her dreams of marriage and freedom contributes to her stress. For the audience too, the dream was destroyed after the Chinese invasion and the conversion of friendship into hatred. The reviewer in *Filmfare* saw *Bandini* as a very good film. The camerawork and imaginative dedicated and painstaking direction were singled out for praise. Nutan was praised very strongly and the rest of the members of the cast were seen as subordinate to her performance. The music was seen as delightful. The reviewer was clearly bowled over by the director whose finest hour the film was seen to be, and also a shining hour for Hindi films enveloped in a suffocating cocoon of mediocrity. The portrayal of the hero also changed. In place of the strong and stable man, he has emerged as a more frivolous youngster, bursting with energy (Somaaya, 2004). The portrayal of masculinity changed over the years too. From gentle romantic to romantic rebel to aggressive rebel and psychopathic, the cycle is now complete and we now have a gentle romantic but one who is full of aspirations and where the world has become his playground (see Saif Ali Khan in *Kal Ho Na Ho*).

Pyar Tune Kya Kiya was seen as a masala film for the audience of only good cinemas in "A" class centres. The reviewer in *Film Information* noted that it had nothing to offer small centres. The prediction was that it was a loser. *Pyar Tune Kya Kiya* is not a pleasant love story. The heroine discovers that the man she loves is already married. She turns vengeful and attempts to destroy her beloved's life. Somaaya's review (2004) suggests that the rage of the heroine is more to do with herself rather than her circumstances. It is also interesting that the relationship with her father indicates the changing mores of daughter–father relationships. Previously, the heroine would withdraw rather than strike back. It could be that diffidence had previously crushed her confidence and losing gracefully was easier. It is also quite likely that changing times, with relative equality of status and the influence of feminism, have altered these perceptions.

As discussed earlier, *Anjaam* tells the story of Vijay Agnihotri, who obsessively loves Shivani and, unable to take no for an answer, stalks her. The film also gives the heroine a role that is unusual on several levels. The theme of revenge by the wronged woman is not unusual in itself but the manner in which Shivani takes revenge is violent, ruthless, and uncontrolled. Of course there have been other films, such as *Bandit Queen*, *Khoon Bhari Maang*, *Zakhmi Aurat*, *Insaaf ka Tarazu*, etc., with these qualities, but *Anjaam* allows the heroine to take revenge in the jail itself. She is shown to be wearing white, with bloodstains following her miscarriage, which was induced by the sadistic jailer who is masculine and aggressive, and who therefore has to be punished in the same way. Similarly, revenge on Vijay Agnihotri is portrayed in an interesting way. First, she sets out to nurse and nurture him, gaining the praise of the doctor, as well as Vijay's mother; then she seduces him; and ultimately she destroys him by her anger and revenge. This is made palatable with background music of prayers for the goddess Vaishno Devi, who is an incarnation of the goddess Durga, while she is killing the jailer and the stalker.

The stark images of Kali/Durga, interspersed with the music reaching a crescendo, influence the audience into thinking that this avenging murder is somehow acceptable because it is the goddess who is working through the female protagonist and this action is reflective of "possession". The message is also conveyed that women can take on the role of mothers, and later destroyers, if they have been wronged. The message in the film is that Kali is both a mother and a destroyer, so men need to be careful!

Shivani had lost a husband, one child, and her sister due to the direct impact of the stalking; she then loses a foetus in jail; but the sheer bloodiness of her revenge is still shocking.

Damini relates the story of an honest girl married into a rich family who sees her brother-in-law and his friends raping a servant. She is declared to be mad but goes on to fight for justice and thus displays her courage and strength in an effort to uphold the truth against all odds (Prabhu, 2001, p. 189). In spite of the predominantly male backdrop, she embodies the essential values of Indian womanhood.

In a survey of audience attitudes towards the role of women in Hindi films, Prabhu (2001, p. 184) found that the predominant image of women in their minds is that of educated women but submissive wives or daughters. The expectations of the audience and the directors' portrayal start to converge. The stereotypes of good woman, mother, and the vamp or cabaret dancer work at one level, allowing the audience not to be shocked entirely. By the 1980s, violence towards women becomes a part of Hindi film. Prabhu (2001, p. 188) notes that from 1975 to 1982 (the period during which the films she studied were made), there was a transition in role projection of women with relation to personal emotions and decisions which is progressive and path breaking.

In both *Damini* and *Zakhmi Aurat*, the heroine is influenced by Durga. In the former, the heroine escapes from the asylum where she is terrified of being killed and, in spite of being chased, the chase is preceded by a scene of apotheosis (Chatterji, 1998). Chatterji points out that, in *Zakhmi Aurat*, although the woman is angry, she does not sustain this anger and consequently makes herself vulnerable to a similar trauma in the future.

The trend set by earlier violent films such as *Bandit Queen*, *Zakhmi Aurat*, etc., has not entirely dissipated. Parallel cinema has shown women to be creative, active, confident, and self-assured, and men to be weak, vacillating, and inadequate. In the 1990s two Hindi films were released with varying degree of success where women were murderers. These are no different from Bimal Roy's *Bandini*. The heroine in *Bandini* pays the price, whereas in latter films like *Gupt* or *Kaun* she does not. The female protagonists in both films are psychotic but in one case released from the asylum, and in the other living independently where all external contexts have been deliberately removed.

MURDERING *KAUN* AND KEEPING THE SECRET *GUPT*

Until the 1990s the women avenged their dishonour in a goddess-like manner, such as in *Anjaam*. However, the female murderer or psychopath was extremely rare. In an unusual departure from his previous social genre films, Yash Chopra directed *Ittefaq*, with Rajesh Khanna playing Dilip Roy, an escapee from an asylum. Dilip enters a flat with a lonely woman Rekha (Nanda). He is shown as dangerous and the audience has sympathy with Rekha. Dilip then discovers a body in the bathtub. This body is not seen again; the police get involved and Dilip manages to prove that not only he is innocent of murdering his wife but that Rekha has murdered her husband. This 1969 film was linked with the initial success of Rajesh Khanna as a film star who, as noted earlier, then went on to become a major star of the late 1960s and 1970s.

Ittefaq was based on a Gujarati play, which in turn was inspired by another source—*Lamp Post to Murder*. The film was shot in less than a month. Rajesh Khanna was not the first choice to play the lead; neither was the heroine Nanda who was well known for playing sisterly roles and romantic leads, although she did give a good performance.

The script was written in 8 days by Akhtar-Ul-Iman and was shot almost as it appears on the screen (Dwyer, 2002). It ran for over 15 weeks, which was exceptional for a film made on a shoestring budget with no songs. The characters are not glamorous. There is just one set with two main characters and brief appearances by others. In an interview with Somaaya (2002), the film's director Yash Chopra indicated that the film was a quickie to be finished while waiting for another film to be completed. Chopra emphasizes that the film had many firsts to its credit, as it was the first nonsong, 2-hour film without an interval. The film was a success and it did offer an important portrayal of the mentally ill, in this case because the hallucination (seen only once) raises questions in the minds of viewers. Whether it was a real corpse or a genuine hallucination, combined with the traditional image of the heroine who was well known for playing the doting sister and lovable individual, the point on which the film turns makes the mental illness essential to the suspense.

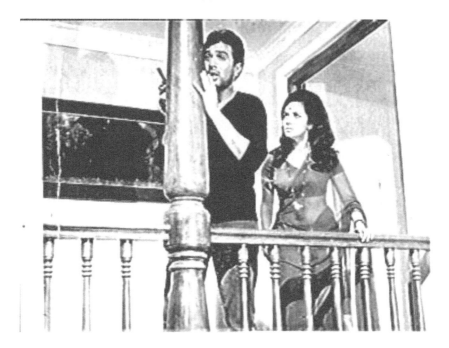

Figure 12.1   *Ittefaq* (courtesy of National Film Archive of India)

The producer of *Ittefaq*, B. R. Chopra, tackled a similar theme in *Dhund*, in which Danny Denzogpa plays a psychopathic landowner/hunter and is murdered. He arouses little sympathy because he is verging on the psychotic, abusing those around him and shooting innocent animals; again this film has no songs. The villainous character may provoke some sympathy due to his physical disability as he was confined to a wheelchair, but the portrayal was not sympathetic. It can be argued that his physical and mental disabilities allow him to lose sympathy, which is not uncommon in Hindi films.

However, in the 1990s, Kajol, the daughter of the film star Tanuja and granddaughter of another film star, Shobhna Samarth, emerged as an obsessive psychotic killer in *Gupt*, and the psychopathic behaviour on the part of women in films took on a different sheen. Isha (Kajol) and Sahil (Bobby Deol) had been childhood friends; when she meets him again in college they fall in love. Sahil is also loved by Sheetal, whose father tries but fails to protect her. Sahil's stepfather is keen for him to get married to Sheetal, but is then murdered by Isha. Sahil is convicted of his stepfather's murder and sentenced. He eventually escapes from prison with Sheetal's help, but Isha becomes very jealous. Sahil's family doctor is also murdered and another police inspector is attacked. The police inspector starts to believe Sahil, who continues to maintain his innocence; Isha's father admits to both murders. But the police inspector is attacked while Isha's father is in police custody and this places Isha under suspicion. Her father tells Sahil the truth, that even as a child she had been very possessive towards Sahil and had even killed a dog that had bitten Sahil. Sahil realizes that Isha's next target is Sheetal. The psychopath here is unusual because she is female, had been sent to a "boarding house" on medical advice and has a father who is aware of what is going on.

Gupt was described in a review (see www.imdb.com) as a musical suspense drama made on a lavish scale, with a fast pace and an intelligently written screenplay. The hero, Bobby Deol, was praised for his looks and his acting, and the two female leads were seen as sexy, glamorous, and bewitching and having given excellent performances. The direction and narration were praised. The songs were seen as tuneful with good picturization.

The film *Kaun* deals with three characters who are not given any names. The heroine (Urmila Matondkar) is alone in a house full of antiques and *objets d'art*. The viewer listens with her to the news on TV that a convict has escaped and the public is advised to be cautious because the convict is dangerous and unpredictable. Suddenly the doorbell rings and she hears a male voice (Manoj Bajpai) asking to come in to the house because it is raining heavily outside and his car has stalled. The man wants to telephone the garage. She refuses to allow him in, saying that her husband is asleep. The man persists and then asks for a sandwich. Through the kitchen window he is seen to be the potential villain. The third character appears and says that he is a policeman who has come in response to the phone call from the heroine. The first man gets suspicious as he discovers that the phone is disconnected and decides that the policeman must be a fake. He discovers that the most likely scenario is that the woman herself is the murderer. Both male characters are murdered. Although there is no external context in which to embed the film, especially with regard to the heroine, her presence as a psychopathic murderer is clear. As Shah Rukh Khan in *Darr* had done, she talks to her (nonexistent) mother on the telephone and shows no remorse or guilt at all. These acts of violence are not entirely random ones, but she demonstrates an inordinate capacity to be calm under pressure and yet plays with dolls like a child, reminiscent of Mia Farrow in *Rosemary's Baby*. The acts of stabbing, the bloodshed, and her clothes are all seen to be "modern" representations of an act that until recently was seen only in a predominantly male domain. Urmila Matondkar played a similar role in films like *Ek Hasina Thi*, where she avenges herself on the hero, who had pushed her into admitting a crime for which she was imprisoned. Another film, *Raaz*, has a heroine obsessively chasing the hero, who is not interested in her. Her borderline personality is striking.

In these films there is no apparent evidence that the female protagonists are subjected, suppressed, or subordinate. In all cases the women know what they are doing—in *Gupt*, Isha wants the hero and is prepared to fight and kill for him, whereas in *Kaun* the lack of context makes it even more frightening because the woman kills two men and the reasons for it are unclear except to emphasize her madness. Radner (1998) asks if the psychofemme is the expression of the lunacy of woman crazed by heterosexuality. Is heterosexuality indelibly marked as insane? There is no doubt that in both the Hindi and Hollywood cinema cannon males have been shown to be villainous and sadistic, but this new generation of psychofemmes creates women who refuse the violence of men and take upon themselves the problems of the lunatic violence of men and death, more specifically of murder. *Gupt*, *Anjaam*, and *Kaun* all portray these psychofemmes. *Ek Hasina Thi* and the femme fatale in *Raaz* indicate that the female has now become the ultimate male. These women not only stand for violence, but also carry it out verbally and actually in the sense of proving that they are better than the male. The feminine side has given way to the murderous masculine. This is perhaps in response to the male violence on screen in the same stories, or off screen.

This change in the portrayal of mental illness into psychopathic disorder, which is characterized by irritability, bouts of anger, no remorse or guilt, and no social responsibility among females, is a new development in Hindi cinema.

The portrayal of psychopathy is not unknown in Hollywood films. The prevalence of psychopathic disorder in women in the general population is much lower than that amongst men. The freedom of the narrative and liberty of characterization indicates that these characters may well be unusual and are being deployed to hang the surprise element of the suspense stories in both cases. The fulfilment traditionally emerging from motherhood and family obligations is beginning to shift in the direction of the generation with aspirations to ape America and the west in values and materialism. Shah Rukh Khan won several awards for his portrayals of psychopaths in *Anjaam* and *Baazigar*. The romantic love was under severe threat not from the mentally ill but from wilful personality disordered individuals who had turned up in the complacent middle class lives of lovers aspiring to work harder and become richer. This fear experienced by the middle classes was real and reflected the turning point where middle/upper class young men, reasonably good-looking, well-employed, and charming at times, were turning the safety of the middle class upside down. Although Vijay Agnihotri, Rahul, and Vikram were the boys next door, they did not conform, and this creates fear that creeps into the social setting.

Aaina, released in 1991, tells the story of Amrita Singh, who loves Jackie Shroff but abandons him on the night of the wedding to act in films and become a heroine. In desperation, her parents marry Jackie to their younger daughter, Juhi Chawla, who had silently loved the hero from afar all along.

However, Singh returns and wants to resume her relationship in spite of the fact that Jackie is now her brother-in-law. Not getting her way, she takes an overdose of pills and tries to slash her wrists, providing an interesting insight into borderline personality disorder.

In *Pratighaat* the heroine is disrobed in public, similar to Draupadi, but she vows to avenge her honour as Kali did. However, when she comes to act on her vengeance, she aborts the child she is carrying in order to be free of her maternal obligations and other such ties. She then morphs into Kali in order to behead the villain publicly—a symbol of evil with an axe (Chatterji, 1998). Chatterji argues that *Pratighaat* tries to indict the modern ruling class and enlarges the villainous figure to stand for the system.

Such a play with mythology offers an easier alternative, Chatterji (1998) asserts, to a considered serious critique of democracy in operation. It is more attractive to filmmakers who, on the one hand, are out to make money and, on the other, can offer some patronizing backslapping in order to make a woman-oriented film. Such crude stereotyping and distortion of the female act and body in relation to Hindu mythology make it more identifiable to the viewer, but the ongoing stereotyping is bound to have long-term effects on society and the cinema. Hindi cinema, like cinema around the world, reflects the social ethos of female stereotyping and distortion, which includes marriage, even though there has been a slow but inevitable evolution of the marriage myth over the past few decades. The martyrdom embedded in the Hindu wife is played over and over again and yet tightly controlled by the male. Chatterji points out that symbols of binding and confinement show up in female customs and manners specifically linked to those of the wife. In *Khoon Bhari Mang*, the heroine undergoes plastic surgery to correct a facial disfigurement for which her husband was responsible, and, when he falls for her, she avenges herself. Chatterji observes that the emphasis here is not just on the significance of beauty in the life of a woman-as-wife, but also on the fallibility of an otherwise shrewd and intelligent man who cannot recognize his own wife just because she has had a facelift. Chatterji emphasizes that, within this scenario, the husband–wife relationship is not only reduced to something that lacks both intelligence and conviction, but irritatingly is vulgarized by its cinematographically crude presentation.

The relative increase in the portrayal of bigamous relationships in Hindi cinema in films like *Saajan Chale Sasural*, *Judaai*, and *Gharwali Baharwali* reflects tendencies in real life for heroines to "marry" already married heroes. The need for security and safety is apparent, but the society gets shaken to its foundations; the only way these protagonists can be dealt with is through murder itself—which again frightens the middle classes. The avenge is paramount.

In contrast, Dwyer and Patel (2002) point out that the major hits of the 1990s were the big budget, plush, romantic films. These mark the dominance of the values of the new middle classes and uphold them to the pleasure of the socially mixed audiences both in India and abroad. These authors note that these films revived a form of the feudal family romance in a new, stylish but unmistakable patriarchal structure that is connected to the part they play in the resurgence of Hindutva politics in the 1980s and 1990s. It can also be argued that this connection is not entirely unidirectional.

This allows an expulsion of the "other" into a space that is external and distant. The threat to this security of middle class Hindu folk (particularly comforted by *Maine Pyaar Kiya* and *Hum Aapke Hain Kaun* in the 1990s, which had religious tones and feudal hierarchical settings where everyone knows their place and is happy with his or her status) was shaken by the demolition of Babri Masjid, which brought the concept of the "other" (Muslim in this context) into a very sharp focus. In addition, the hero/ villain distinction became blurred, worrying the middle class audience. The role of the "other" is at a level where their existence is particularly threatening because it confirms the coda of middle class values, treats women like chattel, and takes pride in it but at the same time legitimizes the social expectations of aspiration and achievement.

Hindi films also reflect the caste system in the society. Mythological films are the top notch; stunt films, which provide the labourer with enjoyment, remain bottom of the pile.

Even in romantic films, where middle class values are reflected, the rules of reading of scriptures and the ways of religious rites and rituals are being challenged. The controversy generated in *Mohabbetein* by Amitabh Bachchan performing his religious rituals while wearing shoes was rampant. This led the Kashi Intellectual Forum to ask the Ministry of Information and Broadcasting to take strict action against Amitabh Bachchan (Anon 2000, p. 4). The leader of the Intellectual Forum also threatened to launch an agitation if the scene involving Bachchan was not deleted from the film. Bachchan responded with a letter stating that on the two occasions in question in the film he was actually not wearing shoes. Even while the scenes were being shot in inclement weather, Bachchan insisted that even then all those participating in the shoot, including the film crew, were barefoot. He also insisted that he had taken his shoes off even while he was dubbing the sequence. Religion, rituals, and fundamentalist extreme views now frighten the actors and directors not only in the film but during the shooting itself. Acknowledging that he was "a deeply religious person", Bachchan is reported to have said that he would not dream of any kind of disrespect to religious sentiments.

This marked defensive nature is not unknown regarding the films because their success depends upon the patronage of groups and the government. A similar attack on the director Deepa Mehta and the star of her forthcoming film *Water*, last of a trilogy, led to the shooting being abandoned. The perceived excess of attacks on the media by Hindu organizations has led to a series of problems for producers and actors who, for financial and business reasons, try to avoid any controversy.

The role of the government in providing information and controlling information through television is changing as cable and satellite television access develops; this liberalization is likely to lead to more westernized views and styles, which will incur more protests, punishments, and processions. It is likely that the censorship of cinema too will become more stringent and dictatorial. The type of social norms and the genre of films are likely to influence each other. F. Kazmi (1999) argues that the spate of modern family musicals is a direct result of BJP's climb to power.

CONCLUSIONS

The role of women in Indian life in general and Hindi films in particular has been ambivalent to say the least. They are mothers, courtesans, lovers, and sisters, but the ways the males view them and deal with them vary according to the context. The active characters in the 1950s and 1960s, where the heroines often played the roles of teachers, doctors, and even engineers, became the passive participants in the lives of the male heroes in the 1970s and 1980s. Their existence was peripheral in both visual and characterological terms. In the 1990s, they became obvious by their combination of traditionalism and modernity, which made them progress to becoming psychopathic and psychotic in their own right. The relationship between religious imagery and religious connotations allowed them to get away with murder. The changing role of the female in Hindi films is also a reflection of changing social mores and norms.

CHAPTER THIRTEEN

New century: New villains

Through the late 1960s and early 1970s the political situation in India remained volatile; there was urban working class militancy, a Marxist uprising, as well as a Marxist democratic electorate creating a degree of confusion. The rise of the ex-socialist J. P. Narayan and his challenge to Indira Gandhi were reflected in the rise of Bachchan to tackle the establishment. The fall of Congress, the chaos following Rajiv Gandhi's assassination, the end of the Congress Raj after the electoral defeat in 1994, and the emergence of the third front with the re-emergence of the Hindu nationalist party all reflect some of the psychopathic tendencies observed in the films. The happy consensual marriage was under threat from the obsessive stalker, who may be the globalization/westernization enemy of the Hindu fundamentalist Swadeshi Morcha.

The rise and rise of the BJP led to a transformation of the social order where the middle classes, especially the merchant class, have the visibility of power, but the lower classes and the proletariat have become more subjugated and marginalized, perhaps even institutionalized, under the caste regimes. Such rigidity has allowed Hindi cinema first to froth the romantic idyll, and second to release venom in this idyll. This injection of venom reflects an underlying concern that this idyll cannot last because there is an inherent problem (the serpent in the Garden of Eden), or a fear that the idyll is not going to last. This may be confirmed by the fall of the BJP-led coalition. The feeling of being let down by the lower middle classes and poor classes contributed to the fall of the BJP, confirming that romance does not last. The venom may also be seen as the presence of the "other", which was equated with the insurgency of the CIA in Indira Gandhi's time, and may involve Pakistani agents in the recent times.

Majumdar (2000) argues that the development of the psychotic film (sic) reflects the male splitting. This psychopathic, narcissistic, or borderline personality behaviour adds mental dimension to the physical action. The pure physicality of the villainous act gives way to manipulative, possessive, and obsessive individuals wanting to possess women in a way that was not possible before, and to destroy them if they cannot be possessed in the way the protagonist wants to.

Sethu won the National Best Feature Film in Tamil award in 2000. The citation stated that this was an impressive debut by a director with a commendable grasp of the grammar of mainstream cinema, and that it deserved special mention for combining popular elements with the unconventional. Sethu, the eponymous hero, is the Chairman of the College's student union and is always up to mischief. Even after graduation, hanging around the college he rags junior students. He falls in love with Ahitha, a chaste Brahmin girl, who is engaged to another. Her elder sister has been sent back by her husband because her dowry is inadequate. Sethu gets caught in the middle when the elder sister ends up in a brothel in an attempt to make money. Ahitha responds to Sethu's love, but after he is injured in a fight with the owners of the brothel he is sent to an asylum, where he is kept in chains. He escapes but discovers that Ahitha has killed herself rather than marry her fiancé. Upon seeing this, he returns to the asylum.

Tere Naam, the Hindi remake of *Sethu*, stars the *enfant terrible* of Hindi cinema, Salman Khan. He plays Radhe Mohan, a bully who spends his time on a railway station platform that happens to be next to the college from where he appears to have graduated years ago. His nominees win the elections on his behalf by promising that it will be acceptable to cheat on exams, wink at girls, and so on, all things that can be identified as antisocial. He gets into fights, and teases and rags the newcomers to the college, which is how he meets Nirjara. In their first meeting he asks her to salute him, and then gradually he falls in love with her. Nirjara, the younger daughter of a temple priest, is already engaged to be married. Her brother-in-law demands money from his in-laws. When Radhe hears this he threatens the brother-in-law, who takes the sister back. Meanwhile, Nirjara's fiancé gives up his claim and tells her that she is free to marry Radhe. She declares her love for Radhe, who on his way home is trapped and hurt by thugs he had upset. The psychiatrist in the City Mental Home declares him to be unwell; he recommends to Radhe's brother and sister-in-law that they should pray for his recovery and that he should be transferred to an ashram (generally a holy place) where he will be tied with chains, which will be good for him. In the ashram, which appears to be a collection of caves with two priests doing puja (prayers) as well as keeping the patients chained using mantras and Ayurvedic head oil massage and similar treatments, he gets better but is unable to communicate this. While he is lying ill in the ashram, prayers are in chaste Hindi and Sanskrit, perhaps to appease the ruling Bharatiya Janata Party.

Here is yet another hero who, in spite of his graduation, does not feel that he needs to do any work. His brother taunts him gently but his sister-in-law is generous to a fault and gives him a lot of money. He falls for the charm and simplicity of Nirjara, who is a Brahmin, speaks pure Hindi, and is fully versed in cooking and prayers—a typical male perception of a Bharatiya naari. He cannot understand why she is engaged and threatens her fiancé in order to make him leave her. She is told by her fiancé about the good deeds that Radhe had performed for their family, but before she can say anything to him he has taped over her mouth and kidnapped her, and then violently confesses his feelings. In spite of this mauling, she then "falls" for him. Her father looks aghast when she tells him that she has given everything to Radhe, and she tells him, "no I have only given him my heart . . . which is after all in my body".

The psychiatrist shows Radhe's relatives his own spiritual side as, even before he himself takes any medicine, he takes the prasad (offering after prayers) his mother gives him. The clinic and the hospital are modern, with MRI scans on the viewing box and clean tidy corridors, and yet the traditional ashram is spooky, dark, and gothic, and the treatment is traditional too. It is possible that the auteur of the film was influenced by the Irwadi tragedy where 26 mentally ill people chained to their beds died in a fire.

The shift from the modern to the traditional indicates several things. First, the failure of modernity and the success of tradition are reflected in the BJP-led Indian political climate and philosophy that old indeed is gold. Second, the psychopath was on the verge of being "cured" by the love of a good woman but those who run a brothel attempt to interfere. There is a series of events in the film that all indicate a degree of confusion in the director's mind: the good looking but rough and bully hero versus the chaste Brahmin heroine, the traditional healing versus the modern interventions (which fail), the use of women as prostitutes. These contrasts run through the film. The songs are lavishly produced in wonderful surroundings. The punishment for Indian womanhood is multifaceted. Nirjara's sister very nearly becomes a prostitute in order to "make" money for her in-laws. The heroine herself is domesticated; sent to the College at the insistence of her fiancé (a fellow Brahmin mutters about why he wants her to learn English, as if the only reason for such an eventuality is to learn to speak English). The background music (certainly towards the last half hour of the film when Radhe is in the ashram) consists of very sanskritized chants with a clear subliminal message that a traditional approach to mental illness, with prayers and head massages, will work. It also indicates to the viewer that the scenes set in the ashram, which are reminiscent of Dante's inner circle of hell, can be overcome by prayer (which has to be the Hindu text, although in one scene Radhe's friend Aslam is seen praying to Allah with the Taj Majal in the background). The patients in the ashram are chained as slaves were chained in the Americas. The guru walks around blessing everyone. The patients are worse in their actions and in their behaviour—repetitive and stereotypic as in several other films. *Tere Naam* is unusual in that it raises the viewer's sympathy for a no-gooder psychopath because he has been turned into a vegetable by other psychopaths.

Deewangee, although loosely inspired by a Hollywood film (*Primal Fear*), is an unusual film. Made in 2002, this is the story of Raj (Akshaye Khanna), an eminent lawyer who has never lost a single case. He is approached by Sargam (Urmila Matondkar) to defend her guru Tarang (Ajay Devgan) against the charge of murder. Tarang has been seen running away from the house of a music impresario, Ashwin Mehta (Vijayendra Ghatge), with blood on his clothes but pleads innocent to any crime. He convinces Sargam and Raj that he is being framed and Raj takes on the case. The drama accelerates and although Raj wins the case he is not convinced that justice has been done. He discovers that from a young age (in spite of his relationship with Sargam, who he has loved since school days) Tarang has been reading books about psychiatric disorders in the local library and has convinced everyone that he is mentally ill; his paradoxical relationship with Raj, whom quite clearly he sees as a threat to his own relationship with Sargam, is unusual and entertaining. Learning about how to act like a mentally ill person and con people raises some very interesting questions. It is quite interesting that a reporter for the *Economic Times* saw Ajay Devgan as someone with multiple personalities and likened this with workers in Indian call centres who also have multiple identities in that they acquire foreign accents and foreign names. In some ways it is not surprising that multiple identities are already a norm of social functioning, but the call centres take this to the next level. How realistic and how powerful these identities are only time can tell. In addition, it will be worthwhile exploring in a longitudinal manner how and where these identities spill over. This pretence is more sophisticated than that demonstrated in *Anhonee*.

The other intriguing film of 2002 was another love triangle, *Humraaz*. Again taking its inspiration from a Hollywood film (*A Perfect Murder*) it tells the story of Karan (Akshaye Khanna) and Priya (Amisha Patel) who are in love and run a band; Priya is dispatched to see multibillionaire shipping magnate Raj (Bobby Deol) to seek a job performing on a cruise ship. Raj tries to woo Priya; he succeeds and they get married. However, it becomes clear that Karan is manipulating Priya; the plan is that after the marriage she will murder Raj, inherit his money, and marry Karan.

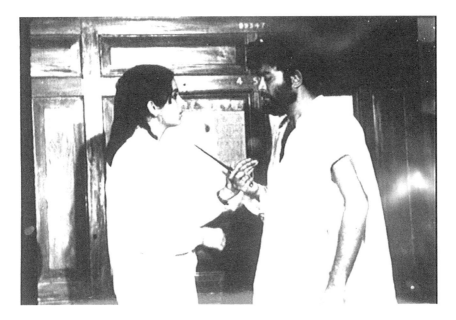

Figure 13.1 Scene from *Anhonee* (courtesy of National Film Archive of India)

However, not surprisingly, she falls in love with Raj and refuses to do what Karan expects, and so the relationship between the trio undergoes a major change. The villains used to hanker after money, plot and cheat, and occasionally murder, but the role of a manipulative creative psychopath such as Karan is an unusual one. The manipulation of a woman who then sees the light transcends both tradition and modern values. An independent professional breadwinner but also demure devoted and docile wife indicates a compartmentalization of values of financial security and spiritual values.

Madhoshi is the story of Anu (Bipasha Basu), who goes mad after watching the 9/11 attacks on the World Trade Center in New York where her sister works; at that precise time she is on the phone to the family to tell them that she is pregnant. This causes Anu to go into shock; her family tries to get her functioning again by arranging her engagement to Arpit (Priyanshu Chatterjee), a maker of international ad films. However, Anu meets Aman (John Abraham), a member of an antiterrorist organization. Enamoured by him (and partly due to her illness), she follows him, but it emerges that he does not exist in reality (thereby confirming the film's tag line of "illusion beyond imagination"). The film was seen as a loose adaptation of *A Beautiful Mind* turned into an intense love story. The scenes between the two leads were reminiscent of their scenes together in *Aetbaar*.

The sequences in the psychiatric ward of the hospital, where Anu continues to have illusory dialogues with Aman, are indeed surprising and shocking. Jha (2004) noted the film to be suffering from a split personality, whereas Adarsh (2004) saw the plot as interesting but acknowledged that although the acting was generally good the film disappointed.

In a review, Khan (2005) sees the film as astonishing (with an implausible plot and clichéd), a tremendous rollercoaster ride, and with an utterly preposterous climax. Once again Khan too is appreciative of the acting skills of main characters, as is Anjali (2004). The portrayal of madness in this context, especially in the post-9/11 world, has changed and the delusions or illusions are related to acts of terrorism and antiterrorism. When Anu first sees Aman he is shooting at people at the railway station; he hands her the revolver and disappears, only to reappear to collect it. The sexual energy of various scenes is striking and gives the film a modern feel and edge.

Another recent film, *Main Aisa Hi Hoon*, is the story of an adult man who has the mind of a 7-year-old. This is more complex than the Hrithik Roshan starrer *Koi Mil Gaya* in lots of ways. Here the hero is a wimpy, whining childlike man who is fighting a messy custody battle for his daughter. Partly inspired by *I am Sam*, starring Sean Penn and Michelle Pfeiffer, Thakur (aka Neel), played by Ajay Devgan, is working in a coffee shop in Shimla where he meets Maya (Esha Deol), who is emotionally unstable and is hooked on to drugs. She falls in love with Neel and becomes pregnant by him but, after giving birth to his daughter Gungun (Rucha Vaidya), she walks out on him. He is trying to raise Gungun with the help of a friend, played by Lillette Dubey. Maya's father from London appears on the scene to take his granddaughter away; with the help of his lawyer Neeti (Sushmita Sen), Neel fights a battle for custody of his child. Neeti is recently divorced herself, and although initially hesitant to take up Neel's case she is converted by his unflinching love for his daughter and his support for her son.

The critics were fairly unanimous in their praise for Ajay Devgan and Sushmita Sen but were concerned about the overall concept, which was perceived to be patchy. A lot of questions are raised by viewers in trying to make sense of the story but being a Hindi film it allows a number of pitfalls—and this film fails to explore human relations (Joy, 2005). The films since 2000 are once again not only heavily influenced by Hollywood formulae but also the technical excellence and competence makes them shine in a number of spheres. Playing the role of someone who is mentally ill or an autistic savant allows actors to shine and gather awards by the handful. One only has to look at Daniel Day-Lewis, Dustin Hoffman, and Russell Crowe to see the proof of this hypothesis. Hrithik Roshan in *Koi Mil Gaya*, Sridevi in *Sadma*, and Pran in *Upkar* uphold this tradition.

In 1996, another film in the tradition of stalking came from the stable of the Bhatt brothers. *Fareb* stars Faraaz Khan, Suman Ranganathan, Milind Gunanji, and Kunika. The story is of a policeman who falls in love with the wife of a man he has been asked to visit following a break-in. After an initial reluctance to do anything, he sees the wife and falls in love with her; he then tries to insinuate himself into the lives of the couple. The first sign of his brutality is when he kills the thief (a similar scenario to that of *Anjaam*). The policeman then ingratiates himself with the heroine, who starts to share her marital secrets with him. The policeman becomes obsessed with her and pays a prostitute to "play" the heroine; because of his fantasies, he beats her. Further confusion reigns till the situation is resolved. Thus the film deals with not only the evil/good dichotomy within the policeman (and we know that psychopathy can work both ways) but also the love/lust between the two relationships.

Another *Fareb* was released in 2005. Here two sisters in real life play two women chasing the same man. Aditya (Manoj Bajpai) is an ad film director married to Neha (Shilpa Shetty), who is a doctor. Her sister Ruja (Shamita Shetty), although married to someone else, falls for her brother-in-law and tries to seduce him. Eventually she succeeds and tries to drive a wedge between Neha and Aditya but is then murdered. The punishment for seduction and "incest" is murder, and the film attempts to deal with it in a half-hearted manner—a problem of marital rift and the stalking of one's brother-in-law indicate that life in urban India is changing rapidly and the old mores and morals don't exist anymore.

These are not representations of the psychopath as villain, but classic psychopaths, where the seeds of psychopathic behaviour have been sown in childhood and there is no repentance, shame, or guilt whatsoever. *Aetbaar* is the story of a doctor, Dr Ranveer Malhotra (Amitabh Bachchan), who loses his young son in a traffic accident and becomes very protective of his daughter, Ria (Bipasha Basu), who, true to form, falls in love with Aryan (John Abraham), who is a lying psychopath. He also lies about the domestic violence that he had suffered in his childhood, and about the fact that his parents are dead, since in fact his mother is still alive and in an old people's home. The surgeon is suspicious of Aryan's motives and then discovers from an old newspaper clipping that Aryan had been imprisoned for murdering his father. However, Ria pays no heed to her father's advice and for a short while moves in with Aryan, where she is shown to be sharing his bed. Gradually, with the help of the police, Dr Malhotra manages to trap Aryan; however, Aryan has recorded the conversation with Dr Malhotra where he had threatened to kill Aryan. As a result he blackmails the doctor. Subsequently the doctor succeeds in getting Aryan imprisoned but, surprise surprise, Aryan escapes; he tries to kill the family but is killed in the process. The hero is interested only in possessing the girl, although he is supposed to have an artistic bent as evinced by his painting of Ria, but he does not hesitate to burn the painting because she thinks it is better than her. Churned out by the Bhatts' production factory, in pre-release publicity the film was described as a spine-chilling thriller. Notwithstanding the fact that the holiday cottage of the Malhotras is in Vancouver, the production values are superb.

The psychopathic behaviours of the hero are a reflection of the stream of Hindi films in the early years of the twenty-first century. The hero is good looking, takes no to mean yes and forces himself on Ria who, like all gullible teenage girls falls for him hook, line, and sinker, never even questioning his stories. It is possible that love is blind and that she hears what she wants to hear. Its images of dark wet streets of the town and the place where Aryan is living, in addition to the story that he works for a car dealer, give a "noir" feel to the film. However, she does not even bother to check whether he actually works there. The hero is in the tradition of those in *Darr*, *Baazigar*, and *Tere Naam*, that is someone who plays the role of Romeo without checking whether Juliet is willing or not.

There is obviously a sense of rebellion inherent in Ria's behaviour and perhaps anger at her father, whom she holds responsible for the death of her brother, but it also indicates an unresolved Electra complex, where the feelings towards the murderous father are projected on to the real psychopath.

CONCLUSIONS

In the early years of the twenty-first century, the political, economic, and social landscape of the country has continued to change rapidly. Within this change lie the roots of economic growth, nuclear status, and an emerging globalized market economy where individuals become products and are used as such. However, the hankering for traditional thinking and way of life, and treatments that are seen as less toxic and less troublesome, indicate that films reflect the reality around them. The portrayal indicates some sympathy, as in *Tere Naam*, but the rule of the psychopath continues.

CHAPTER FOURTEEN

Family fun, frolics, and madness in *Khilona*

In India, the family remains a strong anchor for the individual, especially in rural areas where the joint or extended family is still the norm. The extended network meets regularly at weddings and funerals. The family cares for individuals with mental illness and the way the individual and the illness are handled is crucial in determining the prognosis and the outcome of the illness.

Family is seen as central both to Indian life and to Indian film. Filial loyalty and fraternal solidarity are the hallmark of the Indian family. The psychological identification with the extended family group is so strong that an actual break may be a source of psychic stress and heightened inner conflict. Kakar (1983) cites Schopenhauer's imagery of two hedgehogs on a cold night representing human behaviour (especially in Indian families). By coming close together for warmth, their quills hurt each other—they scuttle away—but when it gets cold they come back together to reach a level of homeostasis where the body temperature is above freezing but the pain inflicted by the quills (i.e., the proximity to each other) is bearable. Kakar suggests that in Indian society the optimum position entails the acceptance of more pain to get greater warmth. Socially, an individual's identity and worth is wrapped up in the reputation of the family. Lifestyle and actions are rarely the product of individual effort, though this is beginning to change in response to urbanization and industrialization. The aspirations of the individual may be wrapped up in the family. Individual initiative is to be seen in the family context. To conform is to invite admiration and to rebel is to invite scorn. Only rarely in Hindi films is the protagonist's family life not described in detail. Family narratives are also related to good/ morality and evil/decadence and connotations of traditional and Indian. Family relationships and obligations, friendships, destiny, patriotism, religion, and controlled sexuality are all part of the film (Thomas, 1985).

Kasbekar (1999) points out that in the 1950s family relationships in Hindi cinema featured the strains and pressures of modern life on the traditional extended joint family structure. The arrival of the new westernized daughter-in-law who "rebels" against the family hierarchy nearly causes the family to break up, but the crisis is resolved through some sacrifice and the errant individual gives in. This approach continued into the early 1970s but was replaced by lost and found members of the family. The big success was when Yash Chopra directed *Waqt* and Nasir Husain, Manmohan Desai, and others followed. With the demise of the studio system in the 1960s stars became more important, like their Hollywood counterparts.

As noted earlier, when one penetrates the bewildering proliferation of social forms and cultural expressions in India, relations and values come down to a level of hierarchy. The father is dominant over his sons, males over females, older brothers over the younger. The stratification is symbolized in the form found in the kinship ideology.

A male grows up recognizing kinship, real or fictional, with other males who are part of his biradari (local caste group), which may or may not coincide with lineage but is the functional basis of the caste system. The relationship between the biradari and the jati (the caste) must be taken into account when attempting to understand the family. The days when families were seen as joint or extended are over.

Kolenda (1967, 1968) demonstrated that in India there were different kinds of family notions of nuclear (husband, wife, and children), joint (up to three generations), or collateral joint (two or more brothers, their wives, and children). Families exist and evolve through time. She argues that family systems develop and break down. Cohn (2000) views this as a complex everchanging picture where it is not clear whether the joint family systems are breaking up. In rural India, the minimal operating definition of a household is those who share a single hearth. Sharing of food includes the joint holding of property, whether land or house or furniture, tools, or goods. However, the use of property is vested in the head of the household, who is generally the oldest male. His authority theoretically is absolute over the property (Cohn, 2000).

Early marriage for a girl serves as a very obvious function, particularly if she is moving into a household belonging to a caste or a religion that has the tradition of joint households, as this allows her to be socialized and less independent. This socialization, maintains Cohn (2000), is important in terms of one of the strains built into this kind of family structure. The ideology of the joint family system is to make the ties among the males of a particular generation strong. Thus, there is considerable social distance between husband and wife at the formal level. Husbands and wives in rural areas do not call each other or refer to each other by name but by their relationship to their children. For example, husband and wife will address each other as "John's mother" or "John's father". The use of the elder son's name also symbolizes one of the main functions of the wife, namely to provide male heirs so that the family line continues.

A wife will generally eat after everyone else, especially the males, has eaten. The children are looked after by a number of people and those who are not burdened by other responsibilities help with the care of the young child. Cohn (2000) points out that even in nuclear families the neighbours and relatives will be involved in childcare, thereby creating a joint family environment. Another interesting observation is that many activities are not necessarily focused on the house, which is seen instead as a place for storage, as a kitchen, or a place for sexual relationships. Males may sleep outdoors, they bathe outside, and conduct their leisure activities outside. Joint families also provide a joint function for business groups. Brothers or cousins act as agents of family business and work in mutual trust with pooled capital. Most urban middle class families support relatives in their households for long periods of time as dependants or while they tend to work or go to school.

The ideology of the joint family persists in different ways and yet the films continue to show both its advantages and disadvantages in a cinematic and dramatic context.

The family often dictates what the individual does in terms of employment or profession and marriage. The marriage is between the families and not the two individuals. Love in the marriage comes forth much later in the relationship. In Hindi films, the wife is often shown as self-sacrificing, martyred, and ill-used by the husband or by fate. She is shown to be indestructible when it comes to protecting her sons, which she does with great ferocity (Vasudev, 1988). The traditional wife, a conservative model of virtue, may win out in the end but the modern cabaret dancer or the courtesan play a significant role in films of a specific era. The paradoxical and ambivalent relationship that an Indian male has with a female is multilayered and works (or does not work) at several levels.

No real relationship can develop with a wife who is a potential mother/goddess and therefore she must be a pure and sexless creature. Vasudev (1988) then questions whether a man can ever have a satisfactory relationship with a woman. The answer is, with the courtesan who, as Vasudev reminds us, has been a significant figure in classical Indian literature and until the 1970s a staple of Indian film. Since she is forever excluded from domesticity she can answer his physical needs and cater to his fantasies (unlike the wife, who is for procreation only). He cannot fall in love with her but inevitably, even if she is a vamp, she falls in love with him; she provides a haven for him where he is allowed to recover from his sorrows but sooner or later she is left pining for him. The classical model was Chandra Mukhi in Sarat Chandra Chatterjee's *Devdas*, which has been filmed several times. Similar characters emerge in *Amar Prem, Sahib, Biwi aur Ghulam, Muqaddar ka Sikander*, and numerous other films. In *Khilona*, as in *Sadhna*, a courtesan is brought home as a pretend wife, but the reasons for doing so are different in the two films: mental illness in the former and a pretend wedding in the latter, to appease the dying mother.

Khilona is the story of a courtesan who is brought home to an orthodox family in order to "cure" a mentally ill son who is a sensitive poet who has developed mental illness after his girlfriend gets married to the villain and then commits suicide. The role of marriage is quite significant, both as the perceived cause and in the management of madness.

As previously mentioned, this film saw marriage as a possible treatment for mental illness. In *Anjaam*, too, the hero's mother is advised to get him married off although no specific psychiatric illness has been identified. In other films also marriage is seen as "curative", whether this is a practical solution to have companionship for the individual or to acquire a carer or whether there are other possible features within the marriage that may be seen as curative or protective. It may be a cure for the illness or simply a way to control the behaviour.

Khilona opens with a woman, Chand (Mumtaz), singing and dancing in the typical setting of a dancing girl's *kotha* (a brothel). As the customers are leaving, Thakur Suraj Singh walks in. Bihari (Shatrughan Sinha), who has been hanging around, welcomes him and makes lewd remarks about Thakur's presence. It turns out that Bihari is Thakur's neighbour and a rich ruffian. We never come to know about his family or his source of income apart from on one occasion where he is shown blackmailing his neighbour.

Chand gets rid of Bihari. Thakur explains to Chand that he was passing by and heard the ghazal, which moved him; Chand admits that she is fond of the poetry of Vijay Kanwal (Sanjeev Kumar), who is her favourite poet, because there is so much pain in his writing. Thakur tells her that now the only pain left in his life is that of madness and he acknowledges that Vijay is his son.

Chand asks if she can see him, even if from a distance. Thakur says that he wants someone to see him from close up, ". . . doctors say that if a young and beautiful girl comes into his life as a wife he might get better". He suggests that he would be willing to pay if Chand would pretend to be Vijay's wife and nurse him back to health. He wants this to be a drama, an experiment. The Madam of the kotha initially refuses to allow this, but Chand manages to persuade her that this will allow her to escape the kotha, even if temporarily.

When the Madam of the kotha, also her adoptive mother, asks her, "How can you live with a mad man?", Chand replies, "Which sane people come here? Drunkards, gamblers, thieves, pickpockets . . . my favourite poet is not likely to be worse than them. His every poem provides inspiration. If I can give new life to such a great poet then this will be my good fortune." Her rationale is that thieves, pickpockets, and addicts who visit her kotha are also insane, thereby indicating the society's definition of deviance and illness.

When Chand goes to the Thakur's house she gets a very cold and hostile reception from Vijay's elder brother Kishore (Ramesh Deo) as well as from Vijay's mother (Durga Khote). The two key messages here are, first, that of a fear of having a courtesan in the house polluting the orthodox Hindi household and, second, that the disapproval may well be to do with the financial implications of the contract. The only person who talks to her is Kishore's wife Laxmi.

Chand is given a room directly opposite to where Vijay is confined and she has to use the outside stairs, the kind of reception an untouchable would get. Thakur takes Chand to her room and she hears Vijay's maniacal laugh. Thakur reassures her that Vijay's room is always locked from the outside and that if Vijay becomes unmanageable she should flash the light of a torch in his eyes. He acknowledges that this step of bringing her to the house is much against his family's wishes and he asks her to be careful of the family's honour. She assures him that she would not do anything that would bring dishonour to the family name or the household.

Thus, not only are boundaries established promptly, it is made clear that the family's honour is paramount; anything she does will have an impact on this. She accepts the boundaries largely because she is keen to get out of the kotha. This could be a reflection of going from one prison to another, not dissimilar to the wedding of a girl who leaves one kind of confined space for another, although in this case the transition is voluntary. The family and its role in managing mental illness has to be seen in this context of expectation and management.

The jointness of the family has also been defined in terms of joint activities, but here there is a clear fragmentation in terms of duties and responsibilities. The Thakur seems to have retired, the eldest son manages the business, and the "middle" son seems to appear and disappear in a guest role literally and figuratively. The sensitive son is unable to cope with the stresses of modern life and is lost initially in a world of his own love and then of his own madness.

As mentioned earlier, the family is an orthodox Hindu family where the daughter-in-law of the house reads from the *Ramayana* in the family temple and prays to the tulsi plant. Chand looks at all this with great longing. Chand goes to get food for Vijay but does not enter the kitchen as if she is aware of the purity of food and her own impurity. When she first meets the family members she greets them with *adaabst* (a Muslim salutation) but on the second day she starts using *namaste* as a greeting, thereby indicating her switch to the Hindu style of greeting. The Thakur arranges a fake wedding, during which Vijay starts to see Chand as his old girlfriend Sapna and screams, and so the fake wedding does not take place. The mother admits that Chand is good looking but she feels she is not worth bringing into the household, establishing her "otherness". Interestingly, Vijay's "otherness" as a sensitive poet and a mad man is accepted by the family. This may be because he is one of their own and also an Orthodox Hindu, whereas she is perhaps Muslim as evinced by her name. We discover much later that not only is she good hearted and pure, but she is also the daughter of a highly placed social reformer, Satnam Dass, a daughter he thought had died in a train accident.

Vijay rushes off dramatically in the middle of the ceremony and has to be physically controlled by Kishore. Chand is horrified at this. Kishore tells the Thakur that he should send Chand back while he arranges for Vijay to be admitted to the madhouse. At this point the mother screams, ". . . [if that happens] send me to the cremation grounds as well. I have told you that while I am alive he will never go to madhouse." Kishore walks off in disgust. Vijay is lying on the floor sobbing. Chand promises Thakur that she is willing to give up her life to help make Vijay better. The mother blesses her. The next day, Chand learns the background to Vijay's illness from the faithful family retainer.

Vijay and Sapna loved each other but her drunkard uncle married her off to Bihari. This reflects another family obligation on the part of the girl. At the wedding reception, Bihari asks Vijay to sing his poetry. Sapna loses her mental balance, leaps off the roof and kills herself. Following the incident, Vijay becomes mad.

Chand enters Vijay's room and convinces him that she is Sapna reincarnated and come to marry him. He puts a garland made of her dupata around her neck (in the Hindu mythology the exchange denotes *gandharva vivah*, love marriage). She nurses him, using love and criticism, and improves his appearance; the family is impressed with the change. Bihari, meanwhile, is trying to lure Radha, the youngest daughter of the Thakur, to run away with him to Bombay to become a film heroine. Chand discovers this and yells at Bihari, but he taunts her for her low status and her profession. She decides to leave the Thakur household but after Vijay's pleas in a song, "You leave breaking my heart as if it were a toy/In whose hands are you leaving me alone", she rushes back.

Like Birju in *Raja*, Vijay too is frightened of thunder and lightning. One night, during a thunderstorm, he "rapes" Chand, thereby confirming the popular notions of madness and violence. The next day he feels guilty and starts to bang his head on the wall. Chand is stunned by the action of rape (which presumably Vijay thought to be his conjugal right) and becomes withdrawn. Seeing blood on Vijay's head, the family call their doctor, who sedates Vijay and recommends that Vijay needs 24-hour observation after this fit. Kishore immediately suggests that Vijay be sent to the madhouse because he may kill himself or kill others. Even his father reluctantly agrees and, as the warders try to remove Vijay, his mother pleads with Chand, "Why would you speak (up)? He is no one to you. Everybody is my son's enemy, he is nobody's brother—he is nobody's son—who has he got in this life anyway? [Meaning that had he been married, the wife would have cared for him.] He doesn't have anyone".

Suddenly Chand takes charge and announces that Vijay will not go to the madhouse. Kishore tries to interfere by saying, "Do you know how extreme his insanity is? If something happens to anyone [i.e., violence] who will be responsible?" Chand volunteers to look after him 24 hours a day. Vijay refuses to face her, repeating, "I am an animal and a sinner." She convinces him that he has not committed a sin.

Uberoi (1993) cautions that family is also a site of exploitation and violence: of men over women; in-laws over brides; of adults over children; even of the young over the elderly. The family is seen as a cultural ideal and a focus of identity. These roles are often pointedly exaggerated in Hindi films. However, the story in *Khilona* is unusual in that it has to deal with Vijay's madness, and Bihari as the villain who is seducing the most vulnerable female of the family. The seduction of the older son by "the evil" Anglo-Indian secretary also adds to this. Amongst all this chaos of the impending pollution the borrowed/false wife, true to her genes, remains pure (even though she's been violated) and holds values of the traditional Hindu daughter-in-law in aspiring to do all things the older daughter-in-law is doing.

The "marriage" here again is interesting to the viewer as the woman is keen to get "married" but the asymmetry in the marital setup, like most marriages in India, is evident. Although it is not entirely clear, the family setup is that of an upper caste Hindu in North India and, as is identified by Karve (1953), the parents of the groom and bride "arrange" the marriage. The relationship as identified in *Khilona* represents the patriarch. Thakur going to the place of the "bride" (the kotha in this instance) also reflects double standards for men and by men, especially when related to women.

Karve (1953) states that, in India, marriage is a sacrament and no normal man or woman should die without receiving this sacrament. If indeed this is the case then at one level pressure to have their "wayward" (i.e., mad) son married may reflect such paternal desire.

The behavioural pattern of the kin-group in the northern family is like that of the family in ancient India. Definite patterns are set for the girls to behave; and the joint family group in a status group is where husband,

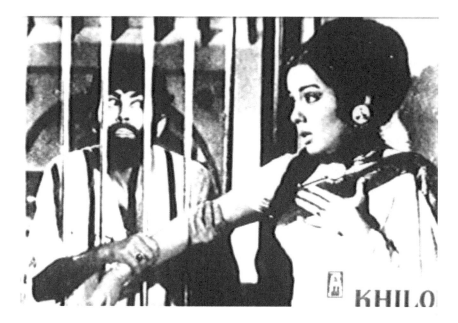

Figure 14.1   Scene from *Khilona* (courtesy of National Film Archive of India)

wife, parents-in-law, daughters-in-law, sons, daughters, sisters-in-law, and brothers-in-law each have an assigned definite place, *vis-à-vis* others. The work they do, and the pleasures they enjoy, are conventions, which they have to follow. Madan (1993) suggests that the distinction between families and households is extremely important and, following on from Shah's (1973) recommendation that households are characterized as simple or complex, also suggests that an addition to simplicity or complexity may be smallness or largeness. Thus, a household can be large and simple or small and complex. These are crucial factors in Madan's view.

Bihari is trying to blackmail Radha as Vijay's younger brother Mohan arrives for Diwali holidays. He is enamoured by Chand and continues to flirt with Chand. She confides in him that she is pregnant with Vijay's child, at which point he leaves the house. Radha is about to elope with Bihari when Chand steps in and calls Vijay, who fights with Bihari.

Bihari jumps off the roof, and seeing this Vijay gets better. However, he is accused of murdering Bihari, but Chand's testimony that Bihari slipped gets Vijay released. No one is willing to believe her that she is carrying Vijay's child; they all accuse her of being a dancing girl and therefore likely to indulge in this behaviour anyway. In the end, Mohan returns and confirms that he had been told about the pregnancy and also that Chand belongs to a good family; finally the family accepts her as a daughter-in-law.

Vijay and his madness are balanced by elder brother Kishore's extramarital affair with his secretary and his embezzling of the family company money. The dancing girl who is born of a good family and has remained pure and unsullied until she is "raped" is, after all, acceptable in the orthodox family where she yearns to be a good Hindu wife—praying in the temple, praying to the tulsi plant, and maintaining the purity of the kitchen. The madness has to be contained within the family; otherwise the honour of the family will be sullied, because if their son is admitted to a madhouse this can be seen as another kind of insult and impurity. There is no explanation for the reluctance to send Vijay to the madhouse, though he lives in a separate room on the roof and is excluded anyway. His nephew, niece, and sister have no point of view; this may reflect their roles in the hierarchy of the household.

The neighbour is obviously trying hard to pollute and hijack the orthodoxy to bring them down but he fails because the imported "other" wants to be accepted and therefore bends over backwards to be a good and dutiful, though fake, daughter-in-law. In one scene Radha is stopped by Chand and she says, "No one knows what will happen tomorrow but at least today I have the same status as Laxmi bhabhi." The desire to belong to an orthodox family with roots and values and rituals suddenly becomes very important to Chand.

The role madness plays in the creative life of sensitive poets and playwrights is well known. In both *Khilona* and *Khamoshi* the sensitive poet becomes mad under the influence of the stresses they experience and in both these instances this is caused by the loss of a girlfriend. The sensitive nature and madness in this context suggest that creative people are more prone to the way losses interact to produce madness.

Although caste and family are tinged with religion, it is the former and not the latter that is attacked as an institution. The changes in the moral values of the society depend upon a number of factors. Under the circumstances, the Thakur household is a microcosm of the society where the household's morality reflects that of the society. As Béteille (1993) observes, social institutions such as the family reproduce themselves partly through the conscious actions of individuals who desire their continued existence.

Arth and *Baseraa* are two other family-based films where mental illness plays a role. *Arth* is an example of a low-budget film aimed at educated middle class urban audiences, which is between art and mainstream cinema. It offers a love triangle with a twist. The reviewer felt that the film was rescued by its unusual denouement and by the fine performances of its two female principals. Shabana Azmi was seen to bring great depth and subtlety to the role conveying both the fragility of the betrayed and the determination of a woman who is discovering her own strength. Smita Patil was effective as the other woman, despite the histrionics of several Lady Macbeth-like mad scenes, which are caused by guilt over having wrecked a marriage. The final encounter is seen as remarkably powerful (Chakrabarty, 2002).

Arth is the story of an ad director and his wife, who was an orphan. The husband is having an affair with an actress, whom he has promised to marry. The actress threatens to tell his wife, at which point he confesses his affair to his wife. Meanwhile the actress has become "schizophrenic" and the wife is asked to visit her. During this visit she meets the actress's mother, who begs her for help, asking her to do something otherwise "they will give her ECT".

The film, allegedly based on the real life story of its director, Mahesh Bhatt, is full of stereotypes of the actress being hysterical, neurotic, and wrongly described as having schizophrenia. The feminist angle is played up when the wife meets a younger man who falls in love with her and wants to marry her; but she wants her independence and sees no reason to get married again. In this film ECT is mentioned as something horrific and possibly punitive. The attitudes of people in India to ECT are variable but lag behind western notions because the image of psychiatry itself lags behind. It is not surprising that Hindi cinema uses ECT as a horrifying tool rather than a therapeutic one.

Arth was described as Mahesh Bhatt ripping off his own life to make a turbulent raw and never-before seen marital drama. The film broke through the taboo topic of infidelity and domestic violence to depict urban lifestyle as ugly and hypocritical. Shabana Azmi made the role of the wife one of the most accomplished performances in Indian cinema. Smita Patil as the mistress did her best, too. The film received more than a fair share of media glare. The reviewer acknowledged the contribution of the cinematography to the film. *Arth* was the first major release and success for its director Mahesh Bhatt. The sheer rawness of emotional revelation, the naked insight into male–female relationships, the honest description of extramarital relationships, the destructive force of illicit sex, and the resulting disquiet leap out of every frame (Banker, 2001). Smita Patil's acting, according to Banker, was hypnotic and her portrayal of the increasingly paranoid psychotic model plagued with typical Indian guilt over wrecking another woman's marriage is brutally honest and true to life. On the other hand, Shabana Azmi's role as a weepy inward-looking character was perfectly realized. Banker sees the film as retaining the power to move and involve its audience in the emotional turmoil of its characters. Shabana Azmi won her second Best Actress National Award for the role.

Arth was noted for the intensity of its performers, who were seen as mesmerizing. Jha (1984) asks the question, on second viewing, whether this is because of the protagonists' emotions or because of Shabana Azmi's interpretation of the role of the wife. The woman clearly rises from the ashes of her ruined marriage to make an independent life (which in the film's context is a manless life) for herself. Jha (1984 n.d. d) points out that it is the viewer's identification with her character that raises the ante. However, he also asks whether it is ever possible for any woman (let alone an attractive one!) to be independent and not be easy game for the men she comes into contact with, and whether a woman can survive on her own in India. Jha sees Bhatt's efforts to be realistic as laboured and many characters to be stereotypes, which he blames on the director's conservatism. Although an interesting film, it does focus on the strong character of the heroine rather than on the neurotic, on the verge of breakdown, other woman. Jha asks, perhaps seriously, whether Bhatt was purging his own soul by making the male protagonist so foolish. It may also be that by making the character of Azmi strong, he has let down the histrionic neurotic one even further. Shalini Pradhan's (1982) review in *Filmfare* points out that ultimately *Arth* is Azmi's film and it is a treat to watch her emotive actions. Hattangady's performance was flawless; Kharbanda was figurative and literally lost between two talented women.

Prabhu (2001, p. 129) sees *Arth* as another film which comments on the patriarchal nature of Indian society and the institution of marriage, highlighting the flimsiness of marriage and the infidelity and vulnerability of the other woman, who is racked with guilt. Both women are being used by the male protagonist in a similar way, for his sexual pleasure. The difference is that Azmi recognizes that she does not need another male in order to feel complete. The insecurity and the hysterical nature of Kavita (played by Smita Patil) demonstrate the narcissistic nature of actors and their preoccupation with themselves, with very little concern for anyone else. Her insecurity is also related to the realization that, if a married man leaves his wife for her, there is no guarantee that he will stay with her in the long term. Prabhu notes that her costumes illustrate her character. By wearing dark and western clothes, her contrast with the Indian woman in saris is clear. This split between the dutiful Bharatiya nari and the westernized vamp has been done to death in Hindi films. *Arth* was seen as a masala film by Chatterji (1998); it happened to be a turning-point film that defined a modern but ordinary housewife's reaction to her husband's adultery. *Abhimaan*, vaguely influenced by *A Star is Born*, explored the wife's development of depression after she miscarries. Combined with an internalized repression of her feelings, in view of the threat experienced by her husband, it is not surprising that the woman develops depression. However, this depression does not fit in with her character, a point also noted by Chatterji.

Somaaya (2000) notes that the real life rivalry between the two actresses (Shabana Azmi and Sunita Patil) reached its peak during the shooting of *Arth*. The two were showing real tension on the sets. Both knew that their roles were not going to be easy. Both were going through their private hell because they were both involved with married men. Somaaya, who admits to being a friend of Shabana Azmi, acknowledges that both actresses affected each other strongly. Thus, life imitates art and art copies life!

In the same mode, *Baseraa* was described as a reflection of ridiculously unrealistic things as a vehicle for getting at psychosocially real things, such as women being required to sacrifice their own happiness for the sake of others and their families. Here, two sisters end up marrying the same man because the older one has developed mental illness and is in an asylum and her children need a mother! Her madness was precipitated by a fall caused by the shock of learning that her younger brother-in-law had died on his wedding night.

She returns home 14 years later (like Rama's return from exile), after she has recovered her memory. Her family is advised that she should be protected from any shock such as learning that her sister is now married to her husband! Thomas (1985) cited that Hindi films can be regarded as moral fables that involve the audience to resolve some disorder in the ideal moral universe; the films are structured around conflicts, contradictions, and tensions within the domain of sexuality. The relationship between the brother-in-law (the husband) and younger sister is charged with sexual energy. However, everyone suffers in silence. The reviewer adds, "Is there a family therapist in the house?" The doctor, although demonstrating scientific rationality, shows a bourgeois morality by encouraging the family to lie and suppress the trauma. "Ultimately although his treatment fails, its ethos of repression triumphs at the cost of superhuman sacrifice performed by the two sisters, which the film invites us to admire", notes the reviewer. The review also points out the role of stairs in the *mise-en-scène* to show the elder sister's fall into madness and ascension of the family to reveal the truth, at which point the sister returns voluntarily to the asylum.

Mirani (n.d.), in an interview with the director of *Baseraa*, reported that the latter wanted a good clean film with an emphasis on emotion, a story with personal appeal. He pointed out that he had touched on more than just a man–woman relationship.

It is not surprising that around the time these films were released several of the top heroines in the Hindi film industry were in bigamous relationships with married actors. The fact is that *Arth* was based on Mahesh Bhatt's personal story, and that *Baseraa* reflected a bigamist marriage, and in both these films the male played a very superficial and virtually sidelined role.

CONCLUSIONS

The relationship between the female as the sufferer and the carer is an intriguing one. Several films show females as long-suffering wives who have looked after learning-disabled, physically disabled, or cruel husbands; but

when it comes to males looking after mentally ill females, somehow circumstances change. The role of females as doctors also highlights how they
are bounded by culture and expectations and what a tight hold the male
patriarchy has on individual females.

CHAPTER FIFTEEN

Electric shock treatment in Hindi cinema

Electric shock treatment or electroconvulsive therapy (ECT) generates a range of feelings of horror and disgust in patients and their carers. Not being aware of the fact that it is relatively safe and that some patients benefit from it, its association with electric shock and the brain makes it extremely difficult for individuals to accept this form of treatment. The audience looks at this mechanism both as a source of terror and perhaps as a punishment to illustrate the villainy of the individual in one form or another. This villainy expresses "the other" that individuals denote. The viewer as "disinterested" or "dispassionate" observer interprets this as a source of punishment for acts, deeds, and behaviours that may be seen as sinful.

In Hollywood films, too, ECT often has an image of horror and terror associated with the feeling that patients are being punished. The classic example is *One Flew Over the Cuckoo's Nest*. This film not only confirms the stereotypes of happy-clappy patients but also the stereotype of the institution where the nurses are all-powerful and the doctors feeble, inadequate, and marginalized. In many Hollywood films, ECT and insulin coma therapy is used as a strategy to induce fear. Gabbard and Gabbard (1999) think that, rather than ECT *per se*, it is the institutional confinement that is more frightening. Like prison movies, institutional confinement movies play on the fear of loss of liberty as well as the fear of being shocked and treated in an inhumane way, so that personal liberties in that particular context tend to disappear. Films showing mental illness use gentle talking treatments along with other fearful treatments such as ECT.

BRIEF HISTORY OF ECT

ECT was first used on a patient by the Hungarian neuropathologist Ladislas Meduna in 1934 to induce an epileptic seizure in order to treat schizophrenia. He gave injections of camphor oil to a man who suffered from a catatonic form of schizophrenia. He demonstrated that after being injected every 3 days, after the fifth injection the patient for the first time was able to look after himself. Following a further three injections, the patient remained well. This discovery of induced seizures became an important treatment technique. In 1938, Cerletti and Bini demonstrated the efficacy and ease of administration of electrically induced seizures; thereafter the technique was taken up all over the world. Around that time the roles of hypnotism and mesmerism were also being examined.

There is considerable evidence in literature (Abrams, 2002; Bhugra & Meux, 1991) to suggest that ECT works very well for a number of patients; specific psychiatric conditions and symptoms, especially mood disorders, severe depression, puerperal psychosis, and delusional depression (where the individual has deep-seated ideas of nihilism), are more responsive. Some cases of acute mania and schizophrenia will also respond. ECT plays an important and useful role in the management of some psychiatric patients, especially if their condition is life-threatening. Some countries have strong views on the use of ECT; for example, parts of Switzerland and Germany have banned its usage.

Even though the introduction of effective drug treatments has revolutionized the management of psychiatric conditions and most of the drugs are easily available and accessible around the world, cinema still has a penchant for exploiting the fears of the audience. In films where medication is given or shown, it is generally in liquid form rather than tablets, capsules, at worst injections and/or ECT.

For both the viewer and the auteur, psychotherapy or talking treatment is more attractive; the psychiatrist or the therapist is functioning as a detective and the process is gentle and caring, whereas ECT is demonized and the psychiatrist/therapist recommending or giving ECT is portrayed in a demonic manner. In Hollywood films too ECT is shown as punishment or a behaviour-altering agent by which the patient is threatened or punished. Coloured lights, peculiar camera angles, and orchestral crescendo on the sound track make the entire process of ECT appear grotesque and frightening. Even in modern hospitals, where anaesthesia for giving ECT should be readily available, often the patient is shown as being held down or tied down with bandages and straps. By focusing on the patient's facial grimaces and the reactions of relatives, directors are able to generate fear of the treatment.

The dramatic aspect of ECT is more prominent and the fear of interfering with the mind (which may already be disturbed in the insane individual) often provides a pivot on which the film narrative can turn. The cathartic cure is implicit in psychotherapy where a flash of insight and a sudden cathartic understanding of the genesis of the problem allow the protagonist to move forward along the storyline. In Hollywood, ECT has sometimes been shown to be effective and useful, whereas no such portrayal has been shown in modern-day Hindi cinema. Occasionally, ECT is used in Hollywood for breakthroughs that are built upon talking treatments.

Gabbard and Gabbard (1999, p. 33) suggest that the treatments which result in patients blaming their upbringing and their parents as possible causes contributing to their ill health and then forgiving them for it are used too often by psychiatrists. It is suggested that this approach meets with film myths of self-help but more specifically with the notion that patients have no responsibility for their illness or their behaviour. It is known that the psychopathic behaviour of some individuals is embedded in the social or antisocial context and may explain the causation of their illness.

ECT adds to the sense of shift from the context where the individual is seen to be punished by this particular therapeutic approach.

IMPLICATIONS FOR PUBLIC ATTITUDES

ECT arouses strong and negative attitudes in the general public. The fear is determined by seeing ECT as a "hard" and "strong" treatment and, especially if it does not work, it makes the stigma even greater. Gabbard and Gabbard (1999, p. 177) reported that at least one patient withdrew his consent to ECT after watching a portrayal of ECT in *One Flew Over the Cuckoo's Nest*. They argue that the average person may (or may not) be adept at distinguishing the reality from its distorted image in the media. It is obvious that the ability of emotionally disturbed individuals who may already be experiencing compromised reality is even more impaired.

There is little doubt that the images of mental illness and mental health professionals portrayed in the cinema do influence help-seeking. Media images continue to work subconsciously even if we consciously reject these images. The cumulative effect of viewing film after film is the creation of a mental warehouse full of internal stereotypes stored in preconscious and unconscious memory banks. The golden-hearted prostitute, the happy vagabond and the mad professor are all stereotypes portrayed widely in Hindi cinema. Patients are likely to expect their doctors and psychiatrists to behave in the same way that they see them behaving on the screen.

Attitudes to ECT are also influenced by past experiences. Those who have had ECT and their carers are likely to have different attitudes from those who have only seen it in cinema or TV, or read about it.

In a study from North India, the attitudes of teenagers to mental illness were revealed to be generally positive and a significant number of students attending college had seen someone with mental illness. Nearly 18% of males and 50% of females believed that mental illness could be cured by marriage. Interestingly, the females were more likely to agree to marry into a family with mental illness, thereby suggesting a reduced social distance. The majority of respondents in the study were able to identify abnormal behaviour as the most important category of symptoms for identifying mental illness (Bhugra, 1993a). In a similar study in the UK with a group of patients who had received ECT, the attitudes were found to be reasonably positive (Bhugra & Meux, 1991). The following is not a comprehensive, but a selective, review of ECT in Hindi cinema.

ECT AND HINDI CINEMA

In some films ECT is genuinely used as a therapeutic effect, whereas in others it is clearly chosen as a horror, evoking a sense of dismay and terror. Somaaya (2004) suggests that the "punishment" for violence is ECT, as illustrated in *Damini*.

In both *Khamoshi* and *Raat aur Din*, ECT is used as a threatening gesture. In *Khamoshi*, Arun Chaudhary is rushed to the ECT suite with no apparent preparation, fasting, or consent. In the prelude to the scene, the chief psychiatrist responds to the matron and assistant psychiatrist while doing the rounds and establishes his humanity by claiming, "I am not in favour of shock treatment!" He reflects the attitude of psychoanalysts towards this form of physical treatment. He is told that it is impossible to control Arun, thereby suggesting to the viewer that the only way of controlling his behaviour is by ECT. He goes on to ask the question "How is his behaviour?", to which the reply is, "Irritable." At this point, physical signs are asked for and responded to, such as:

Temperature?	99 degrees;
Pulse?	110;
Volume?	Weak and low;
No sleep?	Major problem is his stubbornness.

Stubbornness is neither a symptom of any major condition in the psychiatric annals nor a condition needing treatment. It remains a trait that does not require treatment, least of all ECT.

By identifying stubbornness as the cause, the childish nature of Arun's behaviour is established where the parental physician and matronly nurse decide to "punish" Arun and control his behaviour. The next step for Arun's management is discussed in the corridor: "How is Arun?", "No different"; "By putting pressure on patient's nerves he can be killed . . .". The assistant psychiatrist suggests, "We will have to start other treatment."

The chief psychiatrist asks, "Electric shock?", to which the assistant replies, "Maybe we should do it."

The rationale against the use of ECT is not that it is not indicated or that it is not likely to be helpful. There is a sense of let down in the chief psychiatrist's voice. His concern is: "Alas, after electric shock I won't be able to prove my treatment." He also questions implicitly the ability of the current therapist, Bina. Rather than question Bina's approach or what kind of additional help she may require for Arun's management, the chief psychiatrist sighs and says, "If it was Radha it would be different." Thus, he gives a subconscious nod to the miracle-working therapist. He begs Radha to take responsibility and virtually blackmails her. Radha is convinced only after Arun tries to strangle Bina and, when she is separating the two, he slaps Radha. Arun is expressing paranoid ideas and is possibly acting on those ideas, whereas Radha is unaware of the underlying suspiciousness. Radha explains to Sulekha that Arun has acute mania. It suggests that in spite of models of the psychoanalysis being offered there is no supervision available. The attitude of the psychoanalyst is shown as that of controlling the patient.

Interestingly, as primary nurse therapist or as a key member of the staff Radha is kept in the dark about the medical plans to give him ECT. Another nurse tells Radha that Arun has been taken for ECT. The sense of horror in the informant's voice is almost palpable. On getting the news, Radha runs to the ECT section, where Arun is tied down with leather straps. There are flashing lights on the wall and the doctor looks worried. Arun cries, "They will kill me." She unstraps him and the doctor says, "Do you know what you are doing? You'll have to answer for him."

Radha tells Arun not to worry as she is back, and she then takes him to his room. This maternal approach is quintessentially Indian. ECT has not yet happened but the audience has been exposed to the possible horrors of the technique with straps, flashing lights, wooden blocks, and the expressed fear that it could kill Arun. (The mortality rate from ECT is lower than that from dental treatment.) As noted above, there seems to be no mention of anaesthesia.

The aftermath of these actions is also interesting. The chief psychiatrist asks Radha, "At the electric shock, you insulted Dr Rai." Her response, unusual for a nurse, who is generally the handmaiden to the doctors, is that he perceived it as an insult. When the chief psychiatrist chides her for not having explained it nicely, she says that there had been no time. Then, to win him over, she says, "I can assure [you] that even this time your experiment will be successful", thereby making it clear that ECT was an aberration brought about by the assistant psychiatrist.

In *Raat aur Din*, Baruna is given ECT with flashing lights, in an open room with no preparation and no mention of consent. Here the ECT is "sold" to the husband as a last resort largely because the maximum dose of medication has not helped. Although there is a female nurse in the background, it is the men who are making decisions to treat Baruna and forcibly inject her or give her the ECT.

There are many similarities between her exposure to the shaman who performs basic rituals in front of all the women of the neighbourhood and the family. The shaman is in the process of beating the woman to get rid of the demonic possession. When Pratap (her husband) rushes home, intercedes, and threatens to beat the shaman, he runs away and the women disappear into the background. Similarly, the expressions of complete shock and horror on his face when he realizes the enormity of the act of ECT, lead to another kind of intercession, thereby performing the male role. The similarities between the two rituals confirm that modern day psychiatrists are also shamans, albeit with a different language and repertoire of rites and rituals.

Whereas the shaman holds a burning piece of wood under her nose, talking to the demon who is possessing her, the psychiatrists use a syringe and needle initially, which Baruna chooses to use as weapons not against the doctors but against the nurse. Interestingly, in the act of giving the electric shock it is the nurse who presses the button and Baruna screams; obviously, it is not being done under anaesthesia. When the husband shouts for the doctors to stop, the response from the doctor is "My God! I didn't know you had such a weak heart. You go home and relax. I promise as soon as she wakes she will be in her senses." Notwithstanding major problems in the portrayal of ECT (preparation, consent, anaesthesia or that more than one treatment is required), the false sense of security given that she will be "in her senses" suggests that in this case the wife is the property of her husband and he can intercede any way he chooses. This may be a reflection of the fact that he has entered into a love marriage and ignored his parents' wishes. This may also reflect a dramatic counterpoint in the story.

In the Hollywood film *The Snake Pit*, ECT was portrayed as both barbaric and helpful. As in that film, at least in *Raat aur Din* the attitudes to psychiatry are ambivalent to say the least. Like Olivia de Havilland's portrayal in *The Snake Pit*, Nargis in *Raat aur Din* demonstrates her illness as being almost charming, with gently humorous lines and the mobility of expressions which move very rapidly from sadness to joy to perplexity.

The portrayal of sexuality and charm on the one hand as Peggy, and the traditional Indian womanly form as Baruna on the other, were of sufficient quality to get Nargis the first ever award for best actress in India. While preparing for her role, Nargis watched electric shock therapy being given and she admitted in an interview that the reaction of the patient was something no artist in the world could possible recreate. She said, "Every muscle twitched. I know it can't be done on the screen because I tried hard at home to imitate the effect." Incidentally, according to the author of the article (Bawa, 1980), she decided that the shock treatment (so apt to be a cliché on the screen) was not actually very "cinematic" and that it should not be shown in her film. However, it was, in the sense that her husband's reaction was that of sheer horror.

In several subsequent films the use of electricity and electric shock has a different meaning and context. In the Hollywood arena, ECT and lobotomy have been equated with emasculation.

Next we look at the use of ECT as a dramatic pivot in the story of some Hindi films. These vary from using shock treatment to "remove the memory" or to punish, and on one occasion electric shock causes hemiplegia.

Khandaan is the story of two landlord/farmer brothers who live in a joint family. The older brother is childless but is very fond of his younger brother. His nephew, as a child, climbs on to an electric pole to release a kite that has been caught there. While trying to reach the kite, he gets an electric shock; he acquires hemiplegia and grows up with the disability. His older aunt is visited by her nephew and niece, the children of her brother's marriage with a Goan Christian. The scene is set in raising conflict between traditional rural and modern foreign visited attitudes and behaviour. In the midst of this appears the female lead, who is happy to marry the disabled man. The villainous uncle then kidnaps the infant child of the disabled hero. When trying to liberate the child, the hero receives another electric shock and his hemiplegia disappears. This story does not involve ECT as discussed earlier but electric shock in its literal sense, thereby inducing an element of modern and foreign conveniences epitomized by electricity in the traditional Indian rural settings.

The joint family setting is destroyed by the presence of foreign elements who play the villainous roles to the limit in order to destroy traditional virtues and values. The villain sets up a circus (obviously illustrating the modern concept of entertainment, even though it is as modern as the cinema). However, electricity is a modern convenience to be feared and welcomed in equal proportions in the rural setting. The rural idyll, where social support is available to all at all times, and the family pulls together in the same direction, is disrupted by the arrival of the unwelcome imposed alien guests. This was also one of the last films from the south with the social genre suggesting an end of an era. The romance, the dances, and the usual villainy were there, but the split and the consequences of the villainy were linked with Nehruvian precepts of rural economy and progress through modern gadgets that go wrong.

ECT as a narrative strategy has been used in a number of settings and stories. Bollywood, although not completely unaware of these strategies, does not use these extensively or as appropriately as Hollywood. The use of ECT in the context of institutionalization and asylum is discussed further.

MEMORY LOSS AND TERROR

In *Jewel Thief*, the twist in the tale is that the villain wants to turn the hero Vinay into the villain Amar, a notorious jewel thief. The way to accomplish this is to obliterate his memory by using ECT. Two of his gang members are either doctors or play at being doctors. In a review on the internet (Anon, 2003), *Jewel Thief* was seen as having a Byzantine but engrossing plot with Hitchcock-like psychological overtones (and camera angles). Dev Anand is comparable to the Cary Grant of the colour-saturated 1960s, although most people identified him with Gregory Peck. The picturization of the first song reminds the reviewer of Raj Kapoor and the high modernity in the sets, clothes, and style is noteworthy.

The arrangements for ECT in the bedroom are separated from the viewers and the villain by a curtain. The scene opens with a board with 12 electric bulbs on the walls—two alternate rows of three red bulbs each are lit. The villain asks the doctor how long it will take for Vinay to lose his memory. The doctor replies that, "A person cannot be given more than one electric shock per day. There are some people who lose their memory after one shock and others need six shocks." The villain accepts that within 6 days Vinay will forget all about his past life. The doctor agrees emphatically and confidently that he will not even remember his own name. Vinay is tied to the bed and three people hold him down while he is given an injection; as the music reaches a crescendo he screams and is given a mouth gag. The camera points at the voltameter and Vinay shakes; accompanied by a change to the scenery he hears a voice that keeps telling him that he is Amar. Next, we see his head bandaged with blood on it, suggesting that the ECT may well have caused this bleeding. The villain tells him later that he had been shot at by the police. The doctor then tells the villain, "I thought at least four shocks would be needed but with two shocks only his condition has become compatible with your requirements." Bearing in mind that the villain is managing the ECT, consent obviously is not an issue. However, the claim that ECT can wipe his memory absolutely clean is unrealistic and untrue. In a story this point is a dramatic pivot but it is still mistaken. ECT causes a loss of short-term memory but long-term memory is not affected. The memory loss is patchy, and more importantly it is temporary, so the idea that it will turn him into a new personality is unlikely to say the least.

In *Dastak*, Sharad tells Sushmita Sen about his shock treatment, though no such acts are shown. When she tries to empathize with him and asks him to trust her, his response is: "It is not you who is speaking, it is the world to which I am mad. The [same] world years ago made me sit in a dark room and gave me electric shock. The voice is yours but the words are theirs." The paranoia against the world emanates from their treatment of him, especially the violence from his father, whom he eventually murders. The difference is diagnostic and the treatment with shock therapy is again a dramatic cliché.

In a more recent film, *Raja*, released in 1995, the elder brother (Birju) of the eponymous hero is thrown on an electric grid, following a road accident, where he receives a shock that makes him physically disabled and adversely affects his mental capacity. Even though he behaves like a child and plays with children, he still manages to pull a fast one over someone in the street, which impresses the psychiatrist who meets and recognizes him 15 years later. Seen as "Once a mad man, always a mad man", the villains manage to get him admitted to a hospital, where we see him receiving ECT. The scene opens with a red light on the wall and Birju tied to the bed with electrodes on his ears that appear more like headphones than electrodes; his mouth is gagged with the piece of a bandage and we see two "episodes" of shock, each lasting approximately 7 seconds. On hearing the news his brother Raja runs to the asylum, which has gothic staircases with no other patients or staff visible. Raja runs around calling for his brother, who is squatting in the corner of an almost empty room cowering and crying, "They will kill me, take me home Raja." Never mind that there is no apparent clinical condition that requires ECT, there are no symptoms or signs either. The underlying text may be that this was his punishment as he had dared upset the rich landlords and hence had to suffer. The doctors and the rest of the medical staff represent the controlling social class and are acting on behalf of the rich landlord.

In *Arth*, the heroine (the wronged wife) is asked to help the mistress to avoid ECT (see previous chapter). Images pertaining to technical aspects of psychiatry, such as the EEG machines, make an appearance in *Baharon ki Manzil* and *Karz*. *Karz* is the story of a young singer who, while singing on stage, starts to have flashbacks. He is the reincarnation of a man who soon after his marriage had been murdered by his wife, a woman who is part of a band of villains and is after his wealth. When the singer is seen by doctors, some think he is psychotic. He is seen being investigated, wearing a frightening hat full of electrodes; he starts to remember his past life, drives the villainess mad, and lures her to her death at the same shrine where he had died in the previous incarnation. O'Flaherty (1981) identifies several Hindu themes in the filmic text, that of the mother, the mythic resonances of the older woman reflected in the mythology of Hindu texts, and the portrayal of the goddess.

The portrayal of ECT in Hindi films is not positive. The overview in this chapter is not comprehensive by any means, but where ECT is mentioned or shown in some detail in films it is not for therapeutic reasons, but instead carries a punitive subtext that is extremely strong and obvious. By and large, the characters are male and they are being "punished" for various reasons. It is not straightforward emasculation, as indicated in *One Flew Over the Cuckoo's Nest*, but elements of punishment are clearly evident. The underlying reasons may be that doctors are punishing patients for not getting better, as in *Khamoshi* and *Raat aur Din*, or villains are punishing the goody-goody hero to create a new villain as in *Jewel Thief*. These concepts need to be embedded in the prevailing historical, political, and economic envisions.

CONCLUSIONS

Once an individual is labelled as having a mental illness, then society or other individuals may respond to such an individual by excluding them, pitying them, bullying them, ignoring them, or treating them with respect or psychotherapeutic interventions. On the spectrum of inclusion versus exclusion, the mentally ill individual can be isolated or can be maintained in the community. Social control of mental illness also includes giving the clinician permission to use equal control through physical or psychological means. There is little doubt that ECT as a form of treatment is used rarely but regularly, and that certain social classes are more prone to be given this treatment. The social control system is coercive and involuntary in the use of ECT, whereas in other psychotherapeutic endeavours it may be conciliatory and voluntary. The seeker of therapy envisions therapeutic control as being effective. Both in reality and in its portrayal ECT offers a coercive model of care.

CHAPTER SIXTEEN

Conclusions

Madness in Hindi films has not been ignored. It has been used as a peg in the storyline, as a punishment, and as a crime solver; and psychiatrists have been shown as buffoons, sages, detectives, and punishing fathers. Such repetitiveness influences culture but the changes in the culture of the country at large and culture of the cinema have contributed to an understanding of how an individual behaves. The fact that over the past 50 years or so the portrayal of madness has moved from gentle to psychoanalytic to psychopathic is beyond dispute. The role of the all-forgiving and all-suffering woman needs to be put in the context of the culture where it is expected. Thus, there is no surprise that in films like *Baseraa* the madness appears and disappears according to the degree of sacrifice that is expected from the woman.

Contemporary culture in India is heavily influenced by rapid urbanization and globalization of the media, which is beginning to change not only the body shape of heroes and heroines but their histories and expectations as well. Music in Hindi films has become more western influenced, to the degree that in recent films such as *Kal Ho na Ho* there is an acknowledged remix of the song *Pretty Woman*. The blurring of these cultural boundaries may well be useful and fruitful from the commercial viewpoint, but whether it will be good for the culture remains to be seen. It is likely that the culture will survive with its core intact whereas the fuzzy edges of culture may alter. For example, the influence of MTV and other music channels has led to an increase in the re-recording and remixing of old Hindi film songs, which have been derided by purists. The fact that several producers and directors are aiming their stories at the overseas Non Resident Indian market is worth remembering. By allowing the youngsters to roam and work the world but at the same time keeping their Indian roots intact with very limited room to manoeuvre because of Indian traditions, the producer/directors have clearly chosen to have their cake and eat it too.

There is little doubt that the popularity of Hindi cinema and its reliance on Hollywood for inspiration for stories and music cannot be underestimated. However, the prevalent social and political factors played a major role in the manner in which these were made. The Indianization of western music for Hindi films is well known.

The violence in Hindi films has been influenced by the violence, profanity, and nudity of Hollywood films, which have undoubtedly been more permissive. The moral world and the transition from tradition to modernity can be seen in the way Hindi films have portrayed mental illness. Diagnosis is rarely mentioned but, when it is, more often than not it is clinically wrong. In the 1950s and 1960s, mentally ill individuals were seen as affected, and traditional approaches such as shamans were used. Later, modern diagnoses such as borderline personality disorder and psychopathic personality disorders, which are culturally and socially influenced, have appeared. The modern unity of approach using ECT and medication has often been favoured over talking therapies, which may be seen as less modern. The influence of external factors on the way films are conceived and made deserves to be studied further. First, this would give us an idea of the key factors that may well be contributing to the areas portrayed and the associated stigma. Second, this may enable professionals to help directors and writers to project a more accurate picture, even if it is for entertainment purposes. Third, the social context of mental illness and its prevention and treatment can be influenced using these approaches.

References

Abrams, R. (2002). *Electroconvulsive therapy*. New York: Oxford University Press.

Adarsh, T. (2004). Review of *Madhoshi*. Retrieved 28 September, 2005, from http://www.indianfilm.com

American Psychiatric Association. (2000). *Diagnostic and statistical manual of mental disorders (DSM-IV-TR)*. Washington, DC: APA Press.

Anjali. (2004). Review of *Madhoshi*. Retrieved 28 September, 2005, from http://www.indiainfo.com/reviews/madhoshi.html

Anonymous. (2000, November 27). *Asian Age*. p. 4.

Anonymous. (2003). Review. Retrieved 8 June, 2003, from http://www.imdb.com

Aziz, A. (2003). *Light of the universe: Essays on Hindustani film music*. New Delhi, India: Three Essays Collective.

Babcock, B. A. (1978). Introduction. In B. A. Babcock (Ed.), *The reversible world: Symbolic inversion in art and society* (pp. 13–36). Ithaca, NY: Cornell University Press.

Bakshi, R. (1998). Raj Kapoor. In A. Nandy (Ed.), *The secret politics of our desires* (pp. 92–132). Delhi, India: Oxford University Press.

Banker, A. (2001). *Bollywood*. New Delhi: Penguin India.

Barker, M. (2003). Introduction. In T. Austin & M. Barker (Eds.), *Contemporary Hollywood stardom* (pp. 1–24). London: Arnold.

Barnouw, E., & Krishnaswamy, S. (1980). *Indian film*. New York: Oxford University Press.

Basu, K. (2000). Whither India? The prospect of prosperity. In R. Thapar (Ed.), *India: Another millennium* (pp. 193–211). New Delhi, India: Viking.

Basu, S., Kak, S., & Krishen, P. (1981). Cinema and society: A search for meaning in a new genre. *India International Centre Quarterly*, *8*, 57–75.

Bawa, M. (1980). *Actors and acting* (pp. 70–71). Bombay, India: IBH.

Bedford, E. (1986). Emotions and statements about them. In R. Harré (Ed.), *The social construction of emotions* (pp. 15–31). Oxford, UK: Basil Blackwell.

Benegal, S. (1982). Cited in K. Raha (Ed.), *Indian cinema 1981/1982* (p. 122). New Delhi, India: Directorate of Film Festivals.

Bergstrom, J. (1999). Introduction. In J. Bergstrom (Ed.), *Endless night: Cinema and psychoanalysis, parallel histories* (pp. 1–24). Berkeley, CA: University of California Press.

Bétielle, A. (1993). The family and the reproduction of inequality. In P. Uberoi (Ed.), *Family, kinship and marriage in India* (pp. 435–451). Delhi, India: Oxford University Press.

Bhugra, D. (1989). Attitudes towards mental illness. *Acta Psychiatrica Scandinavica, 80*, 1–12.

Bhugra, D. (1993a). Indian teenagers attitudes to mental illness. *British Journal of Clinical and Social Psychiatry, 9*, 10–11.

Bhugra, D. (1993b). Influence of culture on presentation and management of symptoms. In D. Bhugra & J. Leff (Eds.), *Principles of social psychiatry* (pp. 67–81). Oxford, UK: Blackwell Scientific Publishing.

Bhugra, D. (1999). The colonised psyche: British influence on Indian psychiatry. In D. Bhugra & R. Littlewood (Eds.), *Colonialism and psychiatry* (pp. 46–76). Delhi, India: Oxford University Press.

Bhugra, D. (2002). Psychoanalysis and the Hindi cinema. *South Asian Cinema, 1*, 105–115.

Bhugra, D. (2004). *Culture and self harm.* Hove, UK: Psychology Press.

Bhugra, D. (2005). Mad tales from Bollywood. *Acta Psychiatrica Scandinavica, 112*, 250–256.

Bhugra, D., & Jacob, K. S. (1997). Culture bound syndromes. In D. Bhugra & A. Munro (Eds.), *Troublesome disguises* (pp. 296–334). Oxford, UK: Blackwell Scientific Publishing.

Bhugra, D., & Meux, C. (1991). Consumers' attitudes to ECT. *British Journal of Clinical and Social Psychiatry, 8*, 48–50.

Bisplinghoff, G. D., & Slingo, C. J. (1997). Eve in Calcutta: The Indianisation of a movie madwoman. *Asian Cinema, 9*, 99–111.

Bose, G. S. (1999). The genesis and adjustment of the Oedipus wish. In T. G. Vaidyanathan & J. J. Kripal (Eds.), *Vishnu on Freud's desk* (pp. 21–38). Delhi: Oxford University Press.

Boss, M. (1969). *A psychiatrist discovers India.* London: Oswald Wolff.

Bowers, F. (1956). *Theatre in the East.* New York: Random House.

Burdett, H. C. (1891). *Hospitals and asylums around the world.* London: J. & A. Churchill.

Carroll, J. M. (1980). The difficulty of difference. In J. M. Carroll, *Towards a structural psychology of cinema* (pp. 36–45). The Hague, The Netherlands: Mouton Publishers.

Carstairs, M. (1957). *The twice born: A study of a community of high caste Hindus.* Bloomington, IN: Indiana University Press.

Chakrabarty, B. (2002). Questioning the confines of marriage: *Khushboo* and *Arth*. In J. Jain & S. Rai (Eds), *Films and feminism: Essays in Indian cinema* (pp. 163–169). Jaipur, India: Rawait Books.

Chakravartee, M. (1995). Vision making: American film and Indian culture. *Indian Journal of American Studies, 35*, 33–38.

Chakravarty, S. S. (1998). *National identity in Indian popular cinema.* Delhi, India: Oxford University Press.

Chandra, B., Mukherjee, M., & Mukherjee, A. (2000). *India after independence 1947–2000.* New Delhi, India: Penguin.

Chatterjee, P. (1995a). When melody ruled the day. In A. Vasudev (Ed.), *Frames of mind: Reflections on Indian cinema* (pp. 51–65). New Delhi, India: UBS Publishers and Distributors.

Chatterjee, P. (1995b). A bit of song and dance. In A. Vasudev (Ed.), *Frames of mind: Reflections on Indian cinema* (pp. 197–218). New Delhi, India: UBS Publishers and Distributors.

Chatterji, S. A. (1998). *Subject: cinema, object: woman: A study of the portrayal of women in Indian cinema.* Calcutta, India: Parumita Publications.

Chopra, A. (2001). *Sholay: The making of a classic.* New Delhi, India: Viking.

Cohen, A. (1992). Prognosis for schizophrenia in the third world: A re-evaluation of cross-cultural research. *Culture, Medicine and Psychiatry, 16*, 53–75.

Cohn, B. S. (2000). *India: The social anthropology of a civilisation*. Delhi, India: Oxford University Press.

Cole, W. O. (1996). *A Sikh family in Britain*. London: Canterbury Press.

Das, V. (1999). Tradition, pluralism, identity: Framing the issues. In V. Das, D. Gupta, & P. Uberoi (Eds.), *Tradition, pluralism and identity* (pp. 9–21). Delhi, India: Oxford University Press.

Das Gupta, C. (1991). *The painted face: Studies in India's popular cinema*. New Delhi, India: Roli Books.

Das Gupta, C. (1995). Rasa. In A. Lal & C. Das Gupta (Eds.), *The Indian performing arts in the last twenty-five years* (pp. 219–228). Calcutta, India: Anamika Kala Sangam.

Das Gupta, C. (2002). *India: House full, no intermission*. In A. Vasudev, L. Padgaonker, & R. Doraiswanny (Eds.), *Being and becoming: The cinemas of Asia* (pp. 124–151). Delhi, India: Macmillan.

Datta, S. (2003). *Shyam Benegal*. New Delhi, India: Roli Books.

Davis, D., & Bhugra, D. (2004). *Models of psychopathology*. Maidenhead, UK: Open University Press.

Dayan, F. D. (1976). The tutor code of classical cinema. In B. Nicholas (Ed.), *Movies and method*. Berkeley, CA: University of California Press.

Dennett, D. C. (1981). *Philosophical essays on mind and psychology*. Cambridge, MA: MIT Press.

Desai, M. N. (2004). *Nehru's hero: Dilip Kumar in the life of India*. New Delhi, India: Roli Books.

Deshmukh, B. S. (2004). *A cabinet secretary looks back: From Poona to the Prime Minister's office*. New Delhi, India: HarperCollins India.

Dhar, P. N. (2000). *Indira Gandhi, the emergency and the Indian democracy*. Delhi, India: Oxford University Press.

Dickey, S. (1993). *Cinema and the urban poor in south India*. Cambridge, UK: Cambridge University Press.

Dissanayake, W. (1994). Introduction. In W. Dissanayake (Ed.), *Colonialism and nationalism in Asian cinema* (pp. 9–24). Bloomington, IN: Indiana University Press.

Dissanayake, W., & Sahai, M. (1992). *Sholay*. New Delhi, India: Macmillan.

Dwyer, R. (2002). *Yash Chopra*. London: BFI.

Dwyer, R., & Patel, D. (2002). *Cinema India: The visual culture of Hindi film*. London: Reaktion Books.

Dyer, R. (1986). *Star*. London: Routledge.

Eisenberg, L. (1977). Disease and illness: Distinction between professional and popular ideas of sickness. *Culture Medicine Psychiatry, 1*, 9–23.

Eker, D., & Öner, B. (1999). Attitudes towards mental illness among the general public and professionals, social representations and change. In J. Guimón, W. Fischer, & N. Sartorius (Eds.), *The image of madness: The public facing mental illness and psychiatric treatment* (pp. 1–12). Basel, Switzerland: Karger.

Ernst, W. (1988). *Mad tales from the Raj*. London: Routledge.

Ewens, G. F. W. (1908). *Insanity in India*. Calcutta, India: Thacker, Spink & Co.

Fabrega, H. (1991). Psychiatric stigma in non-western societies. *Comprehensive Psychiatry, 32*, 534–551.

Fazalbhoy, Y. (1939). *The Indian film: A review*. Bombay, India: Bombay Radio Press.

Fenichel, O. (1935). *The psychoanalytic theory of neurosis*. New York: W. W. Norton.

Ford, S., & Chanda, G. S. (2002). Portrayals of gender and generation, east and west: Suzie

Wong in the noble house. In T. Y. T. Luk & J. P. Rice (Eds.), *Before and after Suzie: Hong Kong in western film and literature* (pp. 111–127). Hong Kong: Chinese University Press.

Foucault, M. (French edition 1961, reprinted 1985). *Madness and civilization: A history of insanity in the age of reason* (R. Howard, trans.). London: Tavistock.

Foucault, M. (1973a). *The birth of the clinic: An archaeology of medical perception* (A. M. Sheridan, trans.). London: Tavistock.

Foucault, M. (1973b). *The history of sexuality: Vol. 1. An introduction*. London: Tavistock.

Foucault, M. (1975). Film and popular memory. *Radical Philosophy, 11*, 75–80.

Fracchia, J., Sheppard, C., Canale, D., Ruest, E., Cambria, E., & Merlis, S. (1976). Community perceptions of severity of illness levels of former mental patients. *Comprehensive Psychiatry, 17*(6), 775–778.

Fredrickson, D. (1979). Jung/sign/symbol/film. *Quarterly Review of Film Studies, 4*(2), 167–191.

Freud, S. (1950a). *Collected papers, vol. 1*. London: Hogarth Press.

Freud, S. (1950b). *Collected papers, vol. 2*. London: Hogarth Press.

Friedberg, A. (1990). A denial of difference: Theories of cinematic identification. In E. A. Kaplan (Ed.), *Psychoanalysis and cinema* (pp. 36–45). New York: Routledge.

Gabbard, G., & Gabbard, K. (1999). *Psychiatry and the cinema*. Washington, DC: APA Press.

Garga, B. (1996). *So many cinemas*. Mumbai, India: Eminence Designs.

George, T. J. S. (1994). *The life and times of Nargis*. New Delhi, India: Indus.

Gokulsingh, K. M., & Dissanayake, W. (1998). *Indian popular cinema: A narrative of cultural change*. Hyderabad, India: Orient Longman.

Goldman, R. (1999). Karma, guilt and buried memories. In T. S. Vaidynarthan & J. J. Kripal (Eds.), *Vishnu on Freud's desk* (pp. 250–278). Delhi, India: Oxford University Press.

Gopalan, L. (2002). *Cinema of interruptions*. Delhi, India: Oxford University Press.

Gopalkrishnan, A. (1995). The influence of American cinema. *Indian Journal of American Studies, 25*, 16–19.

Gusdorf, G. (1953). *La parole [On speaking]*. Chicago: Northwestern University Press.

Haldipur, C. V. (1984). Madness in ancient India: Concept of insanity in Charaka Samhita. *Comprehensive Psychiatry, 25*, 335–344.

Hartnack, C. (1999). Psychoanalysis in colonial India. In T. G. Vaidyanathan & J. J. Kripal (Eds.), *Vishnu on Freud's desk* (pp. 81–106). Delhi, India: Oxford University Press.

Heath, S. (1999). Cinema and psychoanalysis: Parallel histories. In J. Bergstrom (Ed.), *Endless night: Cinema and psychoanalysis, parallel histories* (pp. 25–56). Berkeley, CA: University of California Press.

Helman, C. (2000). *Culture, health and illness*. London: Arnold.

Hood, J. W. (2000). *The essential mystery*. New Delhi, India: Orient Longman.

Inden, R. (1999). Transitional class, erotic Arcadia and commercial utopia in Hindi films. In C. Brosiu & M. Butcher (Eds.), *Image journeys: Audiovisual media and cultural change in India* (pp. 41–68). New Delhi: Sage.

Izod, J. (2001). *Myth, mind and the screen*. Cambridge, UK: Cambridge University Press.

Jablensky, A., Sartorious, N., Ernberg, G., Anker, M., Korten, A., Cooper, J. E., et al. (1992). Schizophrenia: Manifestations, incidence and course in different cultures: A WHO ten-country study. *Psychological Medicine, 20*(Suppl.), 1–97.

James, W. (1902). *The varieties of religious experience*. London: Penguin. (Original work published 1890)

Jha, S. (1984, July 1–15). A heart of gold and an invisible chastity belt. *Filmfare*.

Jha, S. (2004). Review of *Madhoshi*. Retrieved 27 September, 2004, from http://www.ians.in

Jha, S. (2005). Review. Retrieved 29 September, 2005, from http://www.nowrunning.com

Jha, S. K. (n.d. a). In A. Varde (Ed.), *Stardust: The 100 greatest films of all time* (p. 64). Mumbai, India: Magna.

Jha, S. K. (n.d. b). In A. Varde (Ed.), *Stardust: The 100 greatest films of all time* (pp. 94–95). Mumbai, India: Magna.

Jha, S. K. (n.d. c). In A. Varde (Ed.), *Stardust: The 100 greatest films of all time* (p. 168). Mumbai, India: Magna.

Jha, S. K. (n.d. d). Arth. In A. Varde (Ed.), *Stardust: The 100 greatest films of all time* (pp. 205–306). Mumbai, India: Magna.

Johnson, K. (2000). *Television and social change in rural India.* New Delhi, India: Sage.

Jones, E. (1961). *Freud and the post-Freudians.* London: Pelican.

Joy, P. (2005, May 8). Review. *The Deccan Herald.*

Jung C. G. (1943). On the psychology of the unconscious. In *Two essays on analytical psychology: The collected works, vol. 7* (2nd ed.). London: Routledge & Kegan Paul, 1966.

Kabir, N. (2001). *Bollywood.* London: Channel 4 Books.

Kak, A. (1980). *Cinema vision India, 1,* 1–3.

Kakar, S. (1983). The cinema of collective fantasy. In A. Vasudev & P. Langlet (Eds.), *Indian cinema superbazaar.* New Delhi, India: Vikas.

Kaplan, E. A. (1990a). From Plato's cave to Freud's screen. In E. A. Kaplan (Ed.), *Psychoanalysis and cinema* (pp. 1–23). New York: Routledge.

Kaplan, E. A. (1990b). Motherhood and representation. In E. A. Kaplan (Ed.), *Psychoanalysis and cinema* (pp. 128–141). New York: Routledge.

Kaplan, E. A. (1990c). *Psychoanalysis and cinema.* New York: Routledge.

Kaplan, E. A. (1991). Problematizing cross-cultural analysis: The case of women in the recent Chinese cinema. In C. Berry (Ed.), *Perspectives on Chinese cinema.* London: BFI.

Karanjia, B. K. (1982). Woman stereotypes: Hallowed heroines. In B. K. Karanjia (Ed.), *A many splendoured cinema* (pp. 198–200). Bombay, India: New Thacker's Fine Arts Press.

Karanjia, B. K. (1990). *Blundering in wonderland.* New Delhi, India: Vikas.

Karnad, G. (1982). In K. Raha (Ed.), *Indian cinema 1981/1982* (p. 121). New Delhi, India: Directorate of Film Festivals.

Karno, M., & Jenkins, J. (1993). Cross cultural issues in the course and treatment of schizophrenia. *Psychiatric clinics of North America, 16,* 339–350.

Karve, I. (1953). *Kinship organisation in India* (Deccan College Monograph Series 11). Poona, India: Postgraduate and Research Institute.

Kasbekar, A. (1999). An introduction to Indian cinema. In J. Nelmes (Ed.), *An introduction to film studies* (pp. 381–416). London: Routledge.

Kasbekar, A. (2001). Hidden pleasures: Negotiating the myth of the female ideal in popular Hindi cinema. In R. Dwyer & C. Pinney (Eds.), *Pleasure and the nation* (pp. 286–308). Delhi, India: Oxford University Press.

Kazmi, F. (1998). How angry is the angry young man? "Rebellion" in conventional Hindi films. In A. Nandy (Ed.), *Secret politics of our desires: Innocence, culpability and Indian popular cinema* (pp. 134–156). New Delhi: Oxford University Press.

Kazmi, F. (1999). *The politics of India's conventional cinema: Imaging a universe, subversing a multiverse.* New Delhi, India: Sage.

Kazmi, N. (1996). *Ire in the soul: Bollywood's angry years.* New Delhi, India: Harper Collins.

Kazmi, N. (1998). *The dream merchants of Bollywood.* New Delhi, India: UBS Publishers and Distributors.

Khan, F. (2005). Review of *Madhoshi.* Retrieved 28 September, 2005, from http://www.hotspotonline.com/moviespot/bolly/reviews/m/madhoshi

Kleinman, A. (1977). Depression, somatization and the new cross cultural psychiatry. *Social Science and Medicine, 11,* 3–10.

Kleinman, A. (1980). *Patients and their healers in the context of their culture.* Berkeley, CA: University of California Press.

Kleinman, A. (1986). Anthropology and psychiatry: The role of culture in cross-cultural research on illness. *British Journal of Psychiatry, 151*, 447–454.

Kolenda, P. (1967). Regional differences in Indian family structure. In R. I. Crane (Ed.), *Regions and regionalism in South Asian studies: An explanatory study* (Monograph and Occasional Paper Series Programme in Comparative Studies on southern Asia). Durham, NC: Duke University Press.

Kolenda, P. (1968). Region, caste and family: A comparative study of the Indian joint family. In M. Singer & B. S. Cohn (Eds.), *Social structure and social change in India.* Chicago: Viking Fund Publications.

Kothari, R. (1995). *State against democracy.* New Delhi, India: Ajanta Publications.

Krutnik, F. (1991). *In a lonely street: Film noir, genre, masculinity.* London: Routledge.

La Planche, J., & Pontalis, J. B. (1973). *The language of psychoanalysis* (D. Michalson-Smith, Trans.). New York: W. W. Norton.

Lebeau, V. (1995). *Introductions in psychoanalysis and cinema* (pp. 1–18). London: Routledge.

Levine, R. E., & Gaw, A. C. (1995). Culture bound syndromes. *Psychiatric Clinics of North America, 18*(3), 523–536.

Littlewood, R. (1990). From categories to contexts: A decade of the "new cross-cultural psychiatry". *British Journal of Psychiatry, 156*, 308–327.

Lynch, O. M. (1990). The social construction of emotion in India. In O. M. Lynch (Ed.), *Divine passions: The social construction of emotion in India* (pp. 3–34). Berkeley, CA: University of California Press.

MacDougall, D. (1998). *Transcultural cinema.* Princeton, NJ: Princeton University Press.

Madan, T. N. (1987). *Non-renunciation: Themes and interpretations of Hindu culture.* Delhi, India: Oxford University Press.

Madan, T. N. (1993). The Hindu family and development. In P. Uberoi (Ed.), *Family, kinship and marriage in India* (pp. 416–434). Delhi, India: Oxford University Press.

Mahmood, H. (1974). *The kaleidoscope of Indian cinema.* New Delhi, India: Affiliated East-West Press.

Majumdar, R. (2000). From subjectification to schizophrenia: The "angry man" and the "psychotic" hero of Bombay cinema. In R. S. Vasudevan (Ed.), *Making meaning in cinema* (pp. 238–266). Delhi, India: Oxford University Press.

Malhotra, I. (2003). *Dynasties of India and beyond.* New Delhi, India: Harper Collins.

Marriott, M. (1976). Hindu transaction: Diversity without dualism. In B. Kapferer (Ed.), *Transaction and meaning: Directions in the anthropology of exchange and symbolic behavior* (pp. 109–142). Philadelphia: ISHI Publishing.

Masood, I. (1982). Hindi film: Mass industry and cinema. In K. Raha (Ed.), *Indian cinema 1981/1982* (pp. 10–15). New Delhi, India: Directorate of Film Festivals.

Masud, I. (1997). *Dream merchants, politicians and partition.* New Delhi, India: Harper Collins.

Mathur, V. (2002). Women in Indian cinema: Fictional constructs. In J. Jain & S. Rai (Eds.), *Films and feminism* (pp. 65–71). Jaipur, India: Rawat Books.

Mayer, J. P. (1972). *Sociology of film: Studies and documents.* New York: Arno Press.

Mehta, V. (1993). *Portrait of India.* New Haven, CT: Yale University Press.

Metz, C. (1982). *The imaginary signifier: Psychoanalysis and the cinema* (C. Brinton, A. Williams, B. Brewster & A. Guzzetti, Trans.). Bloomington, IN: Indiana University Press.

Metz, C. (1985). *Psychoanalysis and cinema.* London: Macmillan.

Mirani, I. (n.d.). Finding the right balance. *Movie*, 19–22 August.

Mishra, V. (1985). Towards a theoretical critique of Bombay cinema. *Screen, 26*(3–4), 133–146.

Mishra, V. (2002). *Bollywood cinema: Temples of desire.* New York: Routledge.

Mitra, A. (1993). *Television and popular culture in India.* New Delhi, India: Sage.

Mitra, A. (1999). *India through the western lens.* New Delhi, India: Sage.

Monaco, J. (2000). *How to read a film*. New York: Oxford University Press.

Morris-Jones, W. H. (1979). *The government and politics of India*. Huntingdon, UK: Eothen Press.

Moscovici, S. (1984). The phenomenon of social representations. In R. Farr & S. Moscovici (Eds.), *Social representations* (pp. 3–70). Cambridge, UK: Cambridge University Press.

Murthy, N. V. K. (1980). *Cinema and society*. Bangalore, India: Bangalore University.

Nair, B. (2002). Female bodies and the male gaze. In J. Jain & S. Rai (Eds.), *Films and feminism*. Jaipur, India: Rawat Publications.

Nair, P. K. (2001). The song in Indian cinema. *South Asian Cinema, 1*, 40–44.

Nandy, A. (1981). The popular Hindi film: Ideology and first principle. *India International Centre Quarterly, 8*, 89–96.

Nandy, A. (1998). *The secret politics of our desire*. Delhi, India: Oxford University Press.

Narain, D. (1957). *Hindu character*. Bombay, India: University of Bombay Press.

Nayyar, O. P. (1960, August 28). Changing trends in film music. *Filmfare*, 39–40.

Nehru J. L. (1947–1964). *Letters to chief ministers (Vols. I–V)* (Vol. 4, p. 188). New Delhi, India: Government of India.

Ninan, S. (1995). *Through the magic window*. New Delhi, India: Penguin.

Obeyesekere, G. (1999). Further steps in relativization: The Indian Oedipus revisited. In T. G. Vaidyanathan & J. J. Kripal (Eds.), *Vishnu on Freud's desk* (pp. 109–136). Delhi, India: Oxford University Press.

O'Flaherty, W. D. (1981). The mythological disguise: An analysis of *Karz*. *India International Centre Quarterly, 8*, 23–29.

Oubert, J. P. (1978). Cinema and suture. *Screen, 18*, 35–47.

Pendakar, M. (1990). India. In J. A. Lent (Ed.), *The Asian film industry* (pp. 229–252). London: Croom Helm.

Persson, P. (2003). *Understanding cinema: A psychological theory of moving imagery*. Cambridge, UK: Cambridge University Press.

Pinney, C. (2001). Introduction: Public, popular and other cultures. In R. Dwyer & C. Pinney (Eds.), *Pleasure and the nation* (pp. 1–34). Delhi, India: Oxford University Press.

Prabhu, M. (2001). *Roles: Reel and real, image of woman in Hindi cinema*. New Delhi, India: Ajanta Books.

Pradhan, S. (1982, May 1–14). *Filmfare, 21*.

Prasad, M. M. (1998). *Ideology of the Hindi film: A historical construction*. Delhi, India: Oxford University Press.

Prasad, M. M. (2000). Signs of ideological re-form in two recent films: Towards real subsumption. In R. S. Vasudevan (Ed.), *Making meaning in Indian cinema* (pp. 145–167). Delhi, India: Oxford University Press.

Premchand, M. (2003). *Yesterday's melodies, today's memories*. Mumbai, India: Jharna Books.

Rabkin, J. (1974). Public attitudes to mental illness. *Schizophrenia Bulletin, 10*, 9–23.

Radner, H. (1998). New Hollywood's new woman: Murder in mind—Sarah and Margie. In S. Neale & M. Smith (Eds.), *Contemporary Hollywood cinema* (pp. 247–262). London: Routledge.

Rai, A. (1997). Thus spoke the sub altern: Post colonial criticism and the scene of desire. *Discourse, 19*, 163–193.

Rajadhyaksha, A., & Willemen, P. (1999). *Encyclopaedia of Indian cinema* (2nd ed.). Delhi, India: Oxford University Press.

Ramanujan, A. K. (1999). The Indian Oedipus. In T. G. Vaidyanathan & J. J. Kripal (Eds.), *Vishnu on Freud's desk* (pp. 109–136). Delhi, India: Oxford University Press.

Ranade, A. (1980). The extraordinary importance of the Indian film song. *Cinema Vision India, 1*, 4–11.

Rangoonwalla, F. (1975). *75 years of Indian cinema*. New Delhi, India: Indian Book. Co.

Rangoonwalla, F. (1979). *A pictorial history of Indian cinema*. London: Hamlyn.

Rao, M. (1989). Victims in vigilante clothing? *Cinema in India, 4*, 24–26.

Ray, R. K. (2001). *Exploring emotional history*. Delhi, India: Oxford University Press.

Raychaudhuri, T. (1999). *Perceptions, emotions, sensibilities*. Delhi, India: Oxford University Press.

Reich, W. (1950). *The mass psychology of fascism*. London: Pelican.

Rivière, J. (1986). Womanliness as a masquerade. In V. Burgin, G. Donald, & C. Kaplan (Eds.), *Formations of fantasy* (p. 35). London: Methuen.

Roberts, G., & Wallis, H. (2002). *Key film texts*. London: Arnold.

Rodowick, D. N. (1991). *The difficulty of difference: Psychoanalysis, sexual difference and film theory*. London: Routledge.

Roffman, P., & Purdy, J. (1981). *The Hollywood social problem film*. Bloomington, IN: Indiana University Press.

Roland, A. (1988). *The concept of self in India and Japan*. Princeton, NJ: Princeton University Press.

Sardar, Z. (1998). Dilip Kumar made me do it. In A. Nandy (Ed.), *Secret politics of our desire* (pp. 19–91). Delhi, India: Oxford Universiry Press.

Sarris, A. (1998). *You ain't heard nothing yet*. New York: Oxford University Press.

Segall, L. M. H., Campbell, D. T., & Herskovits, M. J. (1966). *The influence of culture on visual perception*. Indianapolis, IN: Bobbs Merrill Inc.

Shah, A. (1973). *The household dimension of the family in India*. Berkeley, CA: University of California Press.

Shah, P. (1980). *The Indian film*. Westport, CN: Greenwood Press. (Original work published 1950)

Sharma, N. (1980). Half a century of song. *Cinema Vision India, 1*, 57–65.

Sharma, S., & Varma, L. P. (1984). History of mental hospitals in the Indian subcontinent. *Indian Journal of Psychiatry, 26*, 295–302.

Shaw, W. S. (1932). The alienist department of India. *Journal of Mental Science, 78*, 331–341.

Simmel, G. (1908). Zur philosophie der schauspielers in fragmente und auf sätze. Munich. (Reprinted 1923)

Sims, A. (1999). *Symptoms in the mind*. London: Balliere Tindall.

Singh, N. (1998). *India's culture: The state, the arts and beyond*. Delhi, India: Oxford University Press.

Smart, N. (1989). *The world's religions*. New York: Cambridge University Press.

Smith M. (1998). Theses on the philosophy of Hollywood history. In S. Neale & M. Smith (Eds.), *Contemporary Hollywood cinema* (pp. 3–20). London: Routledge.

Somaaya, B. (2000). *Salaam Bollywood*. South Godstone, UK: Spantech & Lancer.

Somaaya, B. (2002). *Insights and attitudes*. Ahmedabad, India: Sambliau Publishers.

Somaaya, B. (2003). *The story so far*. Mumbai, India: Indian Express Group.

Somaaya, B. (2004). *Cinema: Images and issues*. New Delhi, India: Rupa Books.

Somasundaram, G. (1987). Indian lunacy act 1912: The historical background. *Indian Journal of Psychiatry, 29*, 3–14.

Spratt, P. (1966). *Hindu culture and personality*. Bombay, India: Manaktalas.

Szasz, T. (1962). *The myth of mental illness*. New York: Harper & Row.

Szasz, T. (1981). *The manufacture of mental illness* (New ed.). Syracuse, NY: Syracuse University Press.

Tandon, B. N. (2003). *PMO Diary—I*. Delhi: Konark.

Tandon, B. N. (2006). *PMO Diary—II*. Delhi: Konark.

Tarlo, E. (2001). Paper truths: The emergency and slum clearance through forgotten files. In C. J. Fuller & V. Bénéï (Eds.), *The everyday state and society in modern India* (pp. 68–90). London: Hurst & Company.

Taylor, W. S. (1948). Basic personality in orthodox Hindu culture patterns. *Journal of Abnormal and Social Psychology, 43,* 3–12.

Thapar, R. (2000). Will a millennium be coming our way? In R. Thapar (Ed.), *India: Another millennium?* (pp. IX–XXXI). New Delhi, India: Viking.

Thomas, R. (1985). Indian cinema: Pleasures and popularity. *Screen, 26,* 116–131.

Thoraval, Y. (2000). *The cinemas of India (1896–2000).* New Delhi, India: Macmillan.

Thoulees, R. H. (1933). A racial difference in perception. *Journal of Social Psychology, 4,* 330–339.

Turim, M. (1989). *Flashback in film memory and history.* New York: Routledge.

Uberoi, P. (1993). Introduction. In P. Uberoi (Ed.), *Family, kinship and marriage in India* (pp. 1–42). Delhi, India: Oxford University Press.

Vaidyanathan, T.G. (1999). Introduction. In T. G. Vaidyanathan & J. J. Kripal (Eds.), *Vishnu on Freud's desk* (pp. 1–18). Delhi, India: Oxford University Press.

Valicha, K. (1988a). *The moving image: A study of Indian cinema.* Hyderabad, India: Orient Longman.

Valicha, K. (1988b). *Kishore Kumar: The definitive biography.* New Delhi: Penguin India.

Van den Broek, P., Bauer, P. J., & Bourg, T. (Eds.). (1997). *Developmental spans in event comprehension and representation: Bridging fictional and actual events.* Mahwah, NJ: Lawrence Erlbaum Associates Inc.

Varde, A. (n.d.). Sholay. In A. Varde (Ed.), *Stardust: 100 greatest films of all time* (pp. 277–278). Mumbai, India: Magna.

Vasudev, A. (1988). *The woman: Myth and reality in the Indian cinema.* In W. Dissanayake (Ed.), *Cinema and cultural identity.* Lanham, MD: University Press of America.

Verghese, A., & Beig, A. (1974). Public attitudes towards mental illness: The Vellore study. *Indian Journal of Psychiatry, 16,* 8–18.

Viswanath, G. (2002). *Saffronizing the silver screen: The right winged nineties film.* In J. Jain & S. Rai (Eds.), *Films and feminism: Essays in Indian cinema* (pp. 39–51). Jaipur, India: Rawat Publications.

Waxler, N. (1974). Is outcome for schizophrenia better in non-industrial societies? *Journal of Nervous and Mental Disease, 167,* 77–80.

Wig, N. N. (1994). An overview of cross-cultural and national issues in psychiatric classification. In J. Mezzich, Y. Honda, & M. Kastrup (Eds.), *Psychiatric diagnosis* (pp. 3–10). Berlin: Springer Verlag.

World Health Organization. (1974). *International pilot study of schizophrenia.* Geneva, Switzerland.

World Health Organization. (1992). *International classification of diseases* (10th ed.). Geneva, Switzerland.

Wollen, P. (1972). *Sign and meaning in the cinema* (2nd ed.). New York: Viking. (Original work published 1969)

Wulff, D. M. (1985). The evocation of Bhāva in performances of Bengali Vaisnava Padāvalī Kīrtan. Paper given at conference on emotion, feeling and experience in India, University of Houston, Houston, TX. Cited in O. M. Lynch (Ed.), *Divine passions: The social construction of emotion in India* (pp. 3–34). Berkeley, CA: University of California Press.

Selected filmography

Funtoosh (1956)

Produced by:	Dev Anand
Directed by:	Chetan Anand
Cast:	Dev Anand
	Sheila Ramani
	K. N. Singh
	Kum Kum
	Krishna Dhawan
	Leela Chitnis
	Anwar Hussain
Screenplay:	Uma Anand
Cinematography:	V. Ratra
Lyrics:	Sahir Ludhianvi
Music:	S. D. Burman

Ardhangini (1959)

Produced by:	Amiya Chakraborty
Directed by:	Amiya Chakraborty
Cast:	Meena Kumari
	Raaj Kumar
	Agha

	Shubha Khote
	Durga Khote
	Shiv Raj
Screenplay:	Vishwa Mitter Adil, Shashi Bhushan
Cinematography:	B. M. Sabnis
Lyrics:	Majrooh Sultanpuri
Music:	Vasant Desai

Anuradha (1960)

Produced by:	Hrishikesh Mukherjee
Directed by:	Hrishikesh Mukherjee
Cast:	Balraj Sahni
	Leela Naidu
	Abhi Battacharya
	Nazir Hussein
	Mukri
	Ranu
Screenplay:	Sachin Bhowmick, D. N. Mukherjee, Samir Chowdray
Cinematography:	Jaywant R. Pathare
Lyrics:	Shailendra
Music:	Ravi Shankar

Krorepati (1961)

Produced by:	Om Prakash Saigal
Directed by:	Mohan Segal
Cast:	Kishore Kumar
	Shashi Kala
	Kum Kum
	Anup Kumar
	K. N. Singh
	Radhakishan
Story:	N. K. Suri/M. Saigal
Screenplay:	I. S. Johar
Cinematography:	Y. D. Sarpotdar
Lyrics:	Shailendra & Hamat Jaipuri
Music:	Shanker Jaikishan

Half Ticket (1962)

Produced by:	Kalidas
Directed by:	Kalidas

Cast:	Kishore Kumar
	Madhubala
	Pran
	Manorama
	Tun Tun
Screenplay:	Ramesh Pant
Cinematography:	Purba Bhattacharjee
Lyrics:	Shailendra
Music:	Salil Chaudhury

Bandini (1963)

Produced by:	Bimal Roy
Directed by:	Bimal Roy
Cast:	Nutan
	Ashok Kumar
	Dharmendra
	Tarun Bose
	Asit Sen
	Iftekhar
Screenplay:	M. Ghosh
Cinematography:	Kamal Bose
Lyrics:	Shailendra, Gulzar
Music:	S. D. Burman

Ghazal (1964)

Produced by:	Ved-Madan
Directed by:	Ved-Madan
Cast:	Sunil Dutt
	Meena Kumari
	Prithviraj Kapoor
	Rehman
	Raj Mehra
	Rajendra Nath
Screenplay:	Agha Jaani Kashmiri
Cinematography:	Jagdeesh Chadha
Lyrics:	Sahir Ludhianvi
Music:	Madan Mohan

Woh Kaun Thi (1964)

Produced by:	N. N. Sippy
Directed by:	Raj Khosla

Cast:	Sadhana
	Manoj Kumar
	Parveen Choudhary
	K. N. Singh
	Prem Chopra
	Helen
	Dhumal
Screenplay:	Dhruva Chatterjee
Cinematography:	K. H. Kapadia
Lyrics:	Raja Mehdi Ali Khan
Music:	Madan Mohan

Raat aur Din (1967)

Produced by:	Jaffer Hussain
Directed by:	Satyen Bose
Cast:	Nargis
	Pradeep Kumar
	Firoz Khan
	Leela Mishra
	K. N. Singh
	Anwar Hussain
	Naaz
Screenplay:	Akhtar Hussain, Satyen Bose
Cinematography:	Madan Sinha
Lyrics:	Shailendra/Hasrat Jaipuri
Music:	Shanker Jaikishan

Baharon ki Manzil (1968)

Produced by:	S. H. Rizvi
Directed by:	Y. H. Rizvi
Cast:	Meena Kumari
	Dharmendra
	Rehman
	Farida Jalal
	Kiran Kumar
Screenplay:	Mahmood Sarosh
Cinematography:	Anwar Siraj
Lyrics:	Majrooh
Music:	Laxmikant Pyarelal

Aya Saawan Jhoom ke (1969)

Produced by:	J. Om Prakash
Directed by:	Raghunath Jhalani
Cast:	Dharmendra
	Asha Parekh
	Ravinder Kapoor
	Rajinder Nath
	Nirupa Roy
Screenplay:	Sachin Bhowmick
Cinematography:	K. C. Raja
Lyrics:	Anand Bakshi
Music:	Laxmikant Pyarelal

Ittefaq (1969)

Produced by:	B. R. Chopra
Directed by:	Yash Chopra
Cast:	Rajesh Khanna
	Nanda
	Shammi
	Sujit Kumar
	Bindu
	Madan Puri
Screenplay:	B. R. Films Story Dept
Cinematography:	Kay Gee
Music:	Salil Chaudhary

Khilona (1970)

Produced by:	L. V. Prasad
Directed by:	Chander Vohra
Cast:	Sanjeev Kumar
	Mumtaz
	Ramesh Deo
	Durga Khote
	Shatrughan Sinha
	Jagdeep
Screenplay:	Gulshan Nanda
Cinematography:	Dwarka Divecha
Lyrics:	Anand Bakshi
Music:	Laxmikant Pyrarelal

Pagla Kahin Ka (1970)

Produced by:	Ajit Chakraborty
Directed by:	Shakti Samanta
Cast:	Shammi Kapoor
	Asha Parekh
	Helen
	Prem Chopra
	K. N. Singh
Screenplay:	Sachin Bhowmick
Lyrics:	Hasrat Jaipuri/S. H. Bihari
Music:	Shanker Jaikishan

Lal Patthar (1971)

Produced by:	F. C. Mehra
Directed by:	Sushil Majumdar
Cast:	Raj Kumar
	Raakhee
	Hema Malini
	Vinod Mehra
	Asit Sen
	Ajit
Screenplay:	Nabendu Ghosh
Cinematography:	Dwarka Divecha
Lyrics:	Hasrat Jaipuri/Neeraj/Dev Kohli
Music:	Shanker Jaikishan

Dhund (1973)

Produced by:	B. R. Chopra
Directed by:	B. R. Chopra
Cast:	Zeenat Aman
	Sanjay
	Danny Denzongpa
	Navin Nischol
	Madan Puri
Screenplay:	Akhtar ul-Iman
Cinematography:	Dharam Chopra
Lyrics:	Sahir Ludhianvi
Music:	Ravi

Zanjeer (1973)

Produced by:	Prakash Mehra
Directed by:	Prakash Mehra
Cast:	Amitabh Bachchan
	Jaya Bhaduri
	Ajit
	Pran
	Om Prakash
	Bindu
	Gulshan Bawra
Screenplay:	Salim-Javed
Cinematography:	N. Satyen
Lyrics:	Gulshan Bawra
Music:	Kalyanji Anandji

Doosri Seeta (1974)

Produced by:	B. Khanna, J. L. Bubber
Directed by:	Gogi Anand
Cast:	Ramesh Sharma
	Jaya Bhaduri
	Raza Murad
	A. K. Hangal
	Lalita Pawar
Screenplay:	Gulzar
Cinematography:	K. K. Mahajan
Lyrics:	Gulzar
Music:	R. D. Burman

Deewar (1975)

Produced by:	Gulshan Rai
Directed by:	Yash Chopra
Cast:	Amitabh Bachchan
	Shashi Kapoor
	Parveen Babi
	Neetu Singh
	Nirupa Roy
	Madan Puri
Screenplay:	Salim-Javed
Cinematography:	Kay Gee
Lyrics:	Sahir Ludhianvi
Music:	R. D. Burman

Sholay (1975)

Produced by:	G. P. Sippy
Directed by:	Ramesh Sippy
Cast:	Dharmendra
	Hema Malini
	Sanjeev Kumar
	Amitabh Bachchan
	Jaya Bhaduri
	Amjad Khan
	A. K. Hangal
	Asrani
	Jalal Agha
Screenplay:	Salim-Javed
Cinematography:	Dwarka Divecha
Lyrics:	Anand Bakshi
Music:	R. D. Burman

Mausam (1976)

Produced by:	P. Mallikarjuna Rao
Directed by:	Gulzar
Cast:	Sharmila Tagore
	Sanjeev Kumar
	Om Prakash
	Agha
	Dina Pathak
Screenplay:	Gulzar
Cinematography:	K. Vaikunth
Lyrics:	Gulzar
Music:	Madan Mohan, Salil Chaudhury

Ghar (1978)

Produced by:	N. N. Sippy
Directed by:	Manick Chatterjee
Cast:	Vinod Mehra
	Rekha
	Prema Narayan
	Asit Sen
	Dinesh Thakur
Screenplay:	Dinesh Thakur
Cinematography:	Nandu Bhattacharya

Lyrics:	Gulzar
Music:	R. D. Burman

Hum Paanch (1980)

Produced by:	Boney Kapoor, Surinder Kapoor
Directed by:	Bapu
Cast:	Shabana Azmi
	Mithun Chakraborty
	Amrish Puri
	Sanjeev Kumar
	Deepti Naval
	Naseeruddin Shah
Screenplay:	S. R. Puttanna Kanagal, V. R. Mullapoddi
Cinematography:	Sharad Kadwe
Lyrics:	Anand Bakshi
Music:	Laxmikant Pyarelal

Insaaf ka Tarazu (1980)

Produced by:	B. R. Chopra
Directed by:	B. R. Chopra
Cast:	Zeenat Aman
	Padmini Kolhapure
	Dharmendra
	Raj Babbar
	Deepak Parashar
	Simi Garewal
	Shreeram Lagoo
Screenplay:	Sharad Kumar
Cinematography:	Dharam Chopra
Lyrics:	Sahir Ludhianvi
Music:	Ravindra Jain

Karz (1980)

Produced by:	A. Sheikh, J. Khurana
Directed by:	Subhash Ghai
Cast:	Rishi Kapoor
	Tina Munim
	Simi Garewal
	Raj Kiran
	Jalal Agha

	Premnath
	Durga Khote
Screenplay:	Sachin Bhowmick
Cinematography:	Kamalakar Rao
Lyrics:	Anand Bakshi
Music:	Laxmikant Pyarelal

Baseraa (1981)

Produced by:	Ramesh Behl
Directed by:	Ramesh Talwar
Cast:	Raakhee
	Shashi Kapoor
	Rekha
	Poonam Dhillon
	Raj Kiran
	A. K. Hangal
Screenplay:	G. R. Kamat
Cinematography:	Peter Pereira
Lyrics:	Gulzar
Music:	R. D. Burman

Bemisaal (1982)

Produced by:	Debesh Ghosh
Directed by:	Hrishikesh Mukherjee
Cast:	Amitabh Bachchan
	Raakhee
	Vinod Mehra
	Aruna Irani
	Sheetal
	Deven Verma
Screenplay:	Sachin Bhowmick
Cinematography:	Jaywant Pathare
Lyrics:	Anand Bakshi
Music:	R. D. Burman

Arth (1983)

Produced by:	Kuljit Pal
Directed by:	Mahesh Bhatt
Cast:	Shabana Azmi
	Smita Patil

	Kulbhushan Kharbanda
	Raj Kiran
Screenplay:	Mahesh Bhatt, Sujit Sen
Cinematography:	Pravin Bhatt
Lyrics:	Kaifi Azmi
Music:	Jagjit and Chitra Singh

Sadma (1983)

Produced by:	R. N. Sippy
Directed by:	Balu Mahendra
Cast:	Kamalahasan
	Sridevi
	Shreeram Lagoo
	Gulshan Grover
	Silk Smitha
	Leela Mishra
Screenplay:	Balu Mahendra
Cinematography:	Balu Mahendra
Lyrics:	Gulzar
Music:	Illayaraja

Pratighaat (1987)

Produced by:	Ramaji Rao
Directed by:	N. Chandra
Cast:	Sujata Mehta
	Arvind Kumar
	Charan Raj
	Rohini Hattangadi
	Nana Pateker
Screenplay:	N. Chandra, T. Krishna
Cinematography:	H. Laxmi Narayan
Lyrics:	Ravinda Jain
Music:	Ravindra Jain

Khoon Bhari Maang (1988)

Produced by:	Rakesh Roshan
Directed by:	Rakesh Roshan
Cast:	Rekha
	Kabir Bedi
	Shatrughan Sinha

	Kader Khan
	Saeed Jaffrey
	Sulochana
Screenplay:	Kader Khan, Mohan Kaul
Cinematography:	Pushpal Dutta
Lyrics:	Indivar
Music:	Rajesh Roshan

Shukriya (1988)

Produced by:	Kailash Chopra
Directed by:	A. C. Trilok Chandra
Cast:	Rajeev Kapoor
	Amrita Singh
	Pran
	Beena
	Prem Chopra
	Asrani
Screenplay:	Mohan Kaul, Ravi Kapoor
Cinematography:	Vishwanath Rai
Lyrics:	Verma Malik
Music:	Anu Malik

Zakhmi Aurat (1988)

Produced by:	Ashok Punjabi
Directed by:	Avtar Bhogal
Cast:	Dimple Kapadia
	Raj Babbar
	Roopesh Kumar
	Puneet Issar
	Anupam Kher
Cinematography:	Anil Sehgal
Music:	Bappi Lahiri

Rakhwala (1989)

Produced by:	K. Murali Mohan Rao
Directed by:	D. Rama Naidu
Cast:	Anil Kapoor
	Shabana Azmi
	Farha
	Asrani

	Prem Chopra
	Suresh Oberoi
Music:	Anand-Milind

Damini (1992)

Produced by:	Aly Moorani, Karim Moorani, Bunty Soorma
Directed by:	Raj Kumar Santoshi
Cast:	Rishi Kapoor
	Meenakshi Seshadri
	Kulbhushan Kharbanda
	Rohini Hattangadi
	Viju Khote
	Sunny Deol
	Amrish Puri
Screenplay:	Dilip Shukla
Cinematography:	Ishwar Bidri
Lyrics:	Sameer
Music:	Nadeem-Shravan

Deewana (1992)

Produced by:	Guddu Dhanoa, Lalit Kapoor, Raju Kothani
Directed by:	Raj Kanwar
Cast:	Rishi Kapoor
	Divya Bharati
	Shah Rukh Khan
	Sushma Seth
	Amreesh Puri
	Mohnish Behl
	Alok Nath
Screenplay:	Sagar Sarhadi
Cinematography:	Harmeet Singh
Lyrics:	Sameer
Music:	Nadeem-Shravan

Aaina (1993)

Produced by:	Pamela Chopra
Directed by:	Deepak Sareen
Cast:	Jackie Shroff
	Amrita Singh
	Juhi Chawla
	Sayeed Jaffrey

	Dina Pathak
	Dipak Tijori
Screenplay:	Honey Irani
Cinematography:	Ramesh Bhalla, Nazir Khan
Lyrics:	Sameer
Music:	Dilip Sen, Sameer Sen

Agnisakshi (1993)

Produced by:	Brinda Thackeray
Directed by:	Parto Ghosh
Cast:	Jackie Shroff
	Nana Patekar
	Manisha Koirala
	Divya Dutton
	Ravi Behl
Story:	Ranbir Pushp
Screenplay:	Hriday Lani
Cinematography:	K. V. Ramama
Lyrics:	Sameer
Music:	Nadeem-Shravan

Baazigar (1993)

Produced by:	Ganesh Jain
Directed by:	Abbas-Mustan Burmawalla
Cast:	Shahrukh Khan
	Shilpa Shetty
	Kajol
	Dilip Tahil
	Raakhee
	Johnny Lever
Screenplay:	Javed Siddiqui, Akash Khurana, Robin Bhatt
Cinematography:	Thomas Xavier
Lyrics:	Rani Malik
Music:	Anu Malik

Khalnayak (1993)

Produced by:	Ashok Ghai, Subhash Ghai
Directed by:	Subhash Ghai
Cast:	Sanjay Dutt
	Raakhee
	Madhuri Dixit

	Jackie Shroff
	Neena Gupta
	Anupam Kher
	A. K. Hangal
Screenplay:	Ram Kelkar
Cinematography:	Ashok Mehta
Lyrics:	Anand Bakshi
Music:	Laxmikant Pyarelal

Anjaam (1994)

Produced by:	Maharukh Jakhi
Directed by:	Rahul Rawail
Cast:	Madhuri Dixit
	Shahrukh Khan
	Dipak Tijori
	Johnny Lever
	Kiran Kumar
	Beena
	Kalpana Iyer
Screenplay:	Sutanu Gupta
Cinematography:	Sameer Arya
Lyrics:	Sameer
Music:	Anand-Milind

Dilwale (1994)

Produced by:	Paramijit Baweja
Directed by:	Harry Baweja
Cast:	Ajay Devgan
	Sunil Shetty
	Raveena Tandon
	Paresh Rawal
	Gulshan Grover
	Reema Lagoo
Story:	Karan Razdan
Cinematography:	Damodar Naidu
Lyrics:	Sameer
Music:	Nadeem-Shravan

Raja (1995)

| Produced by: | Ashok Thakeria, Indra Kumar |
| Directed by: | Indra Kumar |

Cast:	Sanjay Kapoor
	Madhuri Dixit
	Paresh Rawal
	Dalip Tahil
	Rita Bhaduri
	Mukesh Khanna
Screenplay:	Rajiv Kaul, Praful Parekh
Cinematography:	Baba Azmi
Lyrics:	Sameer
Music:	Nadeem-Shravan

Daraar (1996)

Produced by:	Sujit Kumar
Directed by:	Abbas-Mustan
Cast:	Rishi Kapoor
	Juhi Chawla
	Arbaaz Khan
	Johnny Lever
	Sushma Seth
Screenplay:	Sachin Bhowmick
Cinematography:	Thomas Xavier
Lyrics:	Majrooh Sultanpuri, Hasrat Jaipuri, Rani Malik, Rahat Indori, Shaheen Iqbal
Music:	Anu Malik

Dastak (1996)

Produced by:	Mukesh Bhatt
Directed by:	Mahesh Bhatt
Cast:	Sushmita Sen
	Sharad Kapoor
	Mukul Dev
	Manjoj Baipai
	Sunil Dhawan
Screenplay:	Sachin Bhowmick
Cinematography:	Bhooshan Patel
Lyrics:	Javed Akhtar
Music:	Rajesh Roshan

Fareb (1996)

Produced by:	Mukesh Bhatt, Nitin Keni
Directed by:	Vikram Bhatt

Cast:	Faraaz Khan
	Suman Ranganathan
	Milind Gunaji
	Ashok Lath
	Kunika
Music:	Jatin-Lalit

Gupt (1997)

Produced by:	Gulshan Rai
Directed by:	Rajit Rai
Cast:	Bobby Deol
	Manisha Koirala
	Kajol
	Prem Chopra
	Raza Murad
	Dilip Tahil
	Raj Babbar
Screenplay:	Shabbir Boxwallah
Cinematography:	Ashok Metha
Lyrics:	Anand Bakshi
Music:	Viju Shah

Yugpurush (1998)

Produced by:	Vijay Metha
Directed by:	Parto Ghosh
Cast:	Nana Patekar
	Jackie Shroff
	Manisha Koirala
	Ashwini Bhave
	Mohnish Behl
Screenplay:	Pradeep Ghatak
Cinematography:	K. V. Ramanna
Lyrics:	Majrooh Sultanpuri
Music:	Rajesh Roshan

Kaun (1999)

Produced by:	Mukesh Udeshi
Directed by:	Ram Gopal Varma
Cast:	Urmila Matondkar
	Manoj Baipai
	Sushant Singh

Screenplay:	Anurag Kashyap/Mukesh Udeshi
Cinematography:	Mazhar Kamran
Music:	Sandeep Chowta

Grahan (2001)

Produced by:	Avinash Adik, Ayesha Shroff, Jackie Shroff
Directed by:	K. Shashilal Nair
Cast:	Jackie Shroff
	Manisha Koirala
	Raghuvaran
	Raj Zutshi
	Anupama Varma
Screenplay:	Sujit Sen
Cinematography:	S. Kumar
Lyrics:	Mehboob, Ila Arun
Music:	Karthik Raja

Pyar Tune Kya Kiya (2001)

Produced by:	Ramgopal Verma
Directed by:	Rajat Mukherjee
Cast:	Urmila Matondkar
	Fardeen Khan
	Suresh Oberoi
	Sonali Kulkarni
	Rajpal Yadav
Screenplay:	Rajat Mukherjee
Cinematography:	Sanjay Kapur
Lyrics:	Nitin Raikwar
Music:	Sandeep Chowta

Deewangee (2002)

Produced by:	Nitin Manmohan
Directed by:	Anees Bazmee
Cast:	Ajay Devgan
	Akshaye Khanna
	Urmila Matondkar
	Seema Biswas
	Farida Jalal
Screenplay:	Anees Bazmee, Neeraj Pathak, Humrayun Mirza
Cinematography:	Pushan Kriplani

Lyrics: Salim Bijnori, Nusrat Badr
Music: Ismail Darbar

Humraaz (2002)

Produced by: Venus Films
Directed by: Abbas and Mustan Burmawallah
Cast: Akshaye Khanna
                  Amisha Patel
                  Bobby Deol
                  Johnny Lever
Screenplay: Shiraz Ahmed, Shyann K. Goel
Cinematography: Ravi Yadav
Lyrics: Sudhakar Sharma
Music: Himesh Reshamiya

Hungama (2003)

Produced by: Ganesh Jain, Pooja Galani
Directed by: Priyadarshan
Cast: Akshaye Khanna
                  Aftaab Shivdasani
                  Paresh Rawal
                  Rimi Sen
                  Shakti Kapoor
                  Rajpal Yadav
Screenplay: Priyadarshan
Cinematography: Thiru
Lyrics: Sameer
Music: Nadeem-Shravan

Tere Naam (2003)

Produced by: Mukash Talreja, Sunil Manchanda
Directed by: Satish Kaushik
Cast: Salman Khan
                  Bhumika Chawla
                  Sachin Khedekar
                  Savita Prabhune
                  Ravi Kissen
                  Anang Desai
Screenplay: Jainendra Jain
Cinematography: S. Sriram

Lyrics: Sameer
Music: Himesh Reshamiya

Aetbaar (2004)

Produced by: Mukesh Bhatt
Directed by: Vikram Bhatt
Cast: Amitabh Bachchan
                     John Abraham
                     Bipasha Basu
                     Supriya Pilgaonkar
                     Tom Alter
                     Amardeep Jha
Screenplay: Robin Bhatt, Sanjeev Duggal
Cinematography: Pravin Bhatt
Lyrics: Dev Kohli, Ibrahim Ashq, Maya Govind, Nasir
                     Faraaz, Chandrashekhar Rajit
Music: Rajesh Roshan

Ek Hasina Thi (2004)

Produced by: Ram Gopal Varma
Directed by: Sriram Raghavan
Cast: Saif Ali Khan
                     Urmila Matondkar
                     Seema Biswas
                     Madan Joshi
Screenplay: Sri Ram Raghaban, Pooja Ladhasurti
Cinematography: C. K. Muraleedharan
Music: Amar Mohile

Madhoshi (2004)

Produced by: Anil Sharma
Directed by: Tanveer Khan
Cast: John Abraham
                     Bipasha Basu
                     Priyanshu Chatterjee
                     Smita Jaykar
                     Nandita Puri
Screenplay: Tanveer Khan
Cinematography: Damodar Naidu
Lyrics: Shakeel Azmi
Music: Roop Kumar Rathod

Fareb (2005)

Produced by:	Rajesh Kumar Singh, Sanjeev Jaiswal
Directed by:	Dipak Tijori
Cast:	Manoj Bajpai
	Shilpa Shetty
	Shamita Shetty
	Milind Gunaji
Screenplay:	Girish Dhanija, Brijesh Jayarajan
Cinematography:	Manoj Soni
Lyrics:	Sayeed Quadri
Music:	Anu Malik

Main Aisa Hi Hoon (2005)

Produced by:	Pammi Baweja
Directed by:	Harry Baweja
Cast:	Ajay Devgan
	Sushmita Sen
	Esha Deol
	Anupam Kher
	Lilette Dubey
	Rucha Vaidya
Screenplay:	Bhavani Iyer
Cinematography:	Ayananka Bose
Lyrics:	Sameer
Music:	Himesh Reshamiya

Appendix

The reviews of various films in this volume have been cited from the following sources:

B4U Hindi Cinema Year Book 2002 (Vol. 2)

Filmfare
  10 July 1953
  6 January 1956
  26 October 1956
  26 August 1960
  21 October 1960
  30 December 1960
  17 May 1963
  19 July 1968
  5 March 1976
  1 March 1978
  16 January 1982
  1 April 1982
  1 May 1982
  16 August 1983
  1 September 1983
  1 June 1984

Film Information
  30 March 1996
  30 November 1996
  3 May 1997
  5 July 1997
  28 March 1998
  8 July 1998
  17 February 2001
  14 July 2001
  28 April 2001
  16 June 2001

Madhuri
  21 March 1980
  9 January 1981

Movie
  July 1983
  August 1985

Picturepost
  July 1966
  April 1976

Screen
  22 August 2003
  17 October 2003

Star and Style
  12 July 1968
  20 September 1968
  20 February 1970
  1 May 1970

Useful websites
  www.imdb.com
  www.indiafm.com
  www.ultraindia.com

Author index

Subject index